Mental Health Nursing

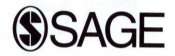

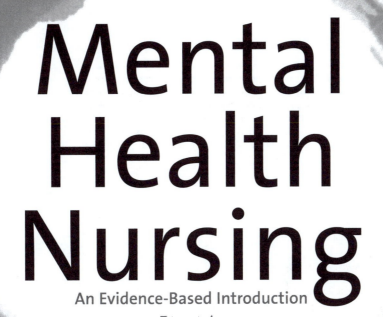

Mental
Health
Nursing

An Evidence-Based Introduction

Edited by

Steven Pryjmachuk

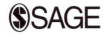

$SAGE

Los Angeles | London | New Delhi
Singapore | Washington DC

First published 2011

SAGE Publications Ltd
I Oliver's Yard
55 City Road
London ECIY ISP

SAGE Publications Inc.
2455 Teller Road
Thousand Oaks, California 91320

SAGE Publications India Pvt Ltd
B 1/ I 1Mohan Cooperative Industrial Area
Mathura Road
New Delhi 110044

SAGE Publications Asia-Pacific Pte Ltd
33 Pekin Street #02-01
Far East Square
Singapore 048763

Library of Congress Control Number: 2010933794

British Library Cataloguing in Publication data

A catalogue record for this book is available from the British Library

ISBN 978-1-84920-071-4
ISBN 978-1-84920-072-1 (pbk)

Typeset by C&M Digitals (P) Ltd, Chennai, India
Printed and bound in Great Britain by TJ International Ltd, Padstow, Cornwall
Printed on paper from sustainable resources

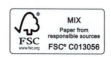

Contents

Contributors

About the Editor

Steven Pryjmachuk PhD is a Mental Health Nurse and Chartered Psychologist with interests in primary and self care in child and adolescent mental health, stress in health care professionals and supporting student learning. He is a Senior Lecturer and the Head of the Mental Health Division in the School of Nursing, Midwifery and Social Work at the University of Manchester.

About the contributors

Clare Baguley MPhil is a Mental Health Nurse and Cognitive Behavioural Therapist with interests in primary mental health care. She is a Lecturer in the School of Nursing, Midwifery and Social Work at the University of Manchester and also works for NHS North West in the IAPT Mental Health Improvement Programme.

John Baker PhD is a Mental Health Nurse with interests in acute mental health nursing, medicines management and the attitudes and clinical skills of mental health workers. He is a Lecturer in the School of Nursing, Midwifery and Social Work at the University of Manchester.

Tim Bradshaw PhD is a Mental Health Nurse with interests in physical health education for people with psychosis and the trans-cultural adaptation of family interventions for people with psychosis. He is a Senior Lecturer in the School of Nursing, Midwifery and Social Work at the University of Manchester where he is also lead for the Bachelor of Nursing (BNurs) Mental Health programme.

Joanne Bramley works for Anxiety UK and is Service User Consultant to the MSc/PgDip in Advanced Practice Interventions for Mental Health in the School of Nursing, Midwifery and Social Work at the University of Manchester.

Jane Briddon BSc (Hons) is a Social Worker and Cognitive Behavioural Therapist in primary mental health care. Her interests include the impact of social/environmental issues on mental health. She is a Lecturer/Practitioner in the School of Nursing, Midwifery and Social Work at the University of Manchester, combining lecturing on the MSc/PgDip in Advanced Practice Interventions for Mental Health with the coordination of Edt*a*, a mental health training agency based within the School.

Simon Burrow MSc is a social worker whose main interests are in dementia care. He is a Teaching Fellow in the School of Nursing, Midwifery and Social Work at the University of Manchester where he is also the programme lead for the Dementia Care pathway of the MSc/PgDip in Advanced Practice Interventions for Mental Health.

Michael Coffey PhD is a Mental Health Nurse with interests in researching multiple perspectives in health and social care. He is a Lecturer in Community Mental Health Nursing at the School of Human and Health Sciences, Swansea University.

Mike Doyle PhD is a Mental Health Nurse with clinical and research interests in forensic mental health care and risk management. He is a Nurse Consultant in Clinical Risk at the North West Adult Forensic Mental Health Services, Greater Manchester West NHS Foundation Trust and a Clinical Lecturer in the School of Community Based Medicine at the University of Manchester.

Sarah Kendal PhD is a Mental Health Nurse with interests in the development of early and preventive mental health interventions, and the promotion of young people's emotional wellbeing. She is a Lecturer in the School of Nursing, Midwifery and Social Work at the University of Manchester.

Hilary Mairs PhD is an Occupational Therapist with interests in psychosocial interventions for people with psychosis and their families. She is a Lecturer in the School of Nursing, Midwifery and Social Work at the University of Manchester where she is also Programme Director for the MSc/PgDip in Advanced Practice Interventions for Mental Health.

Sara Munro PhD is a Mental Health Nurse with interests in acute mental health care, the development of mental health nursing and improving the quality of the patient experience. She is a Nurse Consultant in Acute Mental Health Care for Cumbria Partnership NHS Foundation Trust.

Lucy Rolfe BSc is a qualified Counselling Practitioner and mental health service manager. Her interests are in equality, diversity and service user involvement. She has a background in service development and is currently Wellbeing Co-ordinator at The Lesbian & Gay Foundation.

Noreen Ryan MSc is a Mental Health Nurse with interests in attention deficit hyperactivity disorder (ADHD), neurodevelopmental disorders in children and young people, and non-medical prescribing. She is a Nurse Consultant in Child & Adolescent Mental Health, Bolton Hospitals NHS Foundation Trust.

Ian Wilson MSc is a Mental Health Nurse with interests in complex mental ill-health and substance misuse ('dual diagnosis'). He is a Clinical Teaching Fellow in the School of Nursing, Midwifery and Social Work at the University of Manchester and Dual Diagnosis Trainer/Clinical Nurse at Manchester Mental Health & Social Care Trust.

Preface

If there is one word that sums up the status of British mental health practice during the first decade of the twenty-first century, it is 'change'. Since the millennium we have witnessed a relentless stream of initiatives, reports and demands that have changed the face of mental health practice and that of its principal profession, mental health nursing. To catalogue a few examples, we have seen: the introduction of new mental health legislation; the reorganisation and modernisation of mental health services; critical reviews of the roles of mental health nurses and other mental health professions by governmental and regulatory bodies; service users demanding a greater voice to the extent that 'recovery' is now a dominant theme in mental health care; social inclusion taking precedence over social exclusion; 'evidence-based' practice becoming part of the mainstream; and the introduction of several new nursing roles that have challenged head-on the stereotypical and old-fashioned view that nurses are merely doctors' assistants. And there is no indication that the pace of change will diminish. At the time of writing, we know that nursing is set to become an all-graduate profession across the whole of the UK; a new mental health strategy with a particular focus on inclusion and cross-government working – *New Horizons* – is barely a few months old; the establishment of new mental health practitioners like the 'psychological wellbeing practitioners' has raised questions over the future role of mental health nurses; and 'values-based' practice has surfaced to, depending on your view, either challenge or complement evidence-based practice. Moreover, the fact that this book has been completed in a year in which a General Election has been held (2010) only adds to the likelihood of future change in what we do as mental health nurses.

For many, change can be an anxiety-provoking and pointless endeavour but if the purpose of change is to improve the lot of the significant numbers of people with mental health problems – the very people mental health nursing exists for – then change should be seen as a dynamic, exciting endeavour and one that we should embrace along with the challenges it provides. That is our position: that mental health nursing is in challenging, yet exciting, times and that we can, hopefully, capture some of that excitement and challenge in this book.

The Format of the Book

This book is split into two parts: Part I contains three chapters that provide the necessary background information and context that you need in order to comprehend the remainder (Part II) of the book. In particular, we look at the theoretical perspectives influencing mental health nursing in Chapter 1; the knowledge, values and skills – the *capabilities* – required to be a mental health nurse in Chapter 2; and the composition of the mental health workforce in Chapter 3. Part II contains nine chapters relating to major areas of mental health practice. Because the book is concerned primarily with mental health *nursing*, we have deliberately avoided organising Part II around specific diagnostic categories (as you might find in a *medical* text book), instead preferring to organise the chapters in a way that reflects service provision in many parts of the UK. Thus, we have chapters on: 'common' mental health problems in primary care (Chapters 4 and 5); recovering from psychosis in community settings (Chapter 6); acute mental health (Chapter 7); older people's mental health (Chapter 8); children and young people's mental health (Chapters 9 and 10); substance misuse (Chapter 11); and forensic mental health (Chapter 12).

All of the chapters in both parts of the book commence with a set of **aims** and **learning outcomes** under the heading 'What will I learn?' These aims and outcomes give you an overview of the chapter so that you can identify quickly what content is in that chapter and whether it is relevant to you at any particular point in your studies. All of the chapters contain opportunities for **discussion** and **reflection** in the form of the discussion and reflection points which periodically punctuate the text. The discussion points have been designed to drive debate on particular topics and they can be used formally (e.g. in a classroom session) or informally (e.g. with your peers or in self-directed study groups). The reflection points are designed to be more personal than the discussion points – to generate reflection and thought rather than debate – though many of them could easily be adapted as discussion points if you so wished. In addition, real-life **case scenarios** (more often than not with a reflective element to them) are provided in each of the Part II chapters to get you to think about how you might apply some of the knowledge you have obtained from this book, and elsewhere, to your own nursing practices.

We have tried to write in an informal, yet scholarly, style so that we create a balance between the demands of university-level study and readability and accessibility. We are also cognisant that the UK is made up of four constituent countries and so we have tried, wherever possible, to include Scottish, Welsh and Northern Irish perspectives on the issues and debates that we have covered.

How to Use This Book

While this book can act as a core text for a pre-registration mental health nursing course (and we hope that it will be adopted as such by course leaders), it will not give you all of the answers nor can it possibly cover all of the scenarios you will encounter in your own unique experiences of learning to be a mental health practitioner. Thus, you should not use it to the exclusion of other materials; indeed, we strongly recommend that you get used to using other texts and resources as you progress through your studies. As you will discover, university-level study demands that you see things with a critical eye – that you think about and analyse issues and concepts, and compare and contrast different points of view. This also applies to the notion of **evidence-based practice**. As the title of this book implies, evidence-based practice threads its way throughout this book, in much the same way as it permeates modern healthcare provision. For most of the interventions and practices we discuss, we have, indeed, made reference to 'the evidence' but critical thought in evidence-based practice requires that you do not necessarily take our evidence at face value. The evidence may change, or we may have interpreted the evidence with a bias based on our own theoretical leanings, or we may have accidentally missed some evidence simply because we were unaware it existed. The solution to all of this is, as we have already mentioned, to use additional texts and resources to help you with your studies – in other words, *to read around*. We do give you a helping hand, however, in that we provide lists of further reading and resources at the end of each chapter. Remember that these lists are merely *our suggestions*; they are resources we have been influenced by or resources that we particularly like.

What to Call Those We Work for

When you see a doctor or other healthcare professional, you are often referred to as a 'patient' and, indeed, it is common to hear health professionals talk about patients. Few people object to the use of the term patient in physical health settings but in mental health it can be controversial. There are a variety of reasons why we should, perhaps, avoid the term: it implies passivity and compliance; contributes to the stigmatisation of people with mental health problems; and it can reflect a medicalised (rather than, say, psychosocial) view of mental health and ill-health. There are a several alternatives around, including 'client' (which is popular in social care), 'consumer' (which reflects the influence of consumerism) and 'survivor' (a term that reflects some people's views that they have merely survived, rather than benefited from, their contact with psychiatric services). Perhaps the most popular alternative is **service user**. This term has its roots in consumerism but is a less market-oriented term than 'client' or 'consumer'; it is also a somewhat less emotional term than 'survivor'. Moreover, its use should remind us and the healthcare organisations we work in that we are there primarily to provide a *service* for others rather than to manage or control them (though, as you will discover, there are times when management and control have to be part of that service). Throughout this book, our preference is to use, wherever possible, a completely neutral and generic term like 'person' or 'individual' to describe the people we work with. Sometimes, however, this can be difficult, when clarity is required, for example; in these circumstances, 'service user' will remain our preferred term.

Some Cautions

We need to end with a caution or two. Firstly, healthcare policy changes very quickly and by the time you are reading this book some of the policy we have cited in it may well have been superseded by newer initiatives or reports. While this is unavoidable, it does not necessarily render the policies we have cited or discussed irrelevant. Since most policy develops organically rather than spontaneously, it can be useful to see how it has developed by examining its history. The advice here is to always check that any policy initiative or report you are exploring is up-to-date. As a student in the second decade of the twenty-first century you are lucky to have the Internet and a variety of search tools to help expedite your search for up-to-date material. And while mentioning the Internet, we get onto a second caution: if anything, the Internet changes much faster than healthcare policy. URLs (Web addresses) that are current today may be dead in a year's time. Again, the advice here is to use the tools at your disposal and your initiative to ensure that the information you collect and use is continually up to date.

These are, indeed, exciting times for mental health nursing and we hope that as you immerse yourself into the field, you will find the same creative passion for helping others in mental distress that those of us who have put this book together share.

Steven Pryjmachuk (and the contributors)

Acknowledgements

Thanks to the Scottish Mental Welfare Commission, to Hugh Masters at the Scottish Government, and to Hugh O'Donnell in the School of Nursing and Midwifery at Queen's University Belfast for clarifying aspects of the mental health legislation for Scotland and Northern Ireland, respectively. Thanks also to Liz Mayne, National Lead, Violence and Abuse Policy for the guidance on asking about abuse in Chapter 2.

Special thanks go to those who anonymously reviewed the original Sage proposal and who subsequently and helpfully reviewed early drafts of the chapters.

Thanks also to all of those at Sage for their support (and patience) during the year or so of this book's development.

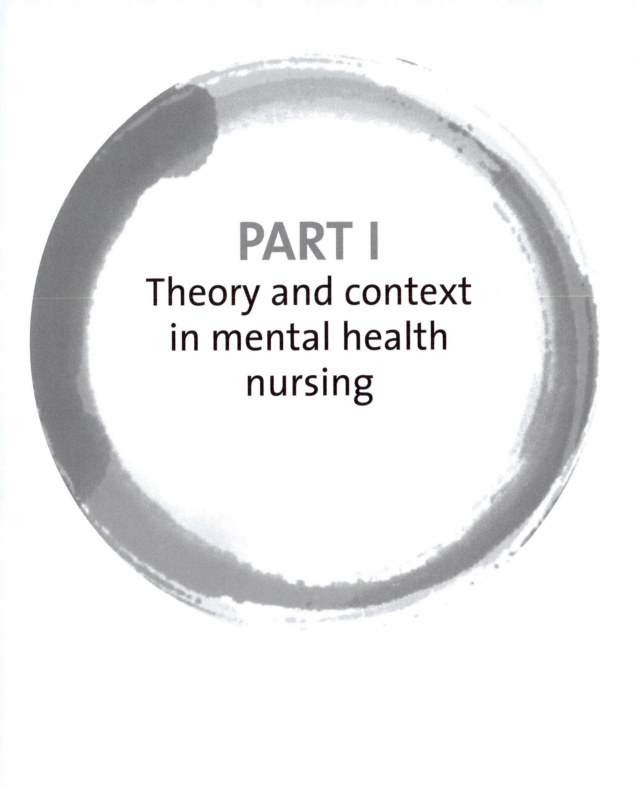

PART I
Theory and context in mental health nursing

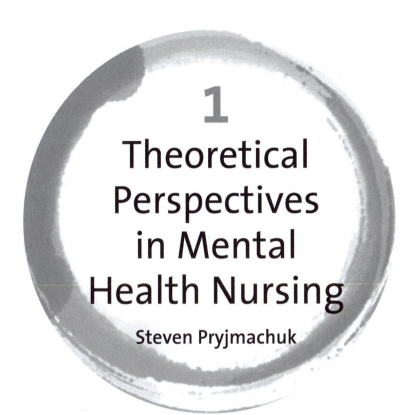

1

Theoretical Perspectives in Mental Health Nursing

Steven Pryjmachuk

What will I learn in this chapter?

The aim of this chapter is to introduce you to the various, often competing, theories and perspectives that have had an influence on contemporary mental health nursing practice. In doing so, it will be necessary to explore the interrelated concepts of 'mental health' and 'mental illness', and to look briefly at the history of mental health nursing, its current state of play, and the directions it may take in the future.

After reading this chapter, you will be able to:

- differentiate between the concepts of mental health and mental illness and explain the interrelationships between the two;
- appreciate how the history of mental health nursing impacts on contemporary mental health nursing practice;
- compare and contrast the variety of competing theoretical perspectives that underpin mental health nursing practice, making particular reference to their respective evidence bases;
- reflect upon the questions surrounding mental health nursing's future direction.

Introduction: What Is Mental Health?

You are obviously reading this because you have an interest in mental health nursing (or, at the very least, mental health), but what exactly is mental health? And why does this book and much of current parlance refer to **mental health** nursing and not **psychiatric** nursing? Indeed, those practising in this area who are on the Nursing and Midwifery Council's statutory register find themselves officially (and legally) **Registered Nurses, Mental Health** and not 'Registered Psychiatric Nurses'. Hopefully, you will find some answers to these questions in this chapter although, as a critical reader (which is what we want modern mental health nurses to be), you do not necessarily have to agree with those answers.

To return to our principal question – what is mental health? – take a few moments to consider the questions below.

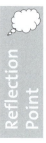

Mental health and ill-health

How do you know if you are mentally healthy? What factors do you think influence someone's mental health?

What's the relationship between 'health' and 'illness'? Is it possible to define illness without defining health or to define health without knowing what illness is?

One answer to our principal question is provided by the World Health Organisation, which defines mental health as 'a state of well-being in which the individual realises his or her own abilities, can cope with the normal stresses of life, can work productively and fruitfully, and is able to make a contribution to his or her community' (WHO, 2001). In using the World Health Organisation's definition to answer our principal question, we may have opened a can of worms however. Consider the reflection point below.

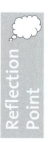

Stress and coping

So, according to the World Health Organisation's definition, is someone mentally 'unhealthy' if they can't cope with the normal stresses of life, work productively or make a contribution to his or her community?

Where does mental *illness* fit into this picture?

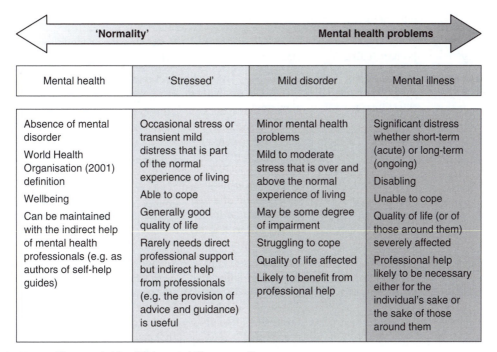

'**Normality**' ←————————————————————————→ **Mental health problems**			
Mental health	'Stressed'	Mild disorder	Mental illness
Absence of mental disorder World Health Organisation (2001) definition Wellbeing Can be maintained with the indirect help of mental health professionals (e.g. as authors of self-help guides)	Occasional stress or transient mild distress that is part of the normal experience of living Able to cope Generally good quality of life Rarely needs direct professional support but indirect help from professionals (e.g. the provision of advice and guidance) is useful	Minor mental health problems Mild to moderate stress that is over and above the normal experience of living May be some degree of impairment Struggling to cope Quality of life affected Likely to benefit from professional help	Significant distress whether short-term (acute) or long-term (ongoing) Disabling Unable to cope Quality of life (or of those around them) severely affected Professional help likely to be necessary either for the individual's sake or the sake of those around them

FIGURE 1.1   The mental health/mental illness continuum

One solution to all of this is to consider mental health and mental illness as the two extremes of a **continuum**. Such a continuum is represented by the double-arrowed bar in Figure 1.1. A continuum is essentially a link between two extremes – normality and mental health problems, in our case – where the transition from one to the other is gradual and seamless. The four discrete columns in Figure 1.1 are an attempt to integrate some commonly used terms into the continuum. Note that although there are solid lines between the discrete columns in Figure 1.1, this is more about a human tendency to 'pigeonhole' people than about defining rigid boundaries between categories. Indeed, it can be very difficult at times to distinguish between the categories, especially at the boundary points: at what point does 'stressed' become a mild disorder and mild disorder become a mental illness, for example?

The right-hand side of the continuum in Figure 1.1 is associated with terms like 'mental illness', 'mental health problems' and 'mental ill health'; terms that are used throughout this book. Another term that fits in with this side of the continuum and one to which we need to give special consideration is **mental disorder**. It needs special consideration because United Kingdom (UK) law uses it to determine who should be forcibly treated or

TABLE 1.1   Definitions of mental disorder across the countries of the UK

Country	Primary legislation	Definition	Exclusions (i.e. cannot be seen as mental disorder)
England and Wales	Mental Health Act 1983, as amended by the Mental Health Act 2007	Section 1(2): 'any disorder or disability of the mind' [Original Section 1(2) of the 1983 Act repealed by the 2007 Act: 'mental illness, arrested or incomplete development of mind, psychopathic disorder and any other disorder or disability of mind']	Section 1(2A): learning disability. Section 1(3): 'Dependence on alcohol or drugs is not considered to be a disorder or disability of the mind' [Original Section 1(3) of the 1983 Act repealed by the 2007 Act: 'promiscuity or other immoral conduct, sexual deviancy or dependence on alcohol or drugs']
Scotland	Mental Health (Care and Treatment) (Scotland) Act 2003	Section 328(1): 'any (a) mental illness; (b) personality disorder; or (c) learning disability, however caused or manifested'	Section 328(2): '(a) sexual orientation; (b) sexual deviancy; (c) transsexualism; (d) transvestism; (e) dependence on, or use of, alcohol or drugs; (f) behaviour that causes, or is likely to cause, harassment, alarm or distress to any other person; (g) acting as no prudent person would act'
Northern Ireland	Mental Health (Northern Ireland) Order 1986	Article 3(1): 'mental illness, mental handicap and any other disorder or disability of mind'	Article 3(2): 'personality disorder, promiscuity or other immoral conduct, sexual deviancy or dependence on alcohol or drugs'

detained under mental health legislation. All four countries of the UK use the term in this way, though its definition varies from country to country (see Table 1.1); learning disability, for example, is a mental disorder in Scotland and Northern Ireland but not in England and Wales.

We can also make some comments about the roles that mental health nurses can play as we move along the continuum outlined in Figure 1.1. While most people would expect mental health nurses to be involved in helping people on the 'mental health problems' side of the continuum, many are surprised to find (and you may be too) that mental health nurses can be – indeed, are – involved in assisting and supporting people with no history of mental health problems in the maintenance of their mental health. They might do this via various **mental health promotion** activities, be they

direct (such as planning and running work-based stress management programmes or working in a primary care service such as a GP clinic or NHS Direct) or **indirect** (such as authoring self-help guides in relation to stress or 'common mental health problems' like anxiety and depression). This important aspect of mental health nursing is often overlooked, perhaps because of the dominant stereotypes relating to what mental health nurses do – stereotypes that almost always involve the dishing out of medication or dealing with disturbed individuals in straitjackets. At this point, it's appropriate to consider where some of these stereotypes may have come from by looking briefly at the history of mental health nursing.

The History of Mental Health Nursing

Attendant or nurse?

The history of British mental health nursing is intrinsically tied up with the history of **psychiatry**. The turning point in psychiatry (hospital psychiatry, at least) was the passing, in England and Wales, of the interrelated and interdependent Lunacy and County Asylums Acts of 1845. These Acts set up the **Lunacy Commission**, a body Roberts (1981) refers to as the 'The Victorian Ministry of Mental Health'. The Lunacy Commission established an obligation for local authorities (the counties and boroughs of the time) to provide asylums for 'pauper lunatics', that is, those without the financial means to obtain care in the privately run madhouses. The Lunacy (Scotland) Act of 1857 underpinned a similar growth in the number of public asylums in Scotland. Interestingly, and in contrast to England and Wales, the Scottish lunacy act formalised the practice of **boarding-out to the community** the 'harmless and chronically insane' (Sturdy & Parry-Jones, 1999), a practice that was, to some extent, a precursor to modern-day community care. Northern Ireland has a shorter history in terms of mental health policy since the province only came into being as a political entity in 1921; prior to 1921, most of Northern Ireland's mental health policy was rooted in the lunacy legislation of pre-partition Ireland (Prior, 1993).

The Lunacy Acts of the mid-nineteenth century essentially created an institutional base for the emerging discipline of psychiatry (Nolan, 1998). Prior to these Acts, those looking after the mentally ill were often referred to as 'keepers', a somewhat dehumanising term (think about it: keepers are often associated with collections of some sort, be they animals or objects). After these Acts, the more humane term **attendant** became a more prevalent description of those who undertook the day-to-day work in asylums. The explicit link with **nursing** started to come about owing to the fact that female attendants were often referred to as nurses and that formal training for attendants implied that nursing was part-and-parcel of what they did. For example, the Royal Medico-Psychological Association (RMPA), which would later become the Royal College of Psychiatrists, formalised training in 1891, awarding those who successfully completed training a 'Certificate of Proficiency in Nursing the Insane'.

The RMPA's dalliance with nursing was not without controversy, however. There was opposition from the asylum attendants themselves, who did not necessarily want to be associated with general nursing. More domineering in the debate, however, was Mrs Ethel Bedford-Fenwick, Matron of St Bartholomew's Hospital, and the force behind a nineteenth-century drive to professionalise nursing via a statutory register. Mrs Bedford-Fenwick had already staked her claim as to what nursing was and what nurses were and her claim did not include asylum workers whom, she argued, should not be called nurses (Nolan, 1998). Since most asylum attendants were male and almost all of Mrs Bedford-Fenwick's 'true' nurses were female, her objections may well have been nothing more than a gender issue (Chatterton, 2004).

Nursing councils

In 1919, Mrs Bedford-Fenwick got her way when statutory nursing registration became law and **General Nursing Councils** were set up for the separate countries of the United Kingdom. The animosity, evident in the likes of Mrs Bedford-Fenwick and her contemporaries, between general nurses and asylum attendants (or **mental nurses** as they would become known) continued in some subtle and not so subtle ways. Mental nurses, along with male nurses (who were, in turn, mainly mental nurses), were only allowed onto a supplementary – some would say, inferior – part of the nursing register, although the RMPA certificate was recognised as a means of admission to this supplementary part. Moreover, in 1925 the General Nursing Councils attempted to wrench control of mental nurse training away from the RMPA, a hostile battle that resulted in two separate systems of training operating until the post-war establishment of the NHS in 1946 (Chatterton, 2004).

Following the establishment of the NHS, the General Nursing Councils reigned supreme until the Briggs Report (DHSS, 1972) led to the Nurses, Midwives and Health Visitors Act 1979 which in turn led to the dissolution of the General Nursing Councils and the creation, in 1983, of the **United Kingdom Central Council for Nursing, Midwifery and Health Visiting** (UKCC) and a national board for nursing education in each of the four countries of the UK. The national boards were significant in being responsible for the '1982' syllabus, essentially a national curriculum for mental nursing (as it was then called). The 1982 syllabus was heavily influenced by the social sciences and it allowed mental health nursing a degree of separation and autonomy from the other branches of nursing (general, children's and learning disability) in that the entire three years of training were focused on mental health and delivered independently from the other branches of nursing.

In 1986, the UKCC's desire to further professionalise nursing led to the establishment of **Project 2000** (UKCC, 1986), a government-backed initiative designed to align nurse education with the education of other health professionals by transferring responsibility for education and training from the hospital-based schools of nursing to the higher education (HE) sector. At its core was the wholesale replacement – by the year 2000 – of the traditional, work-based apprenticeship models of nurse *training* with the academically grounded diploma and degree programmes of nurse *education*. For mental health nursing, Project 2000 brought about another significant change: the introduction of an 18-month **common foundation programme** (CFP), which all nursing students needed to complete before being allowed to specialise in the remaining 18 months of the programme. Many mental health nurse educators were particularly frustrated to find that Project 2000 had essentially halved the time available to learn to be a mental health nurse. Moreover, to some, this was the beginning of an attempt to make the basic training of nurses **generic** – as is the case in many other countries – where specialties such as mental health nursing and children's nursing would only be available after registration.

Reviews of mental health nursing

Elements of a general review of mental health nursing in 1994 (the Butterworth Report; MHNRT, 1994) also permeated nurse education during the 1990s. Most of the institutions training mental health nurses incorporated at least some of this review's recommendations, especially those relating to partnership working (where the patient/client is at the centre of care), the prioritising of patients/clients with severe and enduring mental illness and the use of clinical supervision to underpin high-quality mental health nursing.

In 1998, the UKCC started a review of pre-registration nurse education, partly because it had a statutory duty to periodically do so and partly because some issues around Project 2000 were beginning to emerge, specifically claims that Project 2000 nurses lacked the practical skills expected by employers and the public. The UKCC reported the results of its review in 1999 (UKCC, 1999), the same year that the government issued a major strategy document for nursing, *Making a Difference* (DH, 1999). The consensus in both *Making a Difference* and the UKCC review was that Project 2000's integration of nursing education into HE was largely positive but changes needed to be made to address the concerns of the public and employers as well as those of qualified nurses and nursing students. As such, nurse education changed again in 2001 when HE institutions implemented the so-called 'Making a Difference' curricula. These curricula had to incorporate more opportunities for students to acquire practical skills and involved greater cooperation between healthcare providers (the NHS mainly) and the HE institutions providing nurse education. Perhaps the most significant change, however, was the one that reduced the length of the CFP (now termed simply the 'foundation programme') from 18 to 12 months, consequently increasing the branch programme to two years.

The government's *Making a Difference* strategy document also outlined changes to the **regulation** of nursing and, in 2001, the Nursing and Midwifery Order 2001 provided for the UKCC and the four national boards for nursing education to be replaced with a single body – the **Nursing and Midwifery Council** (NMC).

In 2005, the Chief Nursing Officer for England requested a review of mental health nursing to answer the question 'How can mental health nursing best contribute to the care of service users in the future?' A similar review of mental health nursing (the first of its kind) was undertaken in Scotland shortly afterwards. Both review teams reported the following year (DH, 2006; Scottish Executive, 2006). Like the Butterworth Report of 1994, these two reviews are *general* reviews of mental health nursing; nevertheless, both contained recommendations that have implications for the education and training of mental health nurses. At the time of writing, these two reviews are still very much current and we will revisit them in the next chapter when we attempt to unpick the elements of a 'good' mental health nurse.

More recently, the NMC embarked on another statutorily required periodic review of pre-registration nurse education in 2009; a review that is likely to lead to further changes in the way in which UK nurses are educated and trained. Significant changes that have already been announced include a move to **all-degree** programmes (i.e., the cessation of diploma-level training), the renaming of the specialist branches of nursing to **fields** of nursing

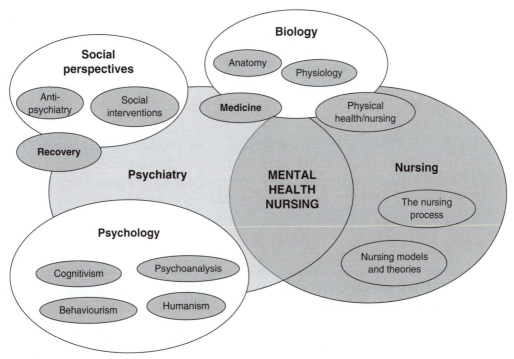

FIGURE 1.2   Theoretical perspectives in mental health nursing

and the **abolition of the first year foundation programme** to be replaced by a combination of generic (core) and field-specific learning across all three years of training.

Theoretical Perspectives in Mental Health Nursing

As we have seen in our historical overview, mental health nursing owes its parentage to both psychiatry and nursing; it is, to use a common saying, the 'bastard offspring' of the two disciplines! This explains why theoretical perspectives from both psychiatry and nursing have permeated mental health nursing (see Figure 1.2) and, to some extent, why the 'generic nurse vs. specialist mental health nurse' debate surfaces every now and then (a debate we will revisit in Chapter 3).

Since psychiatry and its parent, medicine, are not pure sciences, the **psychiatric perspectives** that influence mental health nursing have largely been appropriated from biology, psychology and the social sciences; the **nursing**

perspectives generally come in the guise of nursing theories and models. As you will see, these two perspectives are sometimes complementary and sometimes diametrically opposed.

Psychiatric Perspectives

We mentioned earlier that the psychiatric perspectives on mental health and mental ill health are largely appropriated from biology, psychology and the social sciences. Let's explore the extent to which each of these disciplines has influenced psychiatry and, in turn, mental health nursing practice.

Biological perspectives: the medical model

The practice of medicine, psychiatry's parent discipline, is intrinsically linked to the biological sciences of **anatomy** (the study of the physical structure of organisms) and **physiology** (the study of the functions of the structural parts of organisms). Physical medicine is underpinned by the principle that there is a 'normal' anatomy and physiology that is sometimes rendered 'abnormal' by physical trauma, illness and disease. The practice of physical medicine is thus premised on the identification (**diagnosis**) of these anomalies and the selection of appropriate **treatments** designed to return the body's anatomy and physiology to normality. Throughout medicine's history, this diagnosis–treatment model – **the medical model** – has been the mainstay of medical practice: diagnosing an imbalance in the humours in ancient times will have led to the bloodletting and induced vomiting treatments of those time just as a diagnosis of diabetes leads to treatment with insulin, or a diagnosis of appendicitis leads to an appendectomy, today.

In collaboration with the biological sciences, the medical model has had some remarkable successes over the past 50 years or so. Physical medicine has made significant progress in dealing with the consequences of trauma, illness and disease: it has cured people of terrible diseases such as smallpox; it has enabled people to survive following traumatic injuries; and, through transplantation, it has even extended the lives of those with failing organs. No wonder then that medicine has staked its claim to other aspects of the human condition even when the evidence of abnormality is less than clear-cut. Two good examples are childbirth which, as most midwives will point out, has nothing to do with illness or disease, and madness which, as you will soon discover, can be explained in ways other than that of physiological or anatomical abnormality.

Nevertheless, biological psychiatry[1] works on the same principle as physical medicine but with a specific focus on the brain and nervous system (hence this perspective is sometimes called the **psychophysiological** or **neuropsychological** perspective). Thus dysfunctions in, or damage to, the brain and nervous system lead to observable signs and symptoms that we label 'mental illness' just as dysfunctions in, or damage to, say, the circulatory system or the urinary system might cause physical illnesses associated with those systems. As with physical illness, correcting these dysfunctions involves a range of physical treatments, the most common being the **psychoactive drugs**. Another physical treatment in common use in psychiatry is **electroconvulsive therapy** (ECT). A physical treatment commonly used in the past but which is very rarely used nowadays is **psychosurgery**. Psychosurgery attempts to alleviate mental illness by surgically cutting connections in, or removing parts of, the brain, the most well known form of psychosurgery being the **lobotomy**, a procedure involving surgery to the frontal lobes.

That certain drugs (such as LSD and mescaline) induce states similar to those observed in some mental illnesses, and the observation that psychoactive drugs such as chlorpromazine do appear to alter the course of mental illness in a positive way adds some credibility to the biological perspective. On the other hand, the fact that no specific physiological correlates have been found for any of the mental illnesses (except perhaps some of the dementias) – despite there being plenty of speculation – creates problems for this viewpoint. Nevertheless, there is still a core of biomedical research into mental illness that is driven by the belief that, one day, specific physiological anomalies (such as neurological damage or an imbalance in brain chemicals) will be found for all of the major mental illnesses. We will consider some further criticisms of the biological perspective later on when we discuss psychological and social perspectives on mental illness.

The medical model dominates the delivery and organisation of physical healthcare: medical specialties in most hospitals reflect the physiological systems of the body. Its influence is somewhat less in mental healthcare (and, as you will discover later when we talk about 'recovery', its influence is diminishing further); however, it still impacts significantly on the practices of many mental health professionals including mental health nurses. For example, psychiatrists are still generally seen as the lead clinicians in mental health practice (though, as we will see

---

[1]Biological psychiatry is a bit of an extreme position; while most modern-day psychiatrists embrace elements of the biological perspective (they are trained in medicine, after all), many also integrate psychological and social elements into their practices.

in Chapter 3, this is being challenged by 'new ways of working' in mental health), and the two main classification systems of psychiatric disorders and mental health problems – the *International Classification of Diseases* (ICD) (currently in version 10; WHO, 2007) and the *Diagnostic Statistical Manual* (DSM) (currently in version IV; APA, 2000) – are both products of the medical model.

While the debate about how well the biological perspective can explain mental health and mental ill health is an important one, as nurses we should not ignore the fact that people with mental health problems are *biological* entities. In other words, we need to be aware of the fact that people with mental health problems may also have physical health needs; indeed, there is often a complex interplay between the physical and mental (Seymour, 2003). An understanding of **basic human biology** (and not just of the brain and nervous system) is essential, therefore, if we are to do our best to help people with mental health problems. This will become all the more clear when we focus on the necessary knowledge required to help people with specific kinds of mental health problem in Part II of this book.

Psychological perspectives

Psychology is the study of mind and behaviour (Gross, 2010). Since psychiatry is explicitly associated with the mind and (abnormal) behaviour, it is hardly surprising that its practices have been influenced heavily by psychology. Indeed, as we will see in Chapter 3, there have been some tensions between psychiatrists and those psychologists who work in mental healthcare – clinical and counselling psychologists – within whose remit the mentally unwell come.

There are four main psychological perspectives on mental health and mental ill health: **behaviourism**, **psychoanalysis**, **cognitivism** and **humanism**. In addition, a number of 'hybrid' approaches have emerged as a result of dissatisfaction with one or other of the major perspectives, especially in relation to treatment outcomes. It is perhaps easiest to look at the perspectives and the subsequent hybrids chronologically. With each, we will briefly outline its historical development, its principal proponents, the ways in which it explains mental illness and the implications it has for treatment.

Behaviourism

Behaviourism was developed in the early part of the twentieth century by the American psychologists John B. Watson, B.F. Skinner and Edward Lee

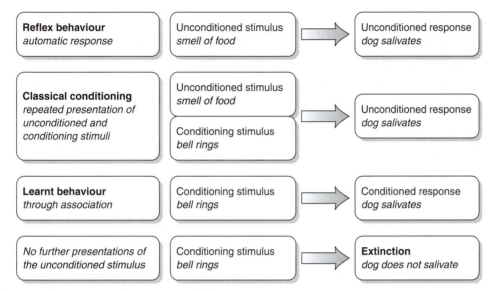

FIGURE 1.3   Classical conditioning in Pavlov's dogs

Thorndike and the Russian physiologist famous for his work with dogs, Ivan Pavlov. It was the dominant force in British psychology right up until the 1950s and remains influential today. Behaviourism focuses only on **observable behaviour**; it sees behaviour merely as a **response** to some external **stimulus** and it is not interested in hypothetical constructs such as the mind. To a behaviourist, all behaviour is **learnt**. Moreover, the ways in which such behaviour is learnt can be manipulated using a variety of techniques known collectively as **conditioning**.

In **classical conditioning**, behaviour is learnt through **association**. Pavlov's studies involving dogs demonstrated that, under certain conditions, an existing response (salivation) could be associated with a new stimulus (a bell ringing) (see Figure 1.3).

Something worth noting from Figure 1.3 is the notion of **extinction**. In classical conditioning, this means that the conditioned response fades when there is no further presentation of the unconditioned stimulus. Extinction is an important aspect of behaviourist theory and is something we will return to shortly.

In **operant conditioning** (sometimes called instrumental conditioning), behaviour is learnt through the principles of **reward** and **punishment**. Operant conditioning is underpinned by the notion that humans are

TABLE 1.2 Factors that determine learning in operant conditioning

Increasing specific behaviours	Decreasing specific behaviours
Positive reinforcement – the addition of something the individual finds rewarding and/or pleasurable, e.g. giving money, food or praise for 'good' behaviour	**Punishment** – something unpleasant is presented in order to discourage behaviour, e.g. physical pain through smacking or electric shock
Negative reinforcement – the removal of something the individual finds annoying or unpleasurable, e.g. a loud noise is removed for 'good' behaviour	**Sanctions** – something pleasant is removed to discourage behaviour, e.g. not earning pocket money
	Extinction – if a specific behaviour is no longer reinforced, then as with classical conditioning, the operantly conditioned behaviour will extinguish

essentially **hedonistic** or pleasure-seeking – that what we find pleasurable (or not, as the case may be) can determine how and what we learn (see Table 1.2).

As you can see from Table 1.2, **reinforcement** increases desired behaviours while **punishment** (and its less contentious cousin, the sanction) and **extinction** are techniques for decreasing unwanted behaviours. Bear in mind also that reinforcement does not have to be tangible – social reinforcers such as praise, acceptance and positive regard can all have a significant impact on the way people behave in society.

Since behaviourists see all human behaviour as learnt behaviour, they see the behaviours associated with what we call 'mental illness' simply as behaviours that have been learnt. Once learnt, these behaviours persist because they have been reinforced or there has been no punishment. Take phobias, discussed in much more detail in Chapter 5, for example. Behaviourists claim that phobias arise because of a learnt association between a specific object/situation and fear, and that they persist because avoidance of the object/situation acts as a negative reinforcer.

Since behaviourists believe that mental health problems are the result of learning, they also believe that these behaviours can be unlearnt or **modified** through conditioning techniques; indeed, a whole new field of 'applied behaviourism' – **behaviour therapy** – emerged during the 1960s and 1970s (see, for example, Wolpe, 1969). Specific behaviour therapies include **aversion therapy**, **systematic desensitisation** (also called **graded exposure**), **flooding** and the **token economy**. Aversion therapy, used extensively in the 1960s and 1970s (particularly to treat 'sexual deviants') is based on classical

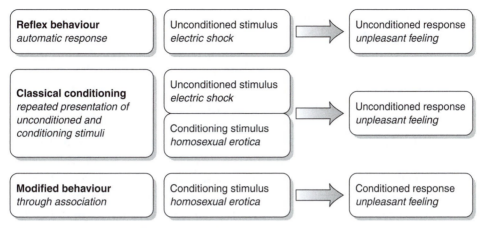

FIGURE 1.4   Aversion therapy for homosexuality

conditioning principles. Figure 1.4 illustrates aversion therapy as a 'cure' for homosexuality.

Aversion therapy has been abandoned as a treatment for sexual deviancy (primarily because it doesn't work but also because of the ethical issues involved in trying to change people's sexuality). It is sometimes still used in the treatment of alcohol misuse. Since certain drugs (e.g. disulfiram) produce a very unpleasant effect when combined with alcohol, the theory goes that people who voluntarily take such drugs and then drink alcohol will associate drinking alcohol with unpleasant effects and will thus avoid alcohol. Unfortunately, adherence to aversive treatment regimens is, understandably, very low (Garbutt, 2009) and, as you will discover in Chapter 11, much more effective ways of helping people who misuse alcohol exist.

Systematic desensitisation, a technique also based on classical conditioning principles, has had some success in the treatment of phobias, as you will discover in Chapter 5. It assumes that a phobic object/situation has somehow become associated with fear and anxiety (as a conditioned response) and that this response can be 'deconditioned' by replacing the anxiety associated with the phobic object/situation with relaxation. This is done via a number of steps (hence why it is sometime called 'graded exposure'), with less anxiety-provoking exposures to the phobic object/situation (such as merely thinking about it) being dealt with first and more severe anxiety-provoking exposures (such as full contact with the object/situation) at later stages in the therapy.

Flooding, another treatment for phobias, works on operant conditioning principles. In flooding, the person with a phobia is forced to confront the phobic object/situation with no opportunity for escape (e.g. someone with a dog phobia would be locked in a room with a dog). Since behaviourists believe phobias persist because avoidance of the object/situation acts as a negative reinforcer, flooding prevents this avoidance and so the phobia extinguishes as a consequence.

The token economy, which peaked in popularity in psychiatry in the 1970s and 1980s, is an operant conditioning approach on a large scale. Tokens are (or, indeed, money is) handed out as a reward for desired behaviours. These tokens can subsequently be exchanged for pleasurable activities. Though the token economy is little used in psychiatry nowadays, the operant conditioning principles underpinning it still form the basis of endeavours such as performance related pay, the 'star charts' common in child rearing (see Chapter 9) and 'contingency management' in substance misuse (see Chapter 11).

That behavioural methods are effective with some mental health problems (phobias and conduct disorders in children being two examples) adds some weight to the behaviourist perspective. However, purely behavioural techniques are relatively ineffective with major mental illnesses such as the psychoses[2] and behaviourism has come in for much criticism (especially in its most extreme form, radical behaviourism) because it fails to appreciate the influence of internal mediating processes (like thoughts, moods and desires) that are an essential part of the human condition. These internal mediating processes are, on the other hand, central to two other psychological perspectives: psychoanalysis and cognitivism.

Psychoanalysis

Psychoanalysis is, to some extent, the antithesis of behaviourism in that its focus is the internal psychological processes the behaviourists deem to be unimportant. It was founded in Europe at the turn of the twentieth century by the Austrian physician Sigmund Freud (hence it is sometimes called **Freudian psychology**), around the same time as behaviourism was being developed in the United States. Several other theorists (Carl Jung, Alfred Adler and Melanie Klein, for example) have built upon the work of Freud to produce their own versions of psychoanalytical therapy and the perspective also encapsulates the briefer and less intensive forms of therapy known as **psychodynamic psychotherapy**.

---

[2]Although cognitive behavioural approaches may have some impact on the so-called 'positive' symptoms of psychosis – see Chapter 6.

Psychoanalysis and its derivatives are principally concerned with the **unconscious** mind. Common to all psychoanalytical theories is the notion of **conflict** between the various parts of the unconscious mind and the emotional energy associated with such conflicts (hence the reason why 'psychodynamic' is often used in psychoanalytical writings). Mental illness thus arises as a result of unresolved subconscious conflicts between various abstract parts of the unconscious mind. These conflicts often arise in childhood, persisting into adulthood and manifesting as mental illness simply because they are unresolved. Perhaps the most well-known conflict is that between the **id** (our real, deep-seated, often irrational desires) and the **superego** (to some extent, the conscience). Treatment centres on resolution of these conflicts, via a prolonged analysis of the individual's experiences and feelings (hence the term 'psychoanalysis'). During psychoanalysis, the therapist interprets various aspects of the individual's experience – their dreams, thoughts, words and feelings – in the hope that the seemingly irrational will become understandable and so the conflicts will resolve.

The observation that childhood experiences often greatly affect our psychological development in later life adds some support to this perspective. Psychoanalysis has, however, fallen out fashion in the UK over the last couple of decades amid concerns over its evidence base. As Fonagy (2003) points out, the evidence base for psychoanalysis is relatively thin and the long-term, intensive nature of much psychoanalytical practice is often at odds with the contemporary emphasis on cost-effective treatments. Nevertheless, many people report a great sense of personal development after undergoing psychoanalysis and psychodynamic psychotherapy – its less rigid cousin – still has many adherents.

Cognitivism

Advances in computer technology during the 1950s and 1960s offered psychologists a new perspective. Analogies between humans and machines were frequently drawn with an emphasis on humans as **information processors** and thus the cognitive school of psychology – cognitivism – was born. Like psychoanalytical theorists, cognitive theorists are interested in the abstract mental processes that underlie our behaviour and thought processes though their focus is not unconscious conflicts but the processes concerned with the acquisition or manipulation of knowledge: the cognitive processes of perceiving, remembering, reasoning, judging, thinking, etc. Moreover, unlike psychoanalytical approaches, cognitive approaches are bound by rigid scientific and experimental methods. The most well-known cognitive theorist is

Jean Piaget, whose theory of cognitive development has had a huge influence on the education policies of the Western world. Cognitivism is currently the dominant perspective in academic psychology and it has been making significant inroads into mental health practice over the last decade or so.

According to the cognitive perspective, mental illness occurs when problems arise in any or all of our cognitive processes and it is our ability to **think** that provides the treatment rationale within this perspective. The control (albeit sometimes limited) that we have over our cognitive processes allows us to 'retune' our thinking and thus produce a world-view that is more healthy to our mental wellbeing. Depression is a good example (and one considered in much more detail Chapter 4). Aaron Beck's cognitive theory of depression (Beck, 1967) argues that depression occurs because of cognitive 'distortions' brought about by **automatic thinking**, **erroneous assumptions and beliefs** and the ways which assign **meaning** to our experiences (see Box 1.1). By tackling these distortions ('retuning' our thinking through **cognitive therapy**), it is possible to change automatic and erroneous beliefs about ourselves and our experiences and consequently change the way we feel about ourselves.

Box 1.1   Principles of Beck's cognitive theory of depression (after Beck, 1967, 1976)

- The interpretation or **meaning** that an individual gives to an event impacts on their emotions and on how they behave.
- The interpretation or meaning is subject to some '**automatic**' ways of thinking.
- People with depression tend to have a negative **schema** – or theme – about the world, brought on through childhood experiences such as the loss of a parent, rejection by peers or criticism by teachers or parents.
- There is a **negative triad** about:
  (1)   the self ('I am defective or inadequate');
  (2)   the person's life experiences ('everything I do ends in defeat or failure'); and
  (3)   the future ('the future is hopeless').
- Cognitive **biases** and **distortions** fuel the negative schema.

The **rational emotive therapy** of Albert Ellis (Ellis, 1962) is another cognitive approach that has many similarities to Beck's cognitive therapy. Interestingly, both Beck and Ellis started off as psychoanalysts before developing their cognitive theories.

Humanism

During the late 1960s and early 1970s, a new school of psychology emerged that questioned whether the objective, cold, rational approach of science was appropriate to a discipline ultimately concerned with human experience. Humanistic psychology places great emphasis on the **subjective** value of our experiences. Major theorists of humanism include Abraham Maslow and Carl Rogers (who we will meet again in the next chapter). Humanistic approaches underlie the majority of modern-day counselling approaches and have been hugely influential in mental health nursing. You might see humanistic approaches referred to as **phenomenological**, **experiential**, **existential** or **personal growth** approaches. Box 1.2 provides some brief descriptions of the meanings of these terms within the context of humanism.

Box 1.2   Terms associated with the humanistic perspective

- **Humanistic:** seeing the person as a **human being**, rather than as an illness or collection of symptoms
- **Phenomenological:** phenomenology is the study of phenomena (the plural of phenomenon), which are simply everyday occurrences or things that happen
- **Experiential:** what a person **experiences** is of primary interest to the practitioner
- **Existential:** concerned with **existence**; a theoretical viewpoint stressing the importance of the individual's own experiences
- **Personal growth:** concerned with the belief that humans have a reservoir of untapped potential and the opportunities for personal growth that arise as a result of tapping this potential can have benefits for not only the individual but society as a whole

---

To a large extent, humanism is a framework for mental *health* rather than mental illness. Humanists believe that increasing the value – the self-esteem – of an individual ultimately leads to greater mental wellbeing. Personal growth is seen as the answer to mental distress in the world. Signs and symptoms of what we call mental illness arise when individuals fail to take responsibility for their own lives, or when they cut themselves off from their own experiences. In therapeutic environments, such personal growth is facilitated through what Rogers (1980) calls the core conditions of the therapist: **unconditional positive regard**, **empathic understanding** and **genuineness** (we will consider these core conditions in more detail in the next chapter).

The fact that many people benefit from humanistic styles of counselling provides some support for this perspective. However, humanism is not without criticism. For example, a focus on personal growth may not be particularly effective with someone experiencing an acute psychotic episode. And while the (unashamed) positioning of the individual at the centre of care may appear laudable, the individual's place in society or any of its structures, such as the family or community, often gets overlooked. Humanism has also been criticised for being too optimistic and perhaps a little unrealistic: Rogers' notion of unconditional positive regard, for example, can be difficult to accept when individuals have done truly evil things and when there is evidence from the cognitive psychologists that we are inherently judgemental when we process information about people.

Reflection Point

Being non-judgemental

Humanistic practitioners often talk of being 'non-judgemental'. How easy do you think this is?

When answering this question, think about when you meet someone for the first time. Do you make assumptions about him or her based on the way they look, they way they speak or the way they act? Do these assumptions make you act in a different way to how you might otherwise act?

What if you read in a service user's case notes that they had been accused of rape? Would your judgement of that person be different from the judgement you would have made had you not read the notes?

Social perspectives

The biological and psychological perspectives discussed thus far have one thing in common: they all focus on the **individual**. However, individuals do not exist in isolation from one another; they exist within social groups such as families, peers, communities and societies. Social perspectives have influenced mental health practices in two main ways: by encouraging practitioners to embed the individual service user's experience into a wider social context, devising appropriate 'social' interventions as a consequence; and challenging the very concept of mental illness itself.

Social interventions

Social interventions can be seen as those interventions that address the individual's role within various social groups. Social interventions as such include group approaches, family approaches and interventions linked to 'normal' life activities such as work, leisure and play, forming relationships, and so on. As you will discover throughout this book, social interventions are becoming increasingly important in the repertoire of interventions available to mental health practitioners.

Family approaches, for example, have been routine in child mental health (see Chapters 9 and 10) for decades because society generally conceptualises children as part of a family unit than as individuals. On the other hand, most adults belong to a family unit or to wider social networks and a growing acknowledgement of this means that family approaches are increasingly being seen as valuable in adult mental health (see, for example, Chapters 6 and 8). The influence of work, another social activity, on an individual's mental health has also come to the fore in recent times, forming a core part of the government's latest mental health strategy, *New Horizons* (see HM Government, 2009). There is also evidence that, in some circumstances, group approaches to mental healthcare may be more effective than individual approaches. Examples include the care of older people with depression or dementia (see Chapter 8), the care of young people who self harm (see Chapter 10), and the care of people with an antisocial personality disorder (see Chapter 12).

Challenging mental illness: anti-psychiatry

Anti-psychiatry (sometimes **critical psychiatry**) essentially began with the publication of *Madness and Civilization*, a history of madness by the French sociologist and philosopher Michel Foucault (see Foucault, 1965). Foucault challenged the fundamental assumption of biological psychiatry by claiming that madness had nothing to with biology but was instead a product of a given society's attitudes and values. Other well-known 'anti-psychiatrists' include R.D. Laing (himself a psychiatrist) and Thomas Szasz, who coined the phrase 'the myth of mental illness' with his book of the same name (Szasz, 1961). Anti-psychiatry argues that mentally ill people are deemed to be mentally ill not because they have, say, an imbalance in brain chemistry but because their behaviours are at odds with what society expects or will tolerate. As such, the mentally ill merely have problems with living or difficulty in conforming to the rules of society. And since society defines madness, psychiatrists (and those who work for them) are seen not as therapists but merely as 'social police'.

This perspective has some credibility. History is littered with examples of those who refuse to conform being seen as deviant or abnormal in some way and society's view of deviance or abnormality can vary both across time and across cultures. Homosexuality, for example, was seen as a treatable mental illness by the psychiatric classifications ICD and DSM for most of the twentieth century (it was removed from DSM in 1973 and from ICD in 1990).

Since it focuses on people as human beings – albeit within the constraints of society's rules and regulations – rather than on illness, anti-psychiatry has some overlap with humanistic perspectives. Other influences in anti-psychiatry include Erving Goffman's work relating to **stigma** (Goffman, 1963) and Thomas Scheff's work on **labelling theory** and madness (see Scheff, 1966). Stigmatisation refers to those 'disqualified from social acceptance' and since it includes those deemed to be mentally ill, it is a concept we will return to throughout this book. Labelling theory is a theory that implies that society's very act of labelling certain people (e.g. as 'criminal', 'immoral' or 'mad') leads to those people developing identities that conform to the label, i.e. the very act of labelling becomes a self-fulfilling prophecy.

More recent commentators who could be said to fit broadly into an anti-psychiatry perspective include: the psychologists Mary Boyle (see Boyle, 2002) and Richard Bentall (see Bentall, 2009), both of whom question the scientific validity of so-called (in their view) mental illnesses such as schizophrenia; the Dutch psychiatrist Marius Romme and Dutch journalist Sandra Escher, whose Hearing Voices movement sees voice hearing not as a symptom of mental illness but as a normal part of the makeup of many individuals; and the lobby group the Campaign for the Abolition of the Schizophrenia Label (see www.caslcampaign.com).

Treating schizophrenia

Below you will find how each of the main perspectives in psychiatry explains schizophrenia. Which do you prefer? Can you think of how treatments might be developed within each of the perspectives?

- **Biological perspective:** Schizophrenia is a genetic condition caused by an imbalance of brain chemicals that affects certain brain systems in particular.
- **Behavioural perspective:** Schizophrenia is simply a set of learnt behaviours.
- **Cognitive perspective:** Schizophrenia arises because of a breakdown in the processing of information. Perhaps internal mechanisms for information processing have become distorted or damaged in some way. Schizophrenia may merely be the human equivalent of computer problems: bugs, viruses, garbled characters on the screen, and so on.
- **Psychodynamic perspective:** Schizophrenia is caused by internal unconscious conflicts, probably arising during the early years of our lives. These conflicts remain unresolved and as a consequence, innate, irrational demands surge into consciousness and manifest as schizophrenia.
- **Humanistic perspective:** A person with so-called 'schizophrenia' is merely exploring their own personality, in particular the 'hidden', deeper parts of the self. It is an experience which, though uncomfortable and distressing at times, can ultimately lead to a greater knowledge of the self – after all, many so-called mentally ill people are extraordinarily creative.
- **Social perspective:** Schizophrenia is not an illness. Some individuals merely refuse to comply with society's rules and regulations and live unmoderated lives, free from the restrictions of society.

If you have had a chance to consider the discussion point above, one of the difficulties you may have encountered is that looking at mental illness from one or other of the specific perspectives listed means you can only partially explain or resolve things. Many theorists and practitioners have been stymied by this limitation and as such two main solutions have emerged, both common in current mental health practice. The first is the establishment of what might be called **hybrid** perspectives, where elements from various perspectives are combined into new theoretical perspectives; the second is **eclecticism**, which is about taking the best elements from each of the perspectives (having no particular loyalty to any of the perspectives) to create your own unique model of practice. We shall discuss hybrid models next but leave eclecticism for a short while as it is best considered when we talk about individual philosophies of mental health nursing a little later.

Hybrid perspectives

The main hybrid perspectives you are likely to come across in mental health practice are **social cognitive theory**, **cognitive analytical therapy**, **interpersonal therapy**, **cognitive behaviour therapy** and the so-called **third wave therapies**. While **the recovery model** can also be seen as a hybrid perspective, it is more of an overall philosophy of mental health practice. Moreover, since recovery is central to much modern-day mental health practice, it will be given special consideration later on in this chapter.

Social cognitive theory

Social cognitive theory (also known as **social learning theory**) is a cognitive theory of learning that emphasises social interactions, in particular the notion of learning through the observation of model behaviour or people (i.e., **role models**). It is, in essence, a hybrid of social and cognitive perspectives, stemming from the work of Albert Bandura in the 1960s. It is still influential today, particularly in consumer and social marketing. A good example is the 2008/9 advertising campaign run by Trident (an anti-gun crime organisation targeting young black Londoners) in which positive black role models were used to illustrate that 'respect' could be garnered, not through guns, but through success in sports, the arts and business.

Social cognitive theory has implications for nursing practice in that it implies that service users may well see nurses as role models.

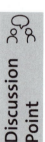

Discussion Point

Nurses as role models

How should you behave in practice if you are to act as a role model? Should nurses be role models? How important do you think each of the following factors is in mental health nursing?

- How you dress
- Your hairstyle
- Your weight
- Whether you smoke cigarettes or not
- Your alcohol intake
- Whether you lose your temper easily
- Whether you use recreational drugs
- Whether you are on time for duty or habitually late
- Whether you have body adornments such as tattoos or piercings

Cognitive – psychodynamic hybrids

Two cognitive – psychodynamic hybrids that have made some inroads into current mental health practice in recent years are **cognitive analytical therapy** (CAT) and **interpersonal therapy** (IPT).

Developed by Anthony Ryle (see Ryle & Kerr, 2002), CAT is a brief therapy designed for use in depression, anxiety and, more recently, personality disorder (see Chapter 12). CAT integrates cognitive therapy principles such as formulation, homework and problem-solving with the analytical elements of psychoanalysis – although the analysis is descriptive and collaborative rather than interpretive as it is in traditional psychoanalysis (Denman, 2001).

IPT, developed by Gerald Klerman (see Klerman et al., 1984) as a treatment for depression, is heavily influenced by interpersonal psychoanalysis, a style of psychoanalysis developed by Harry Stack Sullivan that focuses on interpersonal relationships rather than the intra-psychic conflicts of traditional Freudian psychoanalysis. IPT combines Sullivan's interpersonal psychoanalysis with the structured elements of cognitive behavioural therapy (see the next section) such as time limited therapy, clinical assessment tools and homework.

While the evidence base for CAT is somewhat limited, the evidence for IPT suggests it has potential in the treatment of depression; indeed, it is recommended as a treatment option in both the English National Institute for Health and Clinical Excellence (NICE, 2009) and the Scottish Intercollegiate Guidelines Network (SIGN, 2010) guidance on depression.

Cognitive behavioural approaches

Perhaps the most well-known hybrid approach is **cognitive behaviour therapy** or **CBT**. Unsurprisingly, it is an approach that combines cognitive and behavioural approaches to therapy. Its roots lie in attempts to merge the successes of cognitive approaches like Ellis's rational emotive therapy and Beck's cognitive therapy with the successes of Wolpe's behavioural approaches. CBT has had some remarkable successes, especially with the so called 'common mental health problems' of anxiety and depression (see Chapters 4 and 5), and it is very much a dominant model in current mental health practice. Given its dominance, and the fact that it is permeating areas of mental health practice as diverse as psychosis and self-harm, we will say little more about CBT here since we will make frequent reference to it throughout Part II of this book. Importantly, this does not mean that we have ignored any other therapeutic approaches for which robust evidence exists; CBT crops up so much in the areas and conditions that we look at in Part II of this book simply because its evidence base is significantly better than that of many competing therapies.

The hybrid nature of CBT also seems have sparked a thirst to integrate additional elements into the cognitive behavioural model, resulting in a whole host of what might be called 'third wave' behavioural therapies (behaviour therapy being the first wave and CBT the second; Hayes, 2004). The third wave therapies often have what might be termed an added **spiritual** dimension to them and include: **cognitive behavioural hypnotherapy** (adds hypnosis to CBT); **dialectical behaviour therapy** (DBT; inspired by Buddhist teaching, it adds the notion of 'mindfulness' to CBT); **schema therapy** for personality disorder (adds elements of mindfulness and psychoanalysis to CBT; see also the previous section and Chapter 12) and **acceptance and commitment therapy** (ACT), a therapy that focuses on individuals noticing, accepting and embracing their thoughts and feelings rather than trying to change them as in CBT.

The Recovery Model

While the recovery model is more of a philosophy of mental health-care than a specific theoretical perspective, it does nevertheless draw some of its influence from some of the specific perspectives we have explored thus far, most notably the humanistic and social perspectives. It also draws on the consumer and survivor movements of the 1980s and 1990s as well as concepts related to these movements such as **self-help**, **empowerment** and **advocacy** (Shepherd et al., 2008). In addition, recovery's focus on hope rather than despair and ability rather than disability has some affinity with **positive psychology**, a relatively new development in psychology that focuses on mental wellness rather than illness (see Seligman, 2003).

Recovery is perhaps best understood by examining the principles that underpin it (see Box 1.3). There will, however, be many more opportunities to grasp what recovery means because it is so central to contemporary mental health practice and, as such, is a common theme throughout this book.

> ## Box 1.3 The principles of recovery (adapted from NIMHE, 2005)
>
> - **Choice:** the service user decides if and when to begin the recovery process and directs it.
> - **Avoiding dependency:** the mental health system must be aware of its tendency to promote service user dependency.
> - **Holism:** recovery from mental illness is most effective when a holistic approach is considered including psychological, emotional, spiritual, physical and social needs.
> - **Hope:** service users are able to recover more quickly when hope is encouraged, life roles are defined, spirituality is considered, culture is understood, educational and socialisation needs are identified, and they are supported to achieve their goals via trusting relationships.
> - **Diversity:** individual differences and diversity should be considered and valued.
> - **Eclecticism:** a recovery approach embraces medical/biological, psychological, social and values based approaches to mental health care.
> - **Involving significant others:** involvement of a person's family, partner and friends may enhance the recovery process. The service user should define whom they wish to involve.
> - **Cultural sensitivity:** mental health services are most effective when delivery is within the context of the service user's locality and cultural context.
> - **Community:** community involvement, as defined by the service user, is central to the recovery process.

Shepherd et al. (2008) outline four elements to the recovery process: (1) the instillation of **hope**; (2) the (re)establishment of a **positive identity**; (3) the building of a **meaningful life**; and (4) the taking of **responsibility and control**. In adopting a philosophy of recovery, Shepherd et al. see the role of nurses and other mental health practitioners as guides, facilitators and coaches to service users attempting to progress along the road to recovery.

Recovery is not without its critics. Slade & Hayward (2008), for example, argue that without research evidence of recovery's effectiveness, it is hard to tell what the future holds for recovery. Will it result in the paradigm shift in service provision that its advocates claim? Will it go the way of many other ideas in mental health and simply disappear into obscurity? Perhaps the worst outcome is that nothing changes – that services are renamed to include

'recovery' in their titles without any real change in their function or in the
attitudes of the staff who work for them.

At this point, we have considered what we have called the 'psychiatric'
perspectives on mental health and mental health care (we have essentially
dealt with the left-hand side of Figure 1.2), even though some of these perspectives are in reality diametrically opposed to traditional psychiatry. As
mental health nurses, we also need to deal with our other parent – nursing –
and explore how nursing perspectives have influenced our practices.

Nursing Perspectives

Psychiatric nurses or mental health nurses?

In recent years there has been some debate over whether we are **psychiatric
nurses** (i.e., we practise within psychiatry) or whether we are **mental
health nurses** (i.e., our roles are concerned with mental health rather than
mental illness). Hopefully, by now you will have begun to understand the
origins of this debate and the factors that continue to influence it: our history, the tensions between psychiatry and anti-psychiatry, and the recent
upsurge in conceptualisations and models of psychiatry/mental health that
focus on wellbeing and health rather than disease and ill-health.

As mentioned earlier, by virtue of the NMC, we are legally 'mental health
nurses'. Chambers (2006), in a debate on the topic with du Mont (2006), has
pointed out the irony of this since much of the work we do relates to *mental
illness* rather than mental health. Chambers adds, however, that 'mental health
nurse' is a much more forward-looking title that is less stigmatising and one
that embraces the philosophy of recovery. Du Mont (2006), however, argues
that the since much of what we do is focused on the mentally ill, and since
we are likely to play a greater role in directly treating people with mental
health problems in the future (even to the point of prescribing medication –
see Chapter 3) then we should just be honest and call ourselves 'psychiatric
nurses' or, at the very least, 'mental illness nurses'. An alternative is to adopt
the term that is in frequent use in the United States, **psychiatric/mental
health nurse**, but it's a somewhat inelegant term that has not really caught
on in the UK. One radical proposal is that, like physical health, we split the
profession into two. In physical health, those nurses concerned with the promotion of health – public health nurses – have a separate identity as **health
visitors**, while 'illness nursing' is carried out by general (adult) nurses.

This may be happening already in mental health (nursing) inasmuch as mental health promotion is steadily becoming, as you will see in Chapter 3, the remit of a separate worker, the 'psychological wellbeing practitioner'.

Whatever the debates about the profession – whether we are psychiatric or mental health nurses, or whether what we do is actually *nursing* given the public's stereotypical views of nurses and the recent advances in mental healthcare provision – nursing has had an unquestionable influence on the profession. Its influence has been three-fold: (1) it has reminded us that minds do not exist independently of bodies; (2) it has provided us with **the nursing process**, a specific way of helping people; and (3) it has provided us with a plethora of **nursing models**.

Mind and body

Reminding us that the people we with work with have physical bodies can be a two-edged sword. On the one hand, understanding that there is a connection between physical ill health and mental ill health (especially long term conditions such as heart disease, diabetes and 'medically unexplained symptoms', see Lyons et al., 2006) and vice versa (mentally ill people often have poor physical health, see Osborn, 2001; Seymour, 2003) can only improve the care we give. On the other hand, an overemphasis on the physical can bring about the rigidity and rituals that are often associated with adult (general) nursing. Moreover, such an overemphasis on the physical may be off-putting to many potential applicants for mental health nursing since people wanting to work in mental health generally want to work with the mind rather than the body! The sensible approach here is to have a balance between the two, though arguments about the degree of balance tend to elicit the 'generic nurse vs. specialist mental health nurse' debates we alluded to earlier. Still, few mental health nurses would argue against including basic anatomy and physiology, basic physical nursing care and basic first aid in a mental health nurse preparation programme; many mental health nurses would, however, argue fervently that you do not need to be a generically qualified nurse before you become a mental health nurse, as is the case in many other countries around the world.

The nursing process

The nursing process is a **problem-solving** approach to care. It is frequently described in the British nursing literature as being cyclical and having four

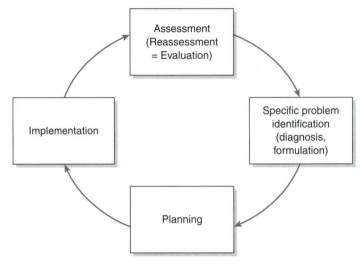

FIGURE 1.5   A modified version of the nursing process

stages: **assessment**, **planning**, **implementation** and **evaluation** (McKenna, 1997). There are two problems with this particular view of the nursing process, however: (1) the leap from assessment to planning is missing an interim stage where the results of the assessment are crystallised in order to guide planning; and (2) since evaluation has many of the same elements of assessment (evaluation can be seen as re-assessment) and requires the same skills, it could be argued that there is really a single stage here and not two. These shortcomings are addressed via a modified version of the nursing process outlined in Figure 1.5.

The missing stage between assessment and planning has been termed 'specific problem identification' (which is quite a useful thing to have in a model based on problem-solving!) but elsewhere in this book you might also find it referred to as **diagnosis** or **formulation**.

Use of the nursing process in mental health nursing is pretty uncontroversial. After all, as you will discover throughout this book, a problem-solving framework is a reasonable one for guiding practice. It has one flaw, however; a flaw that is not fatal but one that yet again opens up the question of mental health nursing's identity. As McKenna (1997) points out, though called the *nursing* process, it is hardly unique to nursing, it being a process that most health-care professionals employ. McKenna adds further that what makes it a *nursing* process is the addition of nursing theory or the practical implementations of those theories, the **nursing models**. And herein lies another problem.

Nursing models

One thing you may notice about the ensuing chapters of this book is the lack of specific reference to nursing models. This is partly because, as Gournay (1995) argued some time back, those nursing models that have been used in mental health are archaic and fall short when it comes to an evidence base. There is perhaps a more compelling argument against their use from those who have contributed to this book. In our experiences of educating and training a variety of mental health professionals – mental health nurses in particular – we know that we can teach students to effectively help people with mental health problems without the need for specific *nursing* theories or models. Notice the emphasis on nursing here: almost all of us (as you will discover) use theoretical models of some sort to aid practice and at the root of most of our models is something akin to the problem-solving approach of the nursing process; it's just that we are not particularly precious about those models being nursing models. This is not to say that nursing models *cannot* be used, however, and we appreciate that many clinical areas and many mental health nurse educators still find nursing models useful, especially as a framework for helping learners undertake assessments with service users. To this end, a summary of the nursing models that have been used by mental health nurses is presented in Table 1.3. If any particular model sparks your interest, or if you find yourself in a practice area that is fixated with a particular model, then further reading will be beneficial – whether you want merely to satisfy your interests or do something a little more rebellious like constructing a case for discontinuation of a particular model in practice.

Models underpinning nursing practice

Discussion Point

Next time you're in practice, ask your colleagues and mentors if they can name any specific models or theoretical frameworks that underpin or influence their practice.

Ask them how rigidly they adhere to the models or frameworks. Have they made adaptations to the model to make it 'fit' better to practise? Can they tell you what the evidence base is for the particular models or frameworks they use?

TABLE 1.3   Nursing models in mental health nursing

Model, originator, locale	Brief details of the model	Comments and criticisms
Activities of Daily Living Roper, Logan & Tierney (see Roper et al., 2000) UK	Assessment and identification of problems in each of several 'activities of daily living': maintaining a safe environment; communication; breathing; eating/drinking; elimination; washing/dressing; controlling temperature; mobilisation; working/playing; expressing sexuality; sleeping; death/dying	Physically oriented model Little applicability to mental health though often used in physically demanding areas of mental health care such as inpatient dementia care
Orem's Self Care Model Dorothea Orem (see Orem, 2001) USA	Identification of self care deficits in the 'universal self-care requisites for health': air; water; food; elimination; activity/rest; solitude/social interaction; hazard prevention; promotion of normality Provision of three levels of support depending on the degree of deficit: total compensation (the person is unable to self care); partial compensation (the person needs help with self care); education and support (the person is taught to self care)	Overlooks some of the profound and complex self care difficulties experienced by those with mental health problems (Gournay, 1995) Illness-oriented approach
Roy Adaptation Model Sister Callista Roy (see Roy & Andrews, 2008) USA	Based on the concept of **adaptation**: the process by which living creatures enhance their survival and development Sees the individual as a set of interrelated biological, psychological and social systems in constant interaction with the environment Goal of nursing is to promote adaptive responses in each of the four adaptive modes: **physiologic-physical** (focuses on the body); **self concept-group identity** (focuses on the psychological and spiritual aspects of the human system); **role function** (focuses on the individual's various roles); **interdependence** (focuses on the individual's close relationships)	Anachronistic (Gournay, 1995) Complex model that is difficult to understand Takes no account of contemporary theories associated with adaptation such as self-efficacy and resilience

TABLE 1.3 (Continued)

Model, originator, locale	Brief details of the model	Comments and criticisms
Interpersonal Relations Model Hildegard Peplau (see Peplau, 1991) USA	Nursing is seen as an interpersonal process, with the nurse adopting a number of roles: **stranger** (useful in building up a relationship); **teacher**; **resource** (supplier of information); **counsellor**; **surrogate** (clarifying where dependence, interdependence and independence are appropriate and acting as an advocate); **leader** (helping the individual maximise their responsibility in achieving their goals) Four phases of the nurse–patient relationship (driven by the individual rather than nurse): (1) **orientation** (the individual and nurse mutually identify the problem); (2) **identification** (the individual identifies with the nurse in order to be helped); (3) **exploitation** (the individual exploits the nurse's skills and resources); and (4) **resolution** (the individual resolves the problems and frees him or herself from the relationship with the nurse)	Developed by a psychiatric nurse Influenced by psychodynamic psychology Little emphasis on the individual's wider social roles (e.g. family, community) Little focus on health promotion or prevention Anachronistic
Tidal model Phil Barker and Poppy Buchanan-Barker (see Barker & Buchanan-Barker, 2005) UK	Uses the metaphor of **water** to enable people with mental health problems to tell their stories and move towards recovery. Key assumptions: • the primary therapeutic focus of mental health care is the 'world of ordinary life', i.e. the community • change is an ongoing constant process and small changes are important • empowerment, in that the helper has to give up the power relationship characterising normal professional–service user relationships • nursing is about caring *with* people rather than caring for them	Developed by a psychiatric nurse Recovery-focused model Can be seen as bordering on the mystical Limited evidence base though qualitative evaluations exist (see Stevenson & Fletcher, 2002)

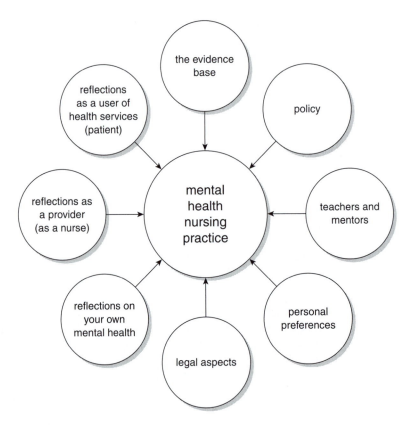

FIGURE 1.6   Eclecticism in mental health nursing

Individual philosophies in mental health nursing: eclecticism

As far as individual nursing practice is concerned, mental health nurses more often than not adopt the perspective(s) that most appeal to them. However, given the current emphasis on evidence-based practice, it is important that we do not let ideological dogma alone dominate our practices. Though there are some practitioners who rigidly adhere to one or other of the theoretical frameworks, these are the exception rather than the rule. Most skilled practitioners take an **eclectic** approach: they have an awareness of the strengths and weaknesses of the various perspectives and models, and they use their professional judgement to select a treatment approach most suitable for a given set of circumstances.

Eclecticism in mental health nursing is normally a combination of: (1) mental health nurses' own experiences; (2) the models and frameworks they have been exposed to by those with influence (such as their teachers and clinical colleagues; government policy and legal requirements also play a role here); (3) the available evidence base; and (4) personal preferences (see Figure 1.6).

Conclusion

In this chapter we have explored the nature of both mental health and mental health nursing. We have set the medical model against a range of other theoretical perspectives with a particular emphasis on recovery as a dominant philosophy of mental health practice and CBT as a dominant therapeutic approach. We have emphasised that these perspectives are dominant not necessarily because they are 'the best' but because they are either, as is the case with recovery, timely in terms of the political appetite of the policymakers and the general public, or because, as is the case with CBT, they have the most robust evidence base when compared to alternatives.

Along our journey we have also raised many questions about the future of mental health nursing. We have considered whether we are, indeed, mental health nurses or whether we are mental illness or psychiatric nurses, and we have questioned the value (or not, as the case may be) of nursing-specific models in a multi-professional environment. Hopefully, by being party to these debates, you have got a taste for modern mental health nursing (or whatever you choose to call it!) and that, as such, your enthusiasm for the profession has grown in what is a very exciting time for mental health nursing.

Further Reading and Resources

Key texts – psychiatric critiques and social perspectives

Boyle M (2002). *Schizophrenia: A Scientific Delusion?*, 2nd edition. London: Routledge.
Modern-day classic questioning the scientific validity of schizophrenia.

Szasz, TS (2010). *The Myth of Mental Illness: Foundations of a Theory of Personal Conduct*, 50th Anniversary edition. London: Harper Perennial.
A 50th Anniversary edition of Szasz's critique of psychiatry, with a new preface for the age of modern psychotropic medication.

Bentall RP (2009). *Doctoring the Mind: Is Our Current Treatment of Mental Illness Really Any Good?* London: Penguin.
Accessible critique of modern psychiatry questioning, like Boyle and Szasz, the validity of psychiatric disorders and the ethics and politics of psychiatric medication.

Key texts – nursing perspectives

Aggleton P & Chalmers H (2000). *Nursing Models and Nursing Practice*, 2nd edition. Basingstoke: Palgrave.
   The key British text on nursing models for those interested in finding out more about specific nursing models.

Nolan P (1998). *A History of Mental Health Nursing*. Cheltenham: Nelson Thornes.
   Classic text for those interested in the history of British mental health nursing.

Stevenson C & Fletcher E (2002). The Tidal Model: the questions answered. *Mental Health Practice*, 5(8), 29–38.
   Simple introduction to the Tidal Model from the Royal College of Nursing's Continuing Professional Development series.

Key texts – general

Appignanesi R & Zarate O (2003). *Freud for Beginners*. New York: Pantheon.
   Fun, cartoon-style introduction to Freudian theory – a theory that can be quite daunting and complex.

Beck AT (1976). *Cognitive Therapy and the Emotional Disorders*. New York: International Universities Press.
   Classic text on cognitive therapy; much of it is still relevant today.

Cooper M, O'Hara M, Scmid P & Wyatt G (2007). *The Handbook of Person-Centred Psychotherapy and Counselling*. Basingstoke: Palgrave Macmillan.
   Comprehensive, modern text on all aspects of person-centred (humanistic) therapy.

Pilgrim D (2009). *Key Concepts in Mental Health*, 2nd edition. London: Sage.
   Accessible text in Sage's 'Key Concepts' series that explores a wide range of key concepts, terms, therapies and approaches in mental health.

Repper J & Perkins R (2003). *Social Inclusion and Recovery: A Model for Mental Health Practice*. London: Ballière-Tindall.
   Key text on the recovery model, written by acknowledged experts in this area, and including service user perspectives.

Shepherd G, Boardman J & Slade M (2008). *Making Recovery a Reality*. London: Sainsbury Centre for Mental Health.
   Key policy document on recovery, written by national experts and published by a leading mental health charity.

Web resources

Campaign for the Abolition of the Schizophrenia Label: www.caslcampaign.com
   Interesting and perhaps radical website of an organisation campaigning for the label 'schizophrenia' to be consigned to the 'diagnostic dustbin'.

The Tidal Model website: www.tidal-model.com
   Official website of the Tidal Model with a whole host of resources about this particular approach to mental health care.

Hearing voices network: www.hearing-voices.org

Website of an organisation committed to helping people who hear voices, providing alternative explanations to the medical viewpoint of 'voices' as auditory hallucinations.

Mental health history timeline: www.studymore.org.uk/mhhtim.htm

The design is basic, but this website offers detailed and thorough information for those interested in the history of mental health practice.

References

APA (American Psychiatric Association) (2000). *Diagnostic and Statistical Manual of Mental Disorders, 4th Edition* (Text Revised) (DSM-IVR) Washington: APA.

Barker P & Buchanan-Barker P (2005). *The Tidal Model: A Guide for Mental Health Professionals.* Hove: Brunner–Routledge.

Beck AT (1967). *Depression: Clinical, Experimental and Theoretical Perspectives.* New York: Hoeber.

Beck AT (1976). *Cognitive Therapy and the Emotional Disorders.* New York: International Universities Press.

Bentall RP (2009). *Doctoring the Mind: Is Our Current Treatment of Mental Illness Really Any Good?* London: Penguin.

Boyle M (2002). *Schizophrenia: A Scientific Delusion?*, 2nd edition. London: Routledge.

Chambers M (2006). The case for 'mental health' nurses. In JR Cutcliffe & M Ward (eds), *Key Debates in Psychiatric/Mental Health Nursing.* Edinburgh: Churchill Livingstone.

Chatterton C (2004). 'Caught in the middle'? Mental nurse training in England 1919–51. *Journal of Psychiatric and Mental Health Nursing,* **11**, 30–35.

Denman C (2001). Cognitive-analytical therapy. *Advances in Psychiatric Treatment,* **7**, 243–256.

DH (Department of Health) (1999). *Making a Difference: Strengthening the Nursing, Midwifery and Health Visiting Contribution to Health and Healthcare.* London: TSO.

DH (Department of Health) (2006). *From Values to Action: The Chief Nursing Officer's Review of Mental Health Nursing.* London: DH.

DHSS (Department of Health and Social Security) (1972). *Report of the Committee on Nursing* (Briggs Report). London: HMSO.

Du Mont P (2006). The case for 'psychiatric' nurses. In JR Cutcliffe & M Ward (Eds), *Key Debates in Psychiatric/Mental Health Nursing.* Edinburgh: Churchill Livingstone.

Ellis A (1962). *Reason and Emotion in Psychotherapy: A Comprehensive Method for Treating Human Disturbances.* New York: Lyle Stuart.

Fonagy P (2003). Psychoanalysis today. *World Psychiatry,* **2**(2), 73–80.

Foucault M (1965). *Madness and Civilization: A History of Insanity in the Age of Reason.* Translated by R Howard. New York: Pantheon.

Garbutt J (2009). The state of pharmacotherapy for the treatment of alcohol dependence. *Journal of Substance Abuse Treatment,* **36**(Suppl 1), S15–S23.

Goffman E (1963). *Stigma: Notes on the Management of Spoiled Identity.* New York: Prentice–Hall.

Gournay K (1995). What to do with nursing models. *Journal of Psychiatric and Mental Health Nursing*, **2**, 325–327.

Gross R (2010). *Psychology: The Science of Mind and Behaviour*, 6th edition. London: Hodder Education.

Hayes SC (2004). Acceptance and commitment therapy, relation frame theory, and the third wave of behavioral and cognitive therapies. *Behavior Therapy*, **35**, 639–665.

HM Government (2009). *New Horizons: A Shared Vision for Mental Health*. London: DH. Available from: www.newhorizons.dh.gov.uk [accessed 14 February 2010].

Klerman GL, Weissman MM, Rounsaville BJ & Chevron ES (1984). *Interpersonal Psychotherapy of Depression*. New York: Basic Books.

Lyons C, Nixon D & Coren A (2006). *Long-term Conditions and Depression: Considerations for Best Practice in Practice Based Commissioning*. London: CSIP/NIMHE.

McKenna H (1997). *Nursing Theories and Models*. London: Routledge.

MHNRT (Mental Health Nursing Review Team) (1994). *Working in Partnership: A Collaborative Approach to Care (Chair: Professor Tony Butterworth)*. London: HMSO.

NICE (National Institute for Health and Clinical Excellence) (2009). *Depression: The Treatment and Management of Depression in Adults (Partial update of NICE clinical guideline 23)*. London: NICE.

NIMHE (National Institute for Mental Health in England) (2005). *NIMHE Guiding Statement on Recovery*. London: NIMHE.

Nolan P (1998). *A History of Mental Health Nursing*. Cheltenham: Nelson Thornes.

Orem DE (2001). *Nursing: Concepts of Practice*, 6th edition. St Louis, MO: Mosby.

Osborn DPJ (2001). The poor physical health of people with mental illness. *Western Journal of Medicine*, **175**, 329–332.

Peplau H (1991). *Interpersonal Relations in Nursing: A Conceptual Frame of Reference for Psychodynamic Nursing*. New York: Springer.

Prior P (1993). Mental health policy in Northern Ireland. *Social Policy & Administration*, **27**(4), 323–334.

Roberts A (1981). The Lunacy Commission: A Study of its Origin, Emergence and Character [website]. London: Middlesex University. Available from: www.studymore.org.uk [accessed 16 November 2009].

Rogers CR (1980). *A Way of Being*. New York: Houghton Mifflin.

Roper N, Logan WW & Tierney AJ (2000). *The Roper–Logan–Tierney Model of Nursing: Based on Activities of Living*. Edinburgh: Churchill Livingstone.

Roy C & Andrews HA (2008). *The Roy Adaptation Model*, 3rd edition. London: Prentice–Hall.

Ryle A & Kerr IB (2002). *Introducing Cognitive Analytical Therapy: Principles and Practice*. Chichester: Wiley.

Scheff TJ (1966). *Being Mentally Ill: A Sociological Theory*. Chicago: Aldine.

Scottish Executive (2006). *Rights, Relationships and Recovery: The Report of the National Review of Mental Health Nursing in Scotland*. Edinburgh: Scottish Executive.

Seligman MEP (2003). *Authentic Happiness: Using the New Positive Psychology to Realise Your Potential for Lasting Fulfilment*. London: Nicholas Brearley.

Seymour L (2003). *Not All in the Mind: The Physical Health of Mental Health Service Users.* London: Mentality. Available from: www.scmh.org.uk [accessed 16 April 2010].

Shepherd G, Boardman J & Slade M (2008). *Making Recovery a Reality.* London: SCMH.

SIGN (Scottish Intercollegiate Guidelines Network) (2010). *Non-pharmaceutical Management of Depression in Adults: A National Guideline Edinburgh*: SIGN.

Slade M & Hayward M (2008). Recovery, psychosis and psychiatry: research is better than rhetoric [Editorial]. *Acta Psychiatrica Scandinavica*, **116**(2), 81–83.

Stevenson C & Fletcher E (2002). The Tidal Model: the questions answered. *Mental Health Practice*, **5**(8), 29–38.

Sturdy H & Parry-Jones W (1999). Boarding-out insane patients: the significance of the Scottish system, 1857–1913. In: P Bartlett & D Wright (eds), *Outside the Walls of the Asylum: The History of Care in the Community, 1750–2000*. London: Athlone Press.

Szasz TS (1961). *The Myth of Mental Illness: Foundations of a Theory of Personal Conduct.* New York: Harper & Row.

UKCC (United Kingdom Central Council for Nursing, Midwifery and Health Visiting) (1986). *Project 2000: A New Preparation for Practice*. London: UKCC.

UKCC (United Kingdom Central Council for Nursing, Midwifery and Health Visiting) (1999). *Fitness for Practice: The UKCC Commission for Nursing and Midwifery Education (Chair: Sir Leonard Peach)*. London: UKCC.

WHO (World Health Organization) (2001). *Strengthening Mental Health Promotion (Fact Sheet No. 220)*. Geneva: WHO. Available from: www.who.int [accessed 10 February 2010].

WHO (World Health Organisation) (2007). *International Classification of Disease, 10th Revision (2007 Version)*. Geneva: WHO. Available from www.who.int [accessed 12 February 2010].

Wolpe J (1969). *The Practice of Behavior Therapy*. New York: Pergamon Press.

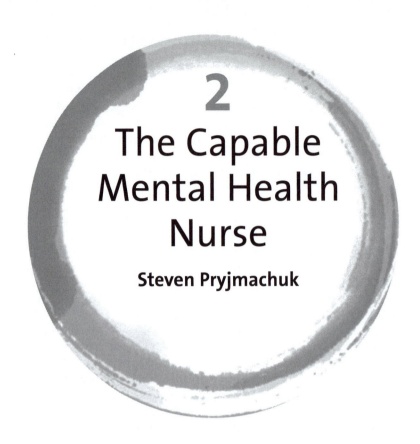

2

The Capable Mental Health Nurse

Steven Pryjmachuk

What will I learn in this chapter?

This chapter focuses on the capabilities required to be an effective mental health nurse. It considers the specific knowledge, skills and personal qualities that are required of a mental health nurse, as well as the external demands (such as government policy) that influence mental health practice.

After reading this chapter, you will be able to:

- identify UK-wide policy relating to mental health practice and mental health nursing in particular;
- understand a variety of concepts associated with competence and capability in mental health practice;
- describe the factors that influence the therapeutic relationship;
- appreciate the specific knowledge, skills and personal qualities required to be an effective mental health nurse.

Introduction

What makes a good mental health nurse?

The question posed above is an important one because it underpins the way in which educators plan and organise the training and education that mental health nurses receive and it can also help potential entrants into the profession decide whether mental health nursing is a suitable career choice or not. It's a rather more complex question than it seems at first sight and it's worth spending a minute or two considering it.

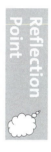

What makes a good mental health nurse?

Ask yourself what makes a good mental health nurse?

What specific qualities and characteristics do you need to be a good mental health nurse? Can those qualities and characteristics be learnt or are people born with them? How many of those qualities and characteristics do you have at the moment? Is there a 'right' personality for being a mental health nurse?

Reflection Point

Now you have had a chance to think about the questions posed in the reflection point above, we need to come clean and admit that, in asking you to answer these particular questions, we are to some extent asking the wrong person! Manufacturers of goods or suppliers of commercial services would not dream of going to market (delivering their product) unless they had done their market research first. In other words, to find out if a product or service was 'good', they would ask potential users of those products or services. Are we then better targeting the questions above at the **users** of mental health services rather than at the providers? Bee et al. (2008) think so. In a recent systematic review of the literature relating to service users' expectations of UK mental health nurses, they found that service users expected mental health nurses to be equipped with both **therapeutic clinical skills** and **generic interpersonal skills**. From the service user perspective, a 'good' mental health nurse is thus one who possesses these skills.

Note that by clinical skills, Bee et al. did not mean technical skills like giving injections or taking blood which are so often associated with physical nursing; they meant the 'professional' skills – such as **information giving** and **problem solving** – that underpin the delivery of user-centred assessment and intervention in mental health care. This specific view of clinical skills does not, however, mean that physical nursing skills are seen as unimportant in mental health care (on the contrary, they can be very important, as you will see in Part II of this book); it merely reminds us that physical nursing skills are merely *one* set of skills in the overall repertoire of skills sets required to be a good mental health nurse[1].

The generic interpersonal skills identified by Bee et al. are another of these skills sets. Generic interpersonal skills are the skills associated with **relationship building**, **engagement** and **communication** and they are underpinned by personal attributes such as **empathy**, **compassion** and **respect**. It is these therapeutic clinical and generic interpersonal skills rather than physical nursing skills that are, in essence, the **core skills** of mental health nursing. Moreover, personal attributes such as empathy, compassion, respect, warmth and genuineness are, as we will see, attributes that reflect the **core values** underpinning mental health nursing.

At this point, we have an inkling of what the core values and core skills of mental health nursing are. It gets a little more complicated than this, however, as identifying what are the attributes of a good mental health nurse or, indeed, a good member of any specific profession brings into play a number of inter-related concepts – not only values and skills, but concepts such as **knowledge**, **attitude**, **competency**, **proficiency**, **capability** and **expertise**. It's helpful to explore these concepts in more detail since they are part of the jargon of modern mental health nursing and, as such, they crop up frequently throughout this book.

Clarifying Some Concepts

Thinking–feeling–doing

We are shaped by what we **know**, what we **feel**, and what we **do**. Psychologists have specific terms for each of these domains: what we know reflects our **cognitive abilities**, what we do is our **behaviour** and what we feel is our **affect** (a more formal term for 'emotions'). When we look at how

---

[1] For an excellent text on physical nursing as applied to mental health care, see Nash (2010) in the Key Texts list at the end of this chapter.

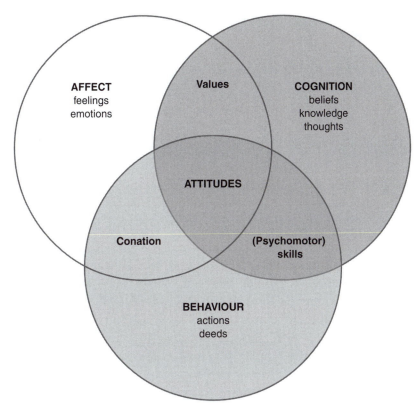

FIGURE 2.1 Interactions between the cognitive, behavioural and affective domains

these psychological domains overlap (Figure 2.1), a number of additional concepts emerge: values, conation, (psychomotor) skills and attitudes.

Let's start with **conation** because it is the term in the diagram you may be least familiar with. Conation refers to the relationship between feelings and behaviour and is related to psychological concepts such as **volition** (will), **drive** and **motivation**. Regarding **skills**, the term can refer to both mental ability and practical ability but when talking about core skills in practice-based disciplines such as nursing, we mostly mean **psychomotor skills** – skills that are a combination of knowledge and behaviour ('psycho' refers to mental processes; 'motor' to the motion produced by muscle activity). We will look at **values** and **attitudes** in more detail shortly but, for now, values can be defined as a combination of feelings and thoughts about some aspect of the world and attitudes as what arises when a behavioural element is introduced.

Discussion Point

Changing people

Think about the three domains in Figure 2.1. Which of the domains do you think is the most open to change? Which is the hardest to change?

These are questions that lots of different agencies and professions have considered over the years, from those desiring positive change for the benefit of society (educators, prison workers, health promoters), to those desiring change for the benefit of private enterprise (marketers and advertisers), to those desiring change for more sinister reasons (oppressive governments and religious cults).

The discussion we had on classical and operant conditioning in Chapter 1 demonstrates that behaviour change is possible even without any direct reference to the conscious mind. Indeed, in lower species, this is a very common occurrence when you think about how animals such as dogs and horses are trained. It might be a little more complicated in humans but behaviour change can occur with little or no cognitive involvement. An example is **taste aversion**, where a specific food is associated with an adverse effect (such as sickness) and the food subsequently avoided even if the food didn't really cause the adverse effect.

Since raw emotional feelings are very hard to change (possibly because of the physiological underpinnings of emotion) the domain least open to change is, perhaps, the affective domain. The autonomic nervous system – particularly the sympathetic branch – controls many of the bodily symptoms we experience in emotions like anger and fear and we largely have little control over it. Indeed, the only control we may have over sympathetic branch arousal is in the way we respond: by either confronting the source of the arousal or escaping from it – the so-called **fight-or-flight** response.

Learning

The cognitive domain is perhaps the most open to change since the very process of acquiring knowledge is in itself a change, a type of change that even has its own name: **learning**! Learning is underpinned by various cognitive processes such as thinking, memorising, problem solving and reasoning – processes that are, in essence, **mental skills** (we shall look at some of these mental skills in more detail later on in this chapter). The cognitive domain also impacts on the acquisition of practical (psychomotor) skills in that acquiring such skills involves an interaction between thinking and doing. This interaction can be very intense at the outset but, as we all know when we think of a task like learning to drive or learning to ride a bike, it becomes easier with practice, especially if feedback is given. You can also 'learn to learn' in that it is possible to enhance mental skills through practice and feedback just as with practical skills.

When the cognitive domain interacts with the affective domain we need to consider **attitudes** and **values**. Whether we can enhance our attitudes and values in the same way as we can enhance our mental and practical skills is open to debate. However, regardless of whether learning can have an impact on our attitudes and values, our attitudes and values undoubtedly influence how and what we learn. This is an important observation for mental health nursing because, if attitudes and values are hard to change, we have to ensure that only those with the 'right' attitudes and values are encouraged into the profession. Given they are so important, let's look at what they are in more detail.

Attitudes and values

Although 'attitude' is often used as a synonym for terms like 'belief', 'value' and 'opinion' there are important differences between these terms. **Beliefs** are merely the things we think are true in the world, whether or not they actually are true (commonly held beliefs – again, whether they are true or not – about specific social groups are called **stereotypes**). **Opinions** are essentially verbal or written expressions of beliefs. As Figure 2.1 illustrates, **values** have more of an emotional feel to them than beliefs and they tend to be enduring and personal (though they are often shaped by culture). Some commonly held values are outlined in Box 2.1.

Box 2.1   Some commonly held values

the family	truth	freedom
wealth	religion	human rights
primogeniture*	fame	equality
community	power	democracy

*Giving precedence to the first-born in a family.

Note that you might not see all of the values in Box 2.1 as values worth holding yourself but since values are personal and since people differ, it is obvious that values will differ among people.

Attitudes are what we get when a behavioural element enters the equation. One of the easiest ways to understand this is to dissect a negative attitude (or **prejudice**, as negative attitudes are sometimes called) such as racism. In racism, there may be stereotypical **beliefs** such as 'blacks are responsible for most crime' or 'they come here and take our jobs'; strong **emotions**, often fear; and **behaviours** such as avoiding 'black' areas or, in more extreme circumstances, being verbally or physically abusive to black people.

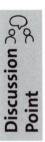

Discussion Point

Tackling racism

In the earlier discussion point, we asked you to look at the three domains in Figure 2.1 and think about which of the three is the hardest to change?

Thinking about people's beliefs, feelings and behaviour – the domains in Figure 2.1 – how might society go about tackling racism?

We will return to attitudes and values later in this chapter when we talk about the core values of mental health nursing, but for now we need to look at some other concepts associated with being a good mental health nurse.

Competence, proficiency and capability

We earlier identified learning as being about the acquisition of knowledge or the changing of cognitions. Learning is, to some extent, concerned with the **process** of education; when we think about the **outcomes** of education (especially professional education), we encounter concepts such as competence, proficiency and capability (see Figure 2.2).

Most people would expect 'good' mental health nurses to be competent. But what exactly does competent mean? **Competence** was defined by the

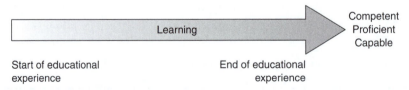

Learning

Competent
Proficient
Capable

Start of educational
experience

End of educational
experience

FIGURE 2.2   Process and outcome in education

predecessor of the Nursing and Midwifery Council (NMC), the UKCC (1999) as 'the skills and ability to practise safely and effectively without the need for direct supervision'. Interestingly, this definition doesn't discriminate between mental and practical skills nor does it seem you need to have any particular values or attitudes to be competent! Fraser and Greenhalgh (2001), however, do include an attitudinal component to competence, defining it as what 'individuals know or are able to do in terms of knowledge, skills and attitudes' (p. 799).

Up until 2001, to get on the nursing register, student nurses needed to demonstrate competence in a range of areas. However, section 5(2)(a) of the Nursing and Midwifery Order 2001 introduced a demand that entrants to the nursing register demonstrate **proficiency** rather than competence in a range of areas which complicates things a little for those of us involved in nurse education. The reason it is complicated is down to Patricia Benner's seminal work on clinical excellence, *From Novice to Expert* (Benner, 1984), work that has had a huge influence on nurse education. Benner argues that there are five levels of clinical expertise (Box 2.2).

As you can see from Box 2.2, the 2001 Nursing and Midwifery Order seems to have upped the ante for entry to the nursing register from Stage 3 'competent' to Stage 4 'proficient'. This may have been a deliberate attempt to improve the standards of newly qualified nurses or, since competent and proficient are often used interchangeably, it may have been an understandable error on the part of the people who drafted the Order. The latter is the most likely since, in preparing for new standards for nurse education across the UK, the NMC (2010) have reverted back to using 'competencies' to describe the expectations of nurses at the point of registration. The NMC have also redefined competence more broadly (and, to some extent, more accurately) as a combination of the 'skills, knowledge and attitudes, values and technical abilities that underpin safe and effective nursing practice' (NMC, 2010, p. 136).

Box 2.2   Benner's five stages of clinical expertise

Stage 1: Novice. Novices are beginners who have little or no experience of the situations in which they need to perform. Novices need sets of rules to help them perform and have little discretion in the decisions they make.

(Continued)

(*Continued*)

Stage 2: Advanced beginner. Advanced beginners demonstrate marginally acceptable performance but still require supervision. Principles to guide actions, based on experience, begin to be formulated.

Stage 3: Competent. Competence develops when the nurse begins to see his or her actions in terms of long-range goals or plans of which she or he is consciously aware. The competent nurse lacks the speed and flexibility of the proficient nurse but does have a feeling of mastery and the ability to cope with and manage the unforeseen in clinical nursing.

Stage 4: Proficient. The proficient nurse learns from experience what typical events to expect in a given situation and how plans need to be modified in response to these events. The proficient nurse's decision making is less laboured because she or he knows which of the many existing attributes and aspects in the present situation are the important ones.

Stage 5: Expert. Because of extensive experience and an analytical approach to those situations, decision making and performance in experts are almost intuitive.

Benner, Patricia. *From Novice to Expert: Excellence and Power in Clinical Nursing Practice, Commemorative Edition*, 1st edition © 2001, pp. 20–34. Adapted by permission of Pearson Education Inc., Upper Saddle River, NJ.

Whether newly qualified nurses need to be competent or proficient is a debate best left to the nursing profession itself but one thing arising from a consideration of Benner's model is the realisation that competence isn't the end stage of clinical expertise: learning in nursing does – indeed, should – go 'beyond competence'. This latter phrase brings into play another concept, one that is central to this chapter: that of **capability**.

Capability

Capability is difficult to define but thinking of it as 'more than competence' can help. Fraser and Greenhalgh (2001) define it as the 'extent to which an individual can apply, adapt and synthesise new knowledge from experience and so continue to improve their performance' (p. 799). Cairns (1996) sees it as the 'capacity to handle the unknown in times of change' (p.8) and Stephenson (1998) argues that capability 'is an integration of knowledge, skills, personal qualities and understanding used appropriately and effectively – not just in familiar and highly focused specialist contexts but in response to new and changing circumstances' (p. 2).

Benner and capability

If capability is 'beyond competence', where does it fit into Benner's model? Is it equivalent to Stage 4 (Proficient) or Stage 5 (Expert)? Is it outside of Benner's model? If so, does Benner's model have any value in understanding capability?

Capability is a concept central to modern mental health practice. In 2001, the Sainsbury Centre for Mental Health published *The Capable Practitioner* (SCMH, 2001), a framework and list of the practitioner capabilities required to implement the English *National Service Framework for Mental Health* (see DH, 1999). The Sainsbury Centre argued that capable mental health practitioners needed more than a prescribed set of competencies but an array of integrated skills and qualities including: (1) having the requisite **knowledge** for effective practice; (2) a **performance** component (in other words, competence), that includes the ability to put theory into practice; (3) an **ethical** component that includes knowledge of culture and values; (4) the ability to be **reflective**, both *in* practice and *on* practice;[2] and (5) a commitment to **lifelong learning**. The Sainsbury Centre's work on *The Capable Practitioner* was further developed, in collaboration with the National Institute for Mental Health in England (NIMHE), into *The Ten Essential Shared Capabilities*[3] (see Box 2.3), a series of broad statements reflecting 'the basic building blocks for all mental health staff whether they be professionally qualified or not and whether they work in the NHS or social care field or the statutory and private and voluntary sector' (NIME/SCMH, 2004, p. 8). The ten essential shared capabilities have been influential in other parts of the UK apart from England; in Scotland, for example, they have contributed to the development of a number of **capability frameworks** including one for acute mental health (NES, 2007) and one for older people (NES, 2008a).

---

[2]See also the discussion later in this chapter on 'reflection on action' and 'reflection in action'.

[3]These essential shared capabilities are often collectively abbreviated to 'ESCs'. In 2007, in a bid to improve generic clinical skills among nursing students, the NMC decided to introduce 'essential skills clusters' into pre-registration nursing curricula (NMC, 2007) which they also – confusingly – refer to as ESCs. If you are a student mental health nurse, you are likely to come across ESC as an abbreviation for *both* the essential shared capabilities and the essential skills clusters, so take care when you see it.

Box 2.3   The ten essential shared capabilities in mental health (NIME/SCMH, 2004)

Working in partnership. Developing and maintaining constructive working relationships with service users, carers, families, colleagues, lay people and wider community networks. Working positively with any tensions created by conflicts of interest or aspiration that may arise between the partners in care.

Respecting diversity. Working in partnership with service users, carers, families and colleagues to provide care and interventions that not only make a positive difference but also do so in ways that respect and value diversity, including age, race, culture, disability, gender, spirituality and sexuality.

Practising ethically. Recognising the rights and aspirations of service users and their families, acknowledging power differentials and minimising them whenever possible. Providing treatment and care that is accountable to service users and carers within the boundaries prescribed by national (professional), legal and local codes of ethical practice.

Challenging inequality. Addressing the causes and consequences of stigma, discrimination, social inequality and exclusion on service users, carers and mental health services. Creating, developing or maintaining valued social roles for people in the communities they come from.

Promoting recovery. Working in partnership to provide care and treatment that enables service users and carers to tackle mental health problems with hope and optimism and to work towards a valued lifestyle within and beyond the limits of any mental health problem.

Identifying people's needs and strengths. Working in partnership to gather information to agree health and social care needs in the context of the preferred lifestyle and aspirations of service users, their families, carers and friends.

Providing service user-centred care. Negotiating achievable and meaningful goals; primarily from the perspective of service users and their families. Influencing and seeking the means to achieve these goals and clarifying the responsibilities of the people who will provide any help that is needed, including systematically evaluating outcomes and achievements.

Making a difference. Facilitating access to and delivering the best quality, evidence-based, values-based health and social care interventions to meet the needs and aspirations of service users and their families and carers.

Promoting safety and positive risk taking. Empowering the person to decide the level of risk they are prepared to take with their health and safety. This includes working with the tension between promoting safety and positive risk taking, including assessing and dealing with possible risks for service users, carers, family members and the wider public.

Personal development and learning. Keeping up to date with changes in practice and participating in lifelong learning, personal and professional development for one's self and colleagues through supervision, appraisal and reflective practice.

Thus, in a nutshell, to be a capable (rather than competent) practitioner, you need the **right knowledge**, the **right attitudes and values**, and the **right skills**. Let's consider each of these in turn by exploring what the core knowledge, the core values and the core skills of mental health nursing might be.

Core Knowledge for Mental Health Nursing

One of the functions of comprehensive, introductory textbooks such as this is to provide student practitioners with the core knowledge required to be an effective practitioner. However, there have to be some cautions here, some of which were alluded to in the Preface.

Firstly, textbooks such as this can contain only the core knowledge of a discipline at a given point in time; the nature of knowledge is such that it develops and advances as time passes, so there is no guarantee that what is presented in this book will be valid when it's being read by you, whether this is a year, five years or ten years from the time of writing. To guard against this, you need to understand that learning is not a static process but a dynamic one that requires you to constantly update and appraise the information available to you. To be an effective practitioner, therefore, you must get into the habit of **reading around**, synthesising the information you collect, and you must embrace **lifelong learning** as a value.

Secondly, since there is currently no standard syllabus for UK mental health nursing (unlike the '1982 syllabus' of the past mentioned in the previous chapter and the curricula for the two sets of 'IAPT' practitioners we will discuss in the next), the core knowledge this book presents to you is deemed to be 'core' simply because we (the editor and contributing authors) believe it to be, though our choices will have been influenced by our expertise as practitioners and educators and by relevant policy and good practice guide-lines. Others may feel we have omitted material they consider to be core, or that we have included material they feel is superfluous, or they may not agree with the specific theoretical stances we have taken. Again, getting into the habit of reading around and synthesising the information you glean from such reading can help you deal with these criticisms.

Finally, the very word 'core' implies that additional (non-core) material is available. While the extent to which you pursue this additional material will depend very much on your interests and career intentions, what we can say with certainty is that you will have to look at additional material at some point in your studies because: (1) you cannot learn everything there is to know about mental health practice from a single resource such as this book; and (2) wide reading underpins yet another skill essential to modern mental health nurses (and one we will discuss in a short while) – the ability to **think critically**. How to identify and acquire such additional material is a skill in itself (and one that most university students have to learn pretty rapidly); we have, nevertheless, given you a helping hand in that there is a list of relevant further reading and resources at the end of each chapter in this book.

Core Values in Mental Health Nursing

In recent years, a number of initiatives and reports across the UK have emphasised and brought into play the essential role that values play in modern mental health practice. Among these initiatives have been the English **Chief Nursing Officer's review of mental health nursing** (DH, 2006a) and the associated best practice competencies and capabili-ties for pre-registration mental health nursing in England (DH, 2006b); the parallel **review of mental health nursing in Scotland** (*Rights, Relationships and Recovery*; Scottish Executive, 2006) and the associated national framework for pre-registration mental health nursing pro-grammes in Scotland (NES, 2008b); the **ten essential shared capabili-ties** (NIMHE/SCMH, 2004); the **Bamford review of mental health and learning disability** in Northern Ireland (DHSSPS, 2007); the **Welsh national service framework for mental health** (*Raising the Standard*; Welsh Assembly Government, 2005); and, most recently, *New Horizons*, the cross-government national mental health strategy (HM Government, 2009).

TABLE 2.1 Values in mental health practice

Value	Details	Emphasised by
Respect	A culture that respects the diversity of individuals	10 ESCs; BPC England; Welsh NSF
Service user centredness	Negotiating achievable and meaningful goals from the perspective of service users and their families	10 ESCs; New Horizons; SMHNF; Welsh NSF
Recovery	Working towards a valued lifestyle within and beyond the limits of any mental health problem, with hope and optimism as the drivers	10 ESCs; BPC England; CNO Review; New Horizons; RRR; SMHNF; Welsh NSF
Equity	Challenging inequality so that all groups in society receive an equitable service; tackling the stigma of mental health so that people with mental health problems are included in society rather than excluded	10 ESCs; Bamford; CNO Review; New Horizons; SMHNF; Welsh NSF
Holism	Taking into account the physical, psychological, social and spiritual needs of an individual	BPC England; CNO Review; New Horizons; SMHNF
Lifelong learning	Keeping up-to-date with changes in practice and participating in personal and professional development	10 ESCs; BPC England; RRR; SMHNF
Partnership working	Developing and maintaining constructive working relationships with service users, carers, families, colleagues, lay people and wider community networks	10 ESCs; BPC England; New Horizons; RRR; Welsh NSF
Rights	Recognising the rights and aspirations of service users and their families; rights to full citizenship	10 ESCs; Bamford; New Horizons; RRR; SMHNF

10 ESCs = 10 Essential Shared Capabilities (NIMHE/SCMH, 2004).
Bamford = Bamford Review of Mental Health and Learning Disability in Northern Ireland (DHSSPS, 2007).
BPC England = Best practice competencies for pre-registration mental health nursing in England (DH, 2006b).
CNO Review = Chief Nursing Officer's review of mental health nursing in England (DH, 2006a).
RRR = Rights, Relationships and Recovery (Scottish Executive, 2006).
SMHNF = Scottish mental health nursing framework (NES, 2008b).
Welsh NSF = (Revised) Adult Mental Health National Service Framework for Wales (Welsh Assembly Government, 2005).

The various values for mental health practice identified by this raft of initiatives and reports are summarised in Table 2.1.

Values-based practice

Evidence-based practice is a notion that has permeated healthcare practice in recent years to such an extent that it is now seen as a fundamental element of modern healthcare practice (it is, as you will discover, a central theme running through this book). The most well- known definition of evidence-based practice is that of Sackett et al. (1996) who state that evidence-based practice[4] is 'the conscientious, explicit, and judicious use of current best evidence in making decisions about the care of individual patients' (p. 71). It is clear from this definition that evidence-based practice involves a **decision making** process and Sackett et al. go on to remark that any such decisions made are the result of both **individual clinical expertise** and the **best available clinical research**. We will not dwell too much on evidence-based practice here since its importance will become evident when you work your way through the chapters in Part II of this book (for a primer on evidence-based practice, see Lindsay, 2007). It is worth bearing in mind, however, that since evidence-based practice is about making *judgements*, and since judgement involves a degree of individuality, evidence-based practice will always involve a degree of subjectivity. A good way of thinking of evidence-based practice is to think not of right or wrong ways of doing things but the best way of doing things given the evidence that is available at the time and the robustness with which that evidence has been appraised.

Values-based practice is a new way of working within healthcare developed by the psychiatrist and philosopher Bill Fulford and based on philosophical theories concerned with the meanings and implications of the language associated with values (see Fulford, 1989). Like evidence-based practice, values-based practice aims to support healthcare decision making. However, while evidence-based practice is about decision making in the context of complex and conflicting health care *information*, values-based practice is about decision making in the context of complex and conflicting *values* in society (remember that not everyone holds the same values). This isn't necessarily easy, however: consider the examples in the reflection point below.

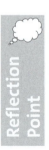

Conflicting values in society

Below are some examples of how conflicting values might create tensions within healthcare practice.

- A nurse with strong religious beliefs asks if someone else in her team can look after a gay man because she finds homosexual practices abhorrent.

---

[4]Sackett et al. actually refer to evidence-based *medicine* (since they were writing for the *British Medical Journal*) but to all intents and purposes evidence-based practice, evidence-based medicine, evidence-based nursing, etc. are one and the same.

- A black service user asks not to be seen by a white nurse because she thinks that the nurse won't understand her specific needs.
- An older person is told by a consultant that she probably won't get a kidney transplant because of her age and that she should resign herself to a life of dialysis.

Can you think of any ways in which you think these tensions might be resolved?

Although the decisions underpinning values-based practice are often complex and difficult, Woodbridge and Fulford (2004) have identified some principles for facilitating values-based practice. These include the adoption of **shared values**, **framework values** and **'good process'**. Shared values are those values that society has in common (freedom and being happy, for example, are two values likely to be held by most of society). Shared values together with the democratic premise – the will of the people – elicit framework values that set clear limits of acceptability. Racist values, for example, are unacceptable because they are incompatible with the shared values of respect and equality, values that have also been enshrined in law through the democratic process. The core values listed in Table 2.1 could be seen as the framework values for mental health practice.

Good process is a little more difficult to grasp. Decision making in healthcare ethics is usually concerned with eliciting good *outcomes* (a 'right' rather than 'wrong' outcome); values-based practice, on the other hand, is more concerned with the decision making *process* than with specific outcomes. The characteristics of good process, identified by Woodbridge and Fulford (2004), are outlined in Box 2.4.

Box 2.4   Good process in values-based practice (from Woodbridge & Fulford, 2004)

Practice skills

1. **Awareness:** being aware of the values in a given situation
2. **Reasoning:** thinking about values when making decisions
3. **Knowledge:** knowing about values and facts that are relevant to a situation
4. **Communication:** using communication to resolve any conflicts or complexity

(Continued)

(*Continued*)

Models of service delivery

5. **User-centred:** considering the service user's values as the first priority
6. **Multidisciplinary:** using a balance of perspectives to resolve conflicts

Values-based practice and evidence-based practice

7. **The 'two feet' principle:** all decisions are based on facts and values; evidence-based practice (facts) and values-based practice therefore work together
8. **The 'squeaky wheel' principle:** values shouldn't just be noticed if there's a problem
9. **Science and values:** increasing scientific knowledge creates choices in health care; this can lead to wider differences in values

Partnership

10. **Partnership:** in values-based practice, decisions are taken by service users working in partnership with providers of care

Looking at Box 2.4, you will see that for values-based practice to occur, practitioners need good intellectual, cognitive and interpersonal skills, and the models of service delivery need to be user-centred and multidisciplinary, with an overarching ideology of **partnership**. Note also that values-based practice and evidence-based practice are complementary, rather than incompatible, aspects of the healthcare decision process. Values-based practice very much underpins the notion of **recovery**, a notion we met first in the previous chapter and one we will meet repeatedly throughout this book.

Core skills in mental health nursing

In the Introduction, we mentioned that service users expected mental health nurses to be equipped with both therapeutic clinical skills and generic interpersonal skills. To a large extent, these two sets of skills are the **core skills** of mental health nursing and we will, as such, explore these in much more detail shortly. A word of warning is required, however. You will not learn these skills from merely reading about them in a book such as this, though books and manuals can certainly help you grasp the theory and principles behind those skills. As with any other skill, such as learning to drive or learning a language, the best way of learning the core skills of mental health nursing is for you to **practise** them. As learners, this should normally be done under the supervision of, and with **feedback** from, those involved in helping you learn such skills (your course tutors, practice mentors and the servicer users you will work with).

Many mental health nurses begin to learn these core skills through **role play**, an activity that is often anxiety-provoking for learners but, importantly, one that allows students to learn in a reasonably safe environment and with lots of opportunities for feedback.

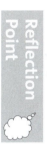

Role play

How does the thought of role play make you feel?

Does it make you feel anxious? If so, try to dissect what the anxious feelings are all about. Are they about making a fool of yourself? Doing it wrong or being a failure? Being put on the spot? Do you think your peers feel the same about role play as you do? Is it worth asking them how they feel about it?

Reflection Point

Of the two skills sets identified by Bee et al. (2008) – therapeutic clinical skills and generic interpersonal skills – it is perhaps best to consider the generic interpersonal skills first because they are a prerequisite for therapeutic clinical skills. The generic interpersonal skills are those that are concerned with the **therapeutic relationship**, from its initial establishment right through until the relationship ends.

Interpersonal skills: the therapeutic relationship

As you can see from Figure 2.3, the interpersonal skills necessary for building, maintaining and ending therapeutic relationships are principally the **communication** skills. These skills, in turn, are underpinned by **personal attributes** and **values** such as **empathy**, **compassion** and **respect**. Environmental factors such as decor and furniture, noise levels and lighting, and the place in which the relationship occurs (home, office, ward, school, etc.) can also impact on the therapeutic relationship.

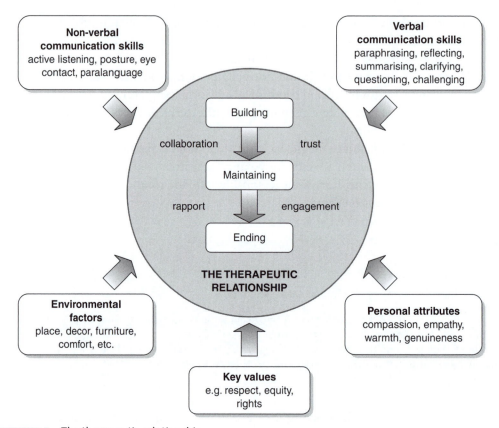

FIGURE 2.3   The therapeutic relationship

Personal Attributes: The 'Core Conditions'

Carl Rogers, whom we discussed briefly in the previous chapter as one of the originators of humanistic psychology, argues (see Rogers, 1980) that three **core conditions** are required in order to help people: (1) **unconditional positive regard**; (2) **empathic understanding**; and (3) **genuineness**.

Unconditional positive regard means that individuals are treated with respect and warmth and in a positive light regardless of their presenting problems. This can create some difficulties for nurses when they are faced with individuals who have done appalling or distasteful things (serious sexual crimes or serious violence, for example) and, in these circumstances, a nurse's ability to reflect on her or his own feelings becomes paramount. Empathic understanding (empathy) is about stepping into the person's world and seeing and feeling the world from their perspective. Empathy is different from sympathy (offering sympathy is a relatively simple skill) in that it is deeper and requires imagination and understanding. Genuineness (or congruence) is about being open and honest with the person seeking help – Rogers (1980) uses the term 'transparent' to describe this trait – being yourself, and not using a professional or personal facade.

According to Aaron Beck, the founder of cognitive therapy, these personal attributes create a climate of **trust**, **rapport** and **collaboration** (see Beck et al., 1979) that promotes **engagement** (on behalf of both the person and the therapist) in the therapeutic relationship. Trust is about having confidence in someone. Beck et al. describe collaboration as a common interest in the person's thoughts, feelings, wishes and behaviour; collaboration, as such, requires mutual trust. Beck et al. also stress the importance of rapport in the therapeutic relationship, which they see as 'harmonious accord between people'.

Communication Skills

The specific interpersonal skills that come into play once a conducive climate for therapy has been established are the skills of communication. **Communication** is the process by which information is passed from one organism to another. While humans differ from other animals in that we have the ability to communicate through spoken and written language (i.e., we can use **verbal** communication), much of our communication is **non-verbal** – that is, it occurs without the use of words.

Michael Argyle, an expert on non-verbal communication, identifies a number of **non-verbal cues** that humans use when interacting with one another (see Box 2.5).

Box 2.5   Aspects of non-verbal communication (after Argyle, 1988)

- The use of the face (**facial expression**)
- **Eye contact**
- The use of **posture**
- **Body space** – our proximity and physical closeness to others
- The use of **gestures** (specific bodily movements)
- The use of **touch**
- **'Artefacts'** – the clothes and emblems we wear and the way we look
- **Paralanguage** – *how* we say things rather than what we say: examples include **vocal intonation** (e.g. emphasising certain words), **vocal buffers** ('ah', 'erm', 'oh') and **vocalisations** such as laughing, crying, groaning and muttering

---

A lack of awareness of these cues can cause problems for those – like nurses – for whom communication is a crucial part of their jobs. For example, misreading eye contact, posture or body space can result in nurses not noticing the signs of escalating aggression (it may even exacerbate such aggression) – signs that are especially important in areas of mental health nursing such as acute and forensic care (see Chapters 7 and 12). Failure to grasp the nuances of paralanguage can, furthermore, lead to embarrassment or misunderstandings. Modern day communication methods like email often lack the nuances of paralanguage (though 'emoticons' such as ☺ or ☹ are occasionally a useful substitute) and there have been many occasions where people have got 'the wrong end of the stick' by misinterpreting what has been written in an email.

Conversely, awareness of these cues can enhance the quality of the interactions. Gerald Egan, whose *Skilled Helper* (Egan, 1975) has influenced a generation of counsellors and therapists (including many mental health nurses), uses the acronym SOLER (see Box 2.6) to identify elements of non-verbal communication that can enhance the therapeutic relationship.

Box 2.6   SOLER (after Egan, 1975)

S – sit squarely to the person (i.e. face them)
O – have an open posture (don't cross arms or legs)
L – lean slightly forward
E – maintain eye contact with the person
R – relax

While awareness of such non-verbal cues usually enhances the quality of interactions, it can sometimes detract from the quality of an interaction in that worrying too much about whether you have got the non-verbal aspects right (whether you have got SOLER right) can make the interaction seem wooden and artificial, so threatening any genuineness, empathy and rapport you are trying to establish. Role play (with supportive feedback) can be helpful in overcoming these worries since it can provide you with an opportunity to practise your verbal and non-verbal skills in a relatively safe environment – it matters less, after all, if you are wooden and artificial in a supportive 'rehearsal' setting than it does if you are working with real service users.

Some behaviours that can enhance the therapeutic relationship use elements of both verbal and non-verbal communication. These include the skill of **active listening**. Active listening (or 'total listening'; McKay et al., 2009) can be demonstrated by the use of appropriate verbal responses – from the simple ('mmm', 'OK', 'aha') to the more complex ('oh yes, I understand', 'go on', 'really!') – and by use of appropriate non-verbal responses such as nodding or shaking of the head, facial expressions, the use of eye contact and the adoption of an attentive posture. These listening skills are particularly important when assessing those who seek your help; used capably they can also convey the empathy and genuineness that are essential to the therapeutic relationship. Table 2.2 lists some verbal skills that are especially useful during the assessment process and for which active listening is an essential component.

Difficult questions

We saw earlier (Table 2.1) that one of the core values of mental health practice is **holism** – a consideration of an individual's physical, psychological, social and spiritual needs and the interrelationships between these dimensions. The assessment processes described in the chapters in Part II are, to a large extent, holistic in that you will have to ask questions other than those that directly relate to signs and symptoms when speaking to people about their mental health. Undoubtedly, this means that you will have to ask difficult questions – about relationships, money, housing and homelessness, substance use, sexual behaviour, domestic violence, childhood abuse and so on. This further reinforces the importance of mental health nurses having the interpersonal skills described above and the therapeutic clinical skills outlined below, and the importance of you seeking supervision whenever you are uncomfortable about, or lack confidence in, a specific area of practice.

One area that is becoming increasingly important in mental health is that of **violence** and **abuse**. The issue of violence is clearly related to forensic mental health care (see Chapter 12) and childhood abuse has always been a central issue when working with children and young people (see Chapters 9 and 10). Violence and abuse, however, have applicability across the whole spectrum of mental health problems. For example, 'elder abuse' is an issue affecting one in four vulnerable older people (Cooper et al., 2008) and there is evidence that childhood abuse may be related to the symptoms of psychosis such as hallucinations and paranoid delusions (Read et al., 2007). As such, there have been calls – reinforced by the Department of Health's violence and abuse policy (see NHS Confederation, 2008; DH, 2008) – that violence and abuse be routinely asked about when assessing in mental health. This is not merely because of the ostensible relationship between violence and abuse and mental health but because service users who have been abused want to be asked – and are more likely to disclose as a result – and those who haven't have

TABLE 2.2 Verbal skills useful in assessment

Skill	Detail	Example
Paraphrasing	Listening to what the person is saying, extracting the meaning into your own words which you then repeat back to the person	Person: 'I'm not sure how I feel really. Some days I'm up and some days I'm down; some days I just don't feel anything.' Nurse: 'OK … so how you feel about your situation varies from day to day.'
Reflecting	Here, you might reflect on your own experiences and try to align them with the person's. Or the person might be encouraged to reflect on his or her feelings or experiences with your help	Person: 'It's awful really. I just feel sick and start sweating and shaking when I think about going out. Can you imagine how that must feel?' Nurse: 'While your feelings might be a bit more intense than anything I've experienced, many of us have felt similar feelings when we've been in the same sorts of situations as you so, yes, I can imagine what it must be like.'
Clarifying	A simple verbal skill that helps you fully understand what the person is telling you	Nurse: 'OK, so have I got this right?' Nurse: 'Tell me a bit more about what you just said. What exactly was it that bothered you?'
Summarising	Useful either at the end of a session or periodically during a session as a way of ensuring that you have listened to, and fully understand, the issues that are important to the person	Nurse: 'So, what you're telling me is that you've found things increasingly difficult since you were made redundant last year and that things came to a head when your mother died two months ago.'

no objections to being asked (Mayne & Holley, 2009). Box 2.7 contains some practical guidance, based on the work of the Department of Health's Violence and Abuse Policy Team (see NHS Confederation, 2008; DH, 2008) as to how the question of abuse might be routinely asked in practice.

Box 2.7 How to ask about abuse

'Have you experienced physical, sexual or emotional abuse at any time in your life?'

Yes ☐　　　　None stated ☐　　　　Not asked ☐

- Record brief details of any disclosure
- If the question is not asked, record the reason

This guidance is based on the work of the Department of Health's Violence and Abuse Policy Team (see NHS Confederation, 2008; DH, 2008). With thanks to Liz Mayne, National Lead, Violence and Abuse Policy.

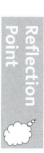

Difficult questions

Given the information in Box 2.7, think how you might phrase questions when you need to find out about a person's:

- substance use
- financial difficulties
- sexual behaviour
- living conditions
- criminal behaviour.

Therapeutic clinical skills

The second set of skills identified by Bee et al.(2008) – therapeutic clinical skills – consist of a wide variety of specific skills that mental health nurses use when intervening or trying to help the people that they work with. These skills both build on and complement the interpersonal skills described above and include: **engagement skills**, the skills necessary to establish a therapeutic relationship with the person seeking help; **challenging skills**, skills that might involve confronting the person seeking help and so require a great deal of insight and empathy; **goal setting**, a skill that can help motivate the person seeking help; **problem solving**, especially in terms of assisting the person seeking help to find their own solutions; **information giving**, the skill of giving routine, yet timely and accurate information and advice; and **ending skills**, the skills required to end the relationship once it has reached its previously agreed or natural end. Because these and other therapeutic clinical skills are so central to helping people with mental health problems, they are considered in much more detail in the each of the chapters in Part II of this book.

Additional skills

There are some additional skills that are useful to mental health nurses though whether or not these skills are core to *mental health* nursing (rather than nursing in general) is open to debate. In particular, there are the **transferable skills**, the skills that are useful in a variety of work environments and which include: **literacy** and **numeracy**; **computer and information technology skills**; oral and written **presentation skills**. Some of these skills are especially important in relation to the legal and professional aspects of nursing – for example, literacy and numeracy have implications for nursing records and for drug administration.

Two additional mental skills that are particularly important in nursing are the related skills of **critical appraisal** and **reflection**. Both might be called a 'meta-skill' in the sense that both can help nurture the interpersonal and therapeutic clinical skills that are the very essence of expert, capable nurses.

Critical appraisal

Critical thinking is essential in modern nursing because the ability to weigh up (appraise) evidence and make judgements about that evidence ultimately leads to better care – care that has beneficial outcomes for users, that is user-centred and cost-effective. The 'evidence' we refer to might be information about a particular service user, a particular intervention or a particular theoretical perspective. In all cases, it is important that you sort out the wheat from the chaff – that you identify which pieces of information are the more robust, have more credibility and have greater utility in the given circumstances. To do this you need to think **objectively** (what is *truly* best for the service user) rather than subjectively (what *you* think is best for the service user). For information gleaned about a particular service user, for example, you might want to question whether what the service user tells you has more credibility than what is written in his or her notes. For information about a particular theoretical perspective, you might want to read around in order to identify the strengths and weaknesses of that perspective and then make up your own mind whether you reject or accept (or partially accept/reject) that perspective. For a particular intervention, you might want to see what research has been carried out on that particular intervention and use some form of **evidence hierarchy** (see Evans, 2003) to grade the research evidence you collect. You don't always need to do this yourself since several organisations – the National Institute for Health and Clinical Excellence (NICE), the Scottish Intercollegiate Guidelines Network (SIGN), the Cochrane Collaboration and the Joanna Briggs Institute (JBI), for example – undertake such activities as a service to the academic and healthcare communities. Bear in mind, however, that although these organisations have a certain authority attached to them and that their outputs may well reflect rigorous and systematic procedures, the nature of critical appraisal means that JBI evidence summaries, Cochrane reviews and NICE and SIGN guidance are also open to critical review.

It is beyond the scope of this book to offer detailed guidance on critical appraisal. Like most skills, it is something that you will learn with practice and guidance. You will certainly get plenty of opportunities to practise since acquiring critical ability is an inherent part of university-level study regardless of the subject area (indeed, you will not succeed at university unless you can grasp this skill) and you will have to demonstrate some degree of critical analysis in most of the essays and assignments you will have to complete as part of your course. Some resources are listed at the end of this chapter for guidance but since critical ability is crucial to university-level study, you will find many, many more materials out there if you search for them or ask your course tutors.

Reflection

The skill of **reflection** is, to a large extent, a critical examination or appraisal of your own thoughts, feelings and actions. Schön (1983) distinguishes between reflection *on* action and reflection *in* action. Reflecting on action happens after the event; reflection in action during the event. Reflection on action is a prerequisite to becoming a competent practitioner; reflection in action, on the other hand, is a deeper skill that is essential if you are to become a capable practitioner. We have given you some opportunities to practise reflection in this book by the use of various 'reflection points' throughout. Again, it is beyond the scope of this book to offer detailed guidance on reflection but since it is so embedded into current British nursing practice, you will find ample opportunities to learn about reflection and practise reflective skills, especially when you are supported through **clinical supervision**. Clinical supervision is closely allied to the notion of reflective practice and is a means by which nursing practice can be enhanced by sharing experiences and reflecting on and learning from those experiences. In its *Clinical Supervision for Registered Nurses* advice sheet, the NMC (2008) outlined a set of principles to underpin clinical supervision for nurses which are reproduced in Box 2.8. For further information on clinical supervision and reflective practice see texts such as Butterworth et al. (1998), Cutcliffe et al. (2001), Bulman & Schutz (2004), Freshwater & Johns (2005) and Johns (2009).

Box 2.8 NMC principles underpinning clinical supervision (NMC, 2008; reproduced with permission)

- Clinical supervision supports practice, enabling registered nurses to maintain and improve standards of care.
- Clinical supervision is a practice-focused professional relationship, involving a practitioner reflecting on practice guided by a skilled supervisor.

(Continued)

(*Continued*)

- Registered nurses and managers should develop the process of clinical supervision according to local circumstances. Ground rules should be agreed so that the supervisor and the registered nurse approach clinical supervision openly, confidently and are aware of what is involved.
- Every registered nurse should have access to clinical supervision and each supervisor should supervise a realistic number of practitioners.
- Preparation for supervisors should be flexible and sensitive to local circumstances. The principles and relevance of clinical supervision should be included in pre-registration and post-registration education programmes.
- Evaluation of clinical supervision is needed to assess how it influences care and practice standards. Evaluation systems should be determined locally.

Conclusion

In this chapter, we have focused on the core knowledge, the core values and the core skills that are required to be an effective – or 'good' – mental health nurse. In the process, we have examined the personal qualities required for mental health nursing, discussed a variety of concepts (such as competence and capability) that influence how mental health nurses are educated and trained, and we have explored the acquisition of interpersonal and therapeutic clinical skills within the overall context of the therapeutic relationship.

Since these sorts of skills cannot be learnt solely from books, the importance of *practice* in their acquisition has been emphasised. 'Practice' can have two meanings and both are relevant here: it can mean rehearsal or trying things out in a supportive environment (through the use of role play, for example) and it can mean learning in a clinical, rather than academic, environment.

By combining ample opportunities for practice (in both senses) with the values that are fitting for modern-day mental health practice and the knowledge you will pick up from this book and from elsewhere, and by adding a degree of critical thought and reflection to your actions, we have no doubt that you will have the makings of a competent, if not a capable mental health nurse.

Further Reading and Resources

Key texts – interpersonal and therapeutic nursing skills

Argyle M (1988). *Bodily Communication*, 2nd edition. London: Methuen.
Classic text on non-verbal communication written by the acknowledged expert in this area. Perhaps a little dated but still relevant.

Freshwater D (2003). *Counselling Skills for Nurses, Midwives and Health Visitors.* Maidenhead: Open University Press.
Good textbook on general counselling skills, written by a leader in mental health nursing.

Callaghan P, Playle J & Cooper L (eds) (2009). *Mental Health Nursing Skills*. Oxford: Oxford University Press.
General, up-to-date textbook on mental health nursing, designed specifically for students and with a particular focus on skills.

Nash M (2010). *Physical Health and Well-Being in Mental Health Nursing: Clinical Skills for Practice*. Maidenhead: Open University Press.
Offers practical guidance to mental health nurses on the somewhat neglected area of physical healthcare.

Woodbridge K & Fulford KWM (2004). *Whose Values? A Workbook for Values-Based Practice in Mental Health Care*. London: Sainsbury Centre for Mental Health.
An excellent workbook on values-based practice, co-written by Bill Fulford, the originator of values-based practice, with plenty of guided exercises. Available free of charge from The Sainsbury Centre for Mental Health (the new name for the Sainsbury Centre) www.centreformentalhealth. org.uk.

Key texts – meta-skills

Butterworth T, Faugier J & Burnard P (eds) (1998). *Clinical Supervision and Mentorship in Nursing*, 2nd edition. Cheltenham: Stanley Thornes.
Key text on clinical supervision in nursing, edited by leading mental health nurses. Still relevant despite being more than a decade old.

Johns C (ed.) (2009). *Becoming a Reflective Practitioner*, 3rd edition. Oxford: Wiley-Blackwell.
Leading textbook on reflective practice in healthcare, edited by the originator of Johns' Model of Structured Reflection.

Freshwater D & Johns C (eds) (2005). *Transforming Nursing through Reflective Practice*, 2nd edition. London: Blackwell.
Johns again, this time in a text co-edited by a leading mental health nurse.

Gambrill E (ed.) (2005). *Critical Thinking in Clinical Practice: Improving the Quality of Judgements and Decisions*, 2nd edition. Hoboken, NJ: Wiley.
Good text on critical thinking for clinicians, though American.

Lindsay B (2007). *Understanding Research and Evidence-Based Practice. Exeter:* Reflect Press. *Easy-to-read primer for those who are a little unsure about the relationships between research and evidence-based practice in healthcare.*

Shermer M (2007). *Why People Believe Weird Things: Pseudoscience, Superstition, and Other Confusions of Our Time.* London: Souvenir Press. *Excellent, easy-to-read text on critical thinking that outlines the reasons why people often ignore the evidence and consequently 'believe weird things'.*

Websites

The Centre for Mental Health (formerly the Sainsbury Centre for Mental Health): www.centreformentalhealth.org.uk *Leading mental health charity that has steered much of the work on capability in mental health practice. Has a wealth of resources on its website, including downloadable copies of its reports.*

Nursing and Midwifery Council: www.nmc-uk.org *Website of the regulatory body for nursing which sets the standards (competencies) required for registration as a nurse in the UK.*

Mental Health in Higher Education: www.mhhe.heacademy.ac.uk *A Higher Education Academy (HEA) initiative (the HEA is an independent organisation promoting teaching and learning in British higher education) that aims to enhance learning and teaching about mental wellbeing and ill-health across the various disciplines in UK higher education.*

National Institute for Health and Clinical Excellence, www.nice.org.uk; the Scottish Intercollegiate Guidelines Network (SIGN), www.sign.ac.uk; the Cochrane Collaboration, www.cochrane.org; and the Joanna Briggs Institute, www.joannabriggs. edu.au *Websites of several leading organisations concerned with the appraisal of healthcare research and evidence.*

NHS Critical Appraisal Skills Programme (CASP), www.phru.nhs.uk/pages/phd/casp.htm *'CASP aims to enable individuals to develop the skills to find and make sense of research evidence, helping them to put knowledge into practice.'*

References

Argyle M (1988). *Bodily Communication,* 2nd edition. London: Methuen.

Beck AT, Rush AJ, Shaw BF & Emery G (1979). *Cognitive Therapy of Depression.* New York: The Guilford Press.

Bee P, Playle J, Lovell K, Barnes P, Gray R & Keeley P (2008). Service user views and expectations of UK-registered mental health nurses: A systematic review of empirical research. *International Journal of Nursing Studies,* **45**, 442–457.

Benner P (1984). *From Novice to Expert: Excellence and Power in Clinical Nursing Practice.* Reading, MA: Addison-Wesley Publishing.

Bulman C & Schutz S (2004). *Reflective Practice in Nursing,* 3rd edition. London: Blackwell.

Butterworth T, Faugier J & Burnard P (eds) (1998). *Clinical Supervision and Mentorship in Nursing,* 2nd edition. Cheltenham: Stanley Thornes.

Cairns L (1996). Capability: going beyond competence. *Capability,* **2**(2), 79–80.

Cooper C, Selwood A & Livingston G (2008). The prevalence of elder abuse and neglect: a systematic review. *Age and Ageing,* **37**(2), 151–160.

Cutcliffe J, Butterworth T & Proctor B (eds) (2001). *Fundamental Themes in Clinical Supervision.* London: Routledge.

DH (Department of Health) (1999). *National Service Framework for Mental Health: Modern Standards and Service Models.* London: HMSO.

DH (Department of Health) (2006a). *From Values to Action: The Chief Nursing Officer's Review of Mental Health Nursing.* London: DH.

DH (Department of Health) (2006b). *Best Practice Competencies and Capabilities for Pre-Registration Mental Health Nurses in England.* London: DH.

DH (Department of Health) (2008). *Refocusing the Care Programme Approach: Policy and Positive Practice Guidance.* London: DH.

DHSSPS (Department of Health, Social Services and Public Safety) (2007). *The Bamford Review of Mental Health and Learning Disability (Northern Ireland): A Comprehensive Legal Framework.* Belfast: DHSSPS.

Egan G (1975). *The Skilled Helper: A Systematic Approach to Effective Helping.* Belmont, CA: Thomson Brooks/Cole.

Evans D (2003). Hierarchy of evidence: a framework for ranking evidence evaluating healthcare interventions. *Journal of Clinical Nursing,* **12,** 77–84.

Fraser SW & Greenhalgh T (2001). Coping with complexity: educating for capability. *British Medical Journal,* **323,** 799–803.

Freshwater D & Johns C (eds) (2005). *Transforming Nursing through Reflective Practice,* 2nd edition. London: Blackwell.

Fulford KWM (1989). *Moral Theory and Medical Practice.* Cambridge: Cambridge University Press.

HM Government (2009). *New Horizons: A Shared Vision for Mental Health.* London: DH. Available from: www.dh.gov.uk [accessed 14 February 2010].

Johns C (ed.) (2009). *Becoming a Reflective Practitioner,* 3rd edition. Oxford: Wiley-Blackwell.

Lindsay B (2007). *Understanding Research and Evidence-Based Practice.* Exeter: Reflect Press.

Mayne L & Holley C (2009). Addressing violence and abuse: 'core business for mental health trusts'. *The Approach [Journal of the Care Programme Approach Association],* **2**(24), 10–13.

McKay M, David M & Fanning P (2009). *Messages: The Communication Skills Book,* 3rd edition. Oakland, CA: New Harbinger.

NES (NHS Education for Scotland) (2007). *A Capability Framework for Working in Acute Mental Health Care: The Values, Skills, and Knowledge Needed to Deliver High Quality Care in a Full Range of Acute Settings.* Edinburgh: NES.

NES (NHS Education for Scotland) (2008a). *Working with Older People in Scotland: A Framework for Mental Health Nurses.* Edinburgh: NES.

NES (NHS Education for Scotland) (2008b). *The National Framework for Pre-registration Mental Health Nursing Programmes in Scotland*. Edinburgh: NHS Education for Scotland.

NHS Confederation (2008). *Briefing 162: Implementing National Policy on Violence and Abuse*. London: NHS Confederation. Available from: www.nhsconfed.org [accessed 21 April 2010].

NIMHE/SCMH (National Institute for Mental Health England/Sainsbury Centre for Mental Health) (2004). *The Ten Essential Shared Capabilities: A Framework for the Whole of the Mental Health Workforce*. London: Department of Health.

NMC (Nursing and Midwifery Council) (2007). Introduction of Essential Skills Clusters for Pre-registration Nursing programmes. NMC Circular 07/2007. London: NMC. Available from www.nmc-uk.org [accessed 21 April 2010].

NMC (Nursing and Midwifery Council) (2008). Clinical supervision for registered nurses [advice sheet]. London: NMC. Available from www.nmc-uk.org [accessed 21 April 2010].

NMC (Nursing and Midwifery Council) (2010). *Standards for Pre-Registration Nursing Education: Draft for Consultation*. London: NMC.

Read J, Hammersley P and Rudegeair T (2007). Why, when and how to ask about childhood abuse. *Advances in Psychiatric Treatment*, **13**, 101–111.

Rogers CR (1980). *A Way of Being*. New York: Houghton Mifflin.

Sackett DL, Rosenberg WMC, Gray JAM, Haynes RB & Richardson WS (1996). Evidence based medicine: what it is and what it isn't [Editorial]. *British Medical Journal*, **312**, 71–72.

Schön DA (1983). *The Reflective Practitioner: How Professionals Think in Action*. New York: Basic Books.

SCMH (Sainsbury Centre for Mental Health) (2001). *The Capable Practitioner: A Framework and List of the Practitioner Capabilities Required to Implement the National Service Framework for Mental Health*. London: SCMH.

Scottish Executive (2006). *Rights, Relationships and Recovery: The Report of the National Review of Mental Health Nursing in Scotland*. Edinburgh: Scottish Executive.

Stephenson J (1998). The concept of capability and its importance in higher education. In J Stephenson & M Yorke (eds), *Capability and Quality in Higher Education*. London: Kogan Page.

UKCC (United Kingdom Central Council for Nursing, Midwifery and Health Visiting) (1999). *Fitness for Practice: The UKCC Commission for Nursing and Midwifery Education*. London: UKCC.

Welsh Assembly Government (2005). *Raising the Standard: The Revised Adult Mental Health National Service Framework and an Action Plan for Wales*. Cardiff: Welsh Assembly Government.

Woodbridge K & Fulford KWM (2004). *Whose Values? A Workbook for Values-Based Practice in Mental Health Care*. London: Sainsbury Centre for Mental Health.

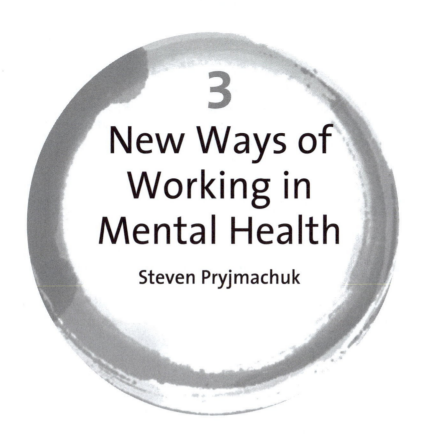

3
New Ways of Working in Mental Health

Steven Pryjmachuk

What will I learn in this chapter?

This chapter focuses on the mental health workforce, the different professional and occupational groups that are responsible for 'mental health work' (work that includes promoting mental health, preventing mental ill health and helping people recover from mental illness). In particular, it will examine how challenges and developments in mental health theory, policy and practice over the last decade or so have led to significant changes, both in the structure of the workforce and in the ways in which its individual workers function.

After reading this chapter, you will be able to:

- explain how the NHS is configured to deliver mental health services across the UK, outlining the similarities and differences in service provision in each of the four countries of the UK;
- outline the similarities and differences between the different types of mental health worker in terms of training, regulation and clinical responsibilities;

- appreciate the variety of factors that have driven new models of service delivery and organisation within UK mental health services, and new ways of working within those services;
- recognise healthcare as a political concern and appreciate the inevitability of change that politics brings about.

Introduction

When 'New Labour' came to power in 1997, it made a number of manifesto pledges. Two of those pledges, now realised, have had a significant impact on health service provision and on those who work for the health service. The first was the pledge to **modernise** the NHS (a process that is still ongoing); the second, a pledge to decentralise government and **devolve** significant powers – including those relating to health – to Scotland, Wales and Northern Ireland.

All four countries of the UK have, as such, seen substantial and significant changes over the last decade or so in the way in which mental health services are organised and delivered. In many cases, these changes have been far-reaching and rapid. Though rapid organisational change is often seen in a negative light – in terms of 'change fatigue' (Garside, 2003) or, ironically, its impact on the *mental health* of the workforce (WHO/ILO, 2002) – many of the changes that have occurred have been positive (McGonagle et al., 2009). Areas where there have been positive changes include: the introduction of **new mental health legislation**; the development of **organisational frameworks to improve standards** of mental health service delivery; the **restructuring of services** within the statutory sector (i.e., the NHS and local authorities); and the establishment of a whole host of 'workstreams' that have targeted activities such as **workforce planning**, the **education and training** of mental health professionals and mental health **research and development**.

Regarding legislation, Scotland passed the Mental Health (Care and Treatment) (Scotland) Act in 2003, while the Mental Health Act 2007 amended the Mental Health Act 1983 in England and Wales (Northern Ireland is expected to update its legislation some time in 2011). Regarding organisational frameworks for standards of mental health service delivery, Scotland was the first to move, publishing *A Framework for Mental Health Services in Scotland* in 1997 (Scottish Office, 1997). England issued its *National Service Framework for Mental Health* a few years later (DH, 1999a), though being a ten-year plan from the outset, it was superseded by a new initiative – *New Horizons* – in late 2009 (see HM Government, 2009). Wales published its framework in 2002, revising it in 2005 (Welsh Assembly Government, 2005), the same year that the Bamford Review (a major review of mental health and learning disability law, policy and service provision in Northern Ireland) issued *A Strategic Framework for Adult Mental Health Services* (see DHSSPS, 2005).

The most significant changes over the last few decades, however, have occurred in the configuration of services and in workforce development, two areas that warrant further discussion.

Configuration of Health Services across the UK

Primary, secondary and tertiary care

Like most NHS-provided healthcare, mental health service provision across the UK can be divided broadly into **primary care** services and **secondary care** services. Primary care services are those services that people with health problems initially seek out and are, as such, sometimes called **first contact** services. The lynchpin of primary care across the UK is the **General Practitioner** (GP; sometimes known as the 'Family Doctor'), but primary care also embraces services such as dentistry, the services provided by pharmacies and pharmacists, health visiting, school nursing and the telephone and online service, NHS Direct. Secondary care services are the more specialised general healthcare services that normally require referral from a primary care practitioner. **Tertiary care** services are the highly specialised services that are provided for particular disorders or groups of people, such as those with cancer or those with mental health problems who commit serious crimes.

A comparison of the three levels of care across a number of factors is contained in Table 3.1 below.

Note that the comparisons provided in Table 3.1, while useful, are generalisations rather than absolutes and exceptions do exist. For instance, although secondary care services are often equated with hospital provision and primary care services with community provision, hospital-based primary care services do exist (accident and emergency services, for example) as do community-based secondary care services (community mental health teams looking after people with ongoing mental health needs, for example). And while autonomy for professionals like nurses tends to be higher in primary care, there may well be circumstances where autonomy is greater in secondary care than it is in primary care (compare a nurse consultant working in acute

TABLE 3.1 Comparing primary, secondary and tertiary care

	Primary care	**Secondary care**	**Tertiary care**
Autonomy	High for all medical and related professionals	Tends to be low for professionals other than doctors	Tends to be low for professionals other than doctors
Base	Often community-based	Often institutional (hospital)	Almost always institutional
Referrals	Direct by patient	Usually a GP but often a range of primary care practitioners	A limited number of primary or secondary care practitioners
Interventions	Low in intensity or invasiveness	High in intensity or invasiveness	Very high in intensity or invasiveness
Nature	Generic	Specialist	Highly specialised
Continuity of care	High (patients often see the same staff)	Low (many staff may be involved)	Often high

mental health with a practice nurse working with a GP who limits her or his activities, for example).

Moreover, rigidly differentiating between services according to the level of care provided can be, at best, artificial and, at worst, unhelpful. As you will discover in Part II of this book, service provision rarely fits neatly into one category. For example, while service provision for common mental health problems (Chapters 4 and 5) has affinity with primary care, reference also has to be made to secondary care because both are an inherent part of the 'stepped care' organisational framework that is used in some parts of the UK. Similarly, the four-tiered organisational framework that underpins services for children and young people with mental health problems (Chapters 9 and 10) incorporates all three levels of care. And while the highly specialised services for those who misuse substances (Chapter 11) and those with mental health problems who come into contact with the criminal justice system (Chapter 12) equate well with the notion of tertiary care, primary and secondary services for these groups of people also exist.

Service Providers

The principal statutory health care provider in **England** is the **NHS Trust**. NHS Trusts are semi-independent public sector bodies that provide services on behalf of the NHS. There are a number of different types of Trust operating across England, each with a specific function and/or structure (see Table 3.2).

TABLE 3.2 NHS Trusts in England

Type of Trust	Details
Primary Care Trust (PCT)	Commissions (on behalf of local populations) primary and secondary care services from a range of primary and secondary care providers*
Acute Trust	Provides general (physical) secondary care services
Mental Health Trust	Provides secondary and tertiary care mental health services. Some may also provide primary care mental health services on behalf of a PCT
Ambulance Trust	Provides emergency and ambulance services
Care Trust	Provides both health and social care in collaboration with a local authority. There are several mental health Care Trusts in England but not all Mental Health Trusts are Care Trusts
Foundation Trust	An NHS Trust that has been given a greater amount of freedom (including financial freedom) in managing its affairs. Decision making is devolved to local communities with the Trust managers being accountable to the Trust's members and governors

*As well as commissioning primary care and community services, PCTs also used to provide the majority of such services. However, following the *Transforming Community Services* initiative (see DH, 2009a), the provider function was removed from most PCTs, with preference being given to a range of alternative providers including other NHS organisations, local authorities and the private and independent sectors.

The National Health Service Reform (Scotland) Act 2004 abolished NHS Trusts in **Scotland**. Since then, health services (including mental health services) have been provided by **NHS Boards** that cover geographical areas similar to the Scottish local authority boundaries. Subdivisions of these boards, the **Community Health Partnerships** (CHPs), work closely with social services and voluntary organisations to provide a range of community and primary care services that includes mental health services.

In October 2009 **Wales** similarly abolished its NHS Trusts replacing them with a number of **Local Health Boards**. Local Health Boards provide secondary care health services (including mental health services) and co-ordinate the provision of primary care and community services (again, including mental health services). Powys Local Health Board is especially interesting as it is scheduled to merge with the local authority some time in 2012 so that Powys County Council will, in effect, become the first modern-day UK council to provide health care.[1] In **Northern Ireland**, health and social care is provided through five integrated **Health and Social Care Trusts**. These trusts provide both primary and secondary health care

---

[1] Some English councils may follow suit and become providers of community and primary care services now that the provider function has been removed from PCTs.

services (including mental health services) as well as a range of social care services.

In talking about how the NHS is configured across the UK, it is important to bear in mind that health is, like education and the economy, an area of our lives that is so important that governments find it hard not to interfere. This has the unfortunate consequence of yielding a never-ending stream of policy initiatives and developments (usually with good intentions) even – as we have seen – when the same political party has been in power for a substantial amount of time. When governments change their colours, it becomes even worse and we strongly suspect that following the General Election outcome of May 2010 you will see more changes in the way in which the NHS is organised across the UK; some predictable, some perhaps not.[2] The message to you, as a potential health-care professional, is that **change is inescapable** and, as such, adaptability to change is a quality that is necessary to help you succeed in a career in mental health care.

Reflection Point

Adaptability to change

Ask yourself how adaptable to change you are.

How would you feel if the team you had gelled with was suddenly broken up due to a 'reorganisation'? What if you were asked to move to a different location? Or work with a different group of service users? Or work in a different way?

How has change affected you in the past? Have you got upset and resisted it? Or have you seen it as a challenge, embracing the change to get the most out of it?

The Mental Health Workforce

Workforce development

The quality of a mental health service is intrinsically linked to the people who work in that service. The education and training, attitudes and values, and skills and abilities of the mental health workforce and its capacity

---

[2]Indeed, just as the writing of this book was completed the new Coalition government announced its intention to transfer the commissioning role from PCTs to GP consortia, effectively sounding the death knell for PCTs.

for working together can all have an impact on a service user's experiences of care and his or her subsequent recovery. Workforce development is thus an essential component of any modern healthcare service, one that encompasses a number of interrelated aspects such as education and training, leadership, new roles and ways of working, research and development, and recruitment and retention. Over the past decade or so several discrete NHS bodies have steered or facilitated development of the mental health workforce, including Workforce Development Consortia (WDC), the National Institute for Mental Health in England (NIMHE), the Care Services Improvement Partnership (CSIP), NHS Education for Scotland (NES) and in Wales the National Leadership and Innovation Agency for Healthcare (NLIAH). Reflecting the rapid pace of change mentioned earlier, some of these bodies existed for only a few years, their work being completed or their relevance questioned as new policy directions emerged. No doubt there will be new bodies in the future and some of those current at the time of writing may well fall victim to changing priorities within the NHS or a change of local or national government. In England, for example, WDC were subsumed into the Strategic Health Authorities in 2005 and NIMHE and CSIP were both subsumed into the National Mental Health Development Unit (NMHDU) in 2009.

One workforce programme that is particularly relevant to this chapter is *New Ways of Working*, an initiative established in 2003 and wound up in 2009 (with the assimilation of NIMHE into the NMHDU). *New Ways of Working* originally came about as a result of psychiatrists' dissatisfaction with the established way of working in mental health but its scope and purpose ultimately had to encompass the whole of the mental health system because psychiatrists are merely one (admittedly important) part of that system (NHS Modernisation Agency/RCPsych/NIMHE, 2004; CSIP/NIMHE, 2007). Although *New Ways of Working* was specific to England, the fact that most of the professional bodies consulted during its development worked across the UK and the fact that Scottish and Welsh representatives sat on its expert panels meant that the initiative was relevant to other parts of the UK (NHS Modernisation Agency/RCPsych/NIMHE, 2004).

To make sense of *New Ways of Working*, however, you need to have an understanding of the people who work in mental health and, at this point, it's necessary to look at the different professions and disciplines involved.

Mental health workers

Mental health service users are often bewildered by the range of workers they come across and they are often confused about the roles and responsibilities of each, especially when workers have similar titles such as psychiatrist and psychologist or occupational therapist and psychological therapist.

Broadly speaking, there are two groups of workers in mental health services. One way of distinguishing the two groups is to say one set is qualified and the other unqualified but this can seem a little pejorative to those deemed unqualified. A better way of distinguishing between the two groups is to group them according to those whose occupational group might have a legitimate claim to the title 'profession' and those that do not. To do this, we first need to take a brief aside and explore the nature of a **profession**. This is not as simple as it seems and has been the subject of intense study over the years, particularly by sociologists.

The professions

The notion of a profession has its roots in the medieval universities of Europe such as Bologna, Paris, Oxford and Cambridge. In these universities there were originally only three disciplines in which the highest degree, a doctorate, could be awarded – divinity (theology), law and medicine[3] – and it is these three discipline that have the greatest claim to being a 'true' profession. During the nineteenth and twentieth centuries, as the Western world became industrialised and more technologically advanced, a whole host of occupational groups started to define themselves as professions: engineering, accountancy, midwifery, social work, teaching and, of course, nursing. Why some occupations are considered to be a profession while others, such as shop work, labouring or secretarial work, are not is a complex question that is beyond the scope of this book (if you are interested, Chapter 1 of Cheetham & Chivers, 2005, provides a comprehensive overview of the history and sociology of professions). Nevertheless, Box 3.1 contains some characteristics commonly associated with the professions that may help you differentiate between the professions and non-professions.

---

[3] *Medicine* has its roots in the ancient universities; *surgery* does not, having its roots in the barber–surgeons of the eighteenth century. Hence physicians specialising in medicine use the (honorary) title 'Dr' while physicians specialising in surgery use 'Mr' (or a female equivalent).

Box 3.1   Characteristics of a profession (after Vollmer & Mills, 1966; Freidson, 1970; Downie, 1990)

- Ownership of a specific body of knowledge (i.e. a theoretical base)
- A prolonged period of training in the body of knowledge, usually in a university setting
- A high degree of autonomy
- Public perception of status and prestige
- A service obligation, in that some form of service is provided to the public at large
- Regulation of members, whether by internal (e.g. through a professional organisation) or external (e.g. through a government or statutory authority) means
- Adherence to a code of conduct
- Explicit organisation of the occupational group via associations, committees, etc
- Unquestionable authority, resulting in a high degree of power
- Monopolistic control over an area of practice (including the rights to restrict entry into the profession)

Nursing as a profession

Given that nursing refers to itself as a profession, how many of the characteristics in Box 3.1 can you identify with nursing? Are there any areas where nursing is weak when compared to medicine, which has had a much longer – and some would say much stronger – claim to be a profession?

Since 2000, healthcare assistants have been allowed to join the Royal College of Nursing (a professional organisation) as associate members but they are generally not considered to be professionals. How do healthcare assistants map against the characteristics listed in Box 3.1?

Is there a difference between professional behaviour and being a professional?

Discussion Point

The mental health professions

In distinguishing between professions and non-professions in the mental health workforce, it's convenient to use **statutory regulation** as the key criterion. In other words, a profession is so only if it is regulated by statute, that is through laws passed by Parliament. In nursing's case, the respective statutes are the **Nurses, Midwives and Health Visitors Act 1997** and the **Nursing and Midwifery Order 2001**. Both of these statutes deal with the regulation

of nurses: the 1977 Act established the Nursing and Midwifery Council's predecessor, the United Kingdom Central Council for Nursing, Midwifery and
Health Visiting; the 2001 Order is technically a 'Statutory Instrument' (a law
that is enacted without full parliamentary debate) and is the law that established the Nursing and Midwifery Council.

Table 3.3 lists the principal mental health professions that are regulated by
statute, also outlining the education and training requirements of each. There are
other healthcare professionals (pharmacists, dietitians and speech therapists, for
example) who might be involved in the care of some people with mental health
problems but we have not included these in the tables as (rightly or wrongly)
they are generally not seen as core members of the mental health team.

Most of the professions listed in Table 3.3 have what are called 'protected titles'
which means that titles like 'registered nurse' are protected by law and only those
qualified to use them can do so legally. All of the professions listed are subject to
a professional code of conduct which, if violated, can bring the practitioner's **fitness to practise** into question which, in turn, may lead to sanctions such as
suspension or removal from the register of the respective regulatory body.

There are some interesting differences among the different professional
groups. Some professions, like nursing and occupational therapy, allow registration (and thus independent practice) on completion of undergraduate
studies; others, like psychiatry and clinical and counselling psychology, insist
on additional postgraduate education and training. Quite why this is the case
is largely historical but it is also connected to complicated arguments over
the point at which someone should specialise. In UK nursing we still have
four pre-registration specialties or 'branches'[4] of nursing: adult, mental health,
children's and learning disability. As such, the 'generic vs. specialist' debate
surfaces every now and then (e.g. Cutcliffe & McKenna, 2006; Holmes, 2006)
with those advocating late specialisation calling for generic basic training
prior to specialist postgraduate training, as is the case in medicine and clinical
psychology, and in nursing in much of the rest of the world. The debate has
been especially acute in Australia where specialist basic training (as is current
in the UK) was replaced with generic basic training in the late 1990s. This
led to mental health nursing becoming a postgraduate specialty and created
something of a crisis in Australian mental health nursing, both in terms of
recruitment into mental health nursing and, more importantly, in terms of
the skills deficits that the new generic nurses had when working in mental
health settings (Stuhlmiller, 2005).

---

[4]When the NMC changes come about in 2011, branches will become 'fields of practice'

TABLE 3.3 The education and training of UK statutorily regulated mental health workers

Profession	Regulatory body	Basic training	Postgraduate training
Arts therapist	HPC	An undergraduate degree in an arts/creative subject such as art, dance, drama, music	[R] Postgraduate training as an arts therapist, such as art therapist or drama therapist
Clinical psychologist	HPC	Undergraduate degree in psychology	[R] Doctoral-level training, usually a professional doctorate such as DClinPsy
Counselling psychologist	HPC	Undergraduate degree in psychology	[R] Postgraduate training in counselling
Mental health nurse	NMC	[R] Undergraduate diploma in nursing (England and Northern Ireland); undergraduate degree in nursing (Scotland and Wales).[a]	Postgraduate qualifications not necessary to practise as a mental health nurse but recommended for the higher nursing grades; doctorate recommended for Nurse Consultant posts
Psychiatrist	GMC	Undergraduate degree in medicine and surgery (e.g. MB ChB), i.e., basic training as a medical doctor	[R†] Two years as a 'Foundation House Officer' (F1/F2 years) followed by 3–6 years as a 'Specialty Registrar' (SpR) Entrance examination for the Royal College of Psychiatrists (RCPsych)
Occupational therapist	HPC	[R] Undergraduate degree in occupational therapy	Postgraduate qualifications not necessary to practise as an OT but recommended for the higher OT grades; doctorate recommended for Consultant OT posts
Social worker	GSCC	[R] Undergraduate or postgraduate degree in social work	Postgraduate qualifications not necessary to practise as a social worker but recommended for the higher social worker grades

[a]From 2011, basic training will be at degree level across the whole of the UK.

[R] = Successful completion of training at this point allows registration with the appropriate regulatory body.

[R†] = Doctors hold 'provisional registration' with the GMC until their F1 year is completed successfully.

HPC = Health Professions Council; NMC = Nursing and Midwifery Council; GMC = General Medical Council; GSSC = General Social Care Council; OT = occupational therapist.

Outside the professions: other mental health workers

As Table 3.4 shows, there are other occupational groups who work in mental health who are not regulated by statute. While some of these (e.g. psycho-therapists and CBT therapists) may indeed refer to themselves as professionals, most of those listed have a somewhat diminished status because they do not have the authority to work unsupervised in NHS settings. CBT therapists and psychotherapists are perhaps an exception but that is largely because these 'quasi-professions' piggy-back on the statutorily regulated professions by insisting on a statutorily recognised professional qualification as a prerequisite for entry.

Included in Table 3.4 are a number of workers that have emerged as a direct result of the NHS modernisation agenda, an agenda that has forced mental health service providers to rethink the services they provide so that they benefit the people who use them rather than the people who work for them. And in doing so, a variety of new ways of working have emerged. We will discuss these new workers in more detail in a short while.

New Ways of Working in Mental Health

Before we discuss these new ways of working in any great detail, take a minute or two to ask yourself who gets the most benefit out of health services.

Reflection Point

Using healthcare services

Think about your own experiences of healthcare – the last time you saw a health professional or had to go into hospital, or the last time you visited a friend or relative in hospital.

What did it feel like to be a patient or visitor rather than a member of the healthcare team? How did the staff treat you? Were you kept waiting or unin-formed? Did you feel that the service was designed with you in mind? Was it convenient for you, your relatives and friends?

If your experiences weren't that positive, what could you do to ensure that the patients and service users you work with in the future don't have the same experiences? If your experiences were positive, what was it about the service that made it so?

TABLE 3.4 The education and training of non-regulated mental health workers

Worker	Regulation	Basic training	Additional training
Assistant practitioner (to one of the healthcare professions in Table 3.3)	Not currently regulated, although the NMC is considering regulation of assistant practitioners in nursing and midwifery	Education and training to foundation degree level	Assistant practitioners can often enter shortened pre-registration training in their supporting profession
CBT therapist	BABCP	One of the 'core' professions listed in Table 3.3	Courses accredited by the BABCP which may be embedded into an academic award such as a diploma or degree
Counsellor (see also counselling psychologist in Table 3.3)	Largely unregulated though the BACP has an informal role and the HPC is considering the regulation of counsellors	No minimum qualification	Completion of training course accredited by BACP
IAPT psychological wellbeing practitioner	Not currently regulated; must work under supervision	People from a wide range of backgrounds with a special interest in therapy; can be gradates or non-graduates	University-based training that follows IAPT's curriculum; embedded into a formal academic award of postgraduate certificate
IAPT high intensity worker	Most of the entry professions are already regulated	Must already be a qualified mental health professional (e.g. occupational therapist, clinical or counselling psychologist, nurse)	Courses accredited by the BABCP (see CBT therapist above); embedded into a formal academic award at minimum postgraduate diploma level

(Continued)

TABLE 3.4 (*Continued*)

Worker	Regulation	Basic training	Additional training
Nursing or healthcare assistant	Not currently regulated, although the NMC is considering regulation of these workers	No qualifications required	Often trained in-house; foundation degree in health or social care for the higher grades (see assistant practitioner above)
Primary care graduate mental health worker	Not currently regulated	An undergraduate degree in an appropriate discipline, usually psychology	University-based training usually embedded into a formal postgraduate award, e.g. postgraduate certificate or diploma
Psychotherapist	Non-statutory regulation by the UKCP; the HPC is considering regulating psychotherapists	Normally an undergraduate degree in a related subject and/or a professional qualification listed in Table 3.3	A broad range of training that takes a minimum of four years and which often requires the individual to undergo psychotherapy themselves
Support worker	Not currently regulated	No qualifications required	Often trained in-house; foundation degree in health or social care for the higher grades (see assistant practitioner above)

NMC = Nursing and Midwifery Council; CBT = Cognitive behaviour therapy; BABCP = British Association of Behavioural and Cognitive Psychotherapies; BACP = British Association of Counselling and Psychotherapy; IAPT = Improving Access to Psychological Therapies; UKCP = UK Council for Psychotherapy.

If, after completing the reflection point above, you felt that the services you experienced were designed to benefit the staff rather than you as a patient or service user (e.g. having office-hours only appointments, or restricting your daily routine or choices), or if you felt dehumanised or patronised, then you are not alone. Experiences such as these have been one of the main drivers in the government's attempts to modernise healthcare provision.

Drivers for change

In mental health, **dissatisfaction with mental health services**, both by service users (SCMH, 1998; MIND, 2004; NES/SRN, 2007) and the staff who work in them (CSIP/NIMHE, 2007), is only one of the reasons for modernisation and change. On top of this there has been, over the last decade or so, a variety of political, social and economic trends that have converged to create the ideal conditions for change in mental health service provision. Among these trends are: a growing acceptance that **mental health and the alleviation of mental distress are too important to society to be neglected** (DH, 1999a; CEPMHPG, 2006); the Labour government's **social inclusion** agenda (see, for example, Social Exclusion Task Force, 2006) and its continuation of former Conservative government policy in relation to **choice** (choice is now embedded into the NHS Constitution; see DH, 2009b); concerns about **professional rivalry** (especially between psychiatrists and clinical psychologists; see Hall, 1996; Norman & Peck, 1999) and allied calls for **joint working** and **inter-professional collaboration** (Kingdon, 1992; Glasby & Lester, 2004); the growth of health consumerism and its influence on the **service user movement** (Wallcraft, 2003; van Tosh et al, 2000); the growing demands for **evidence-based practice**; and, finally, the associated focus on **recovery** brought about in part by the rightful demands of service users that they be at the centre of care.

Focusing on **mental health nursing** in particular, these drivers for change have provided the rationale for both the Chief Nursing Officer's review of mental health nursing in England (DH, 2006) and the national review of mental health nursing in Scotland (Scottish Executive, 2006). Indeed, the English review succinctly brings these drivers together under a common theme of 'newness' (see Box 3.3).

The importance of the drivers identified in Box 3.3 is such that many are cross-cutting themes that run throughout this book (e.g. **new guidance**, from the likes of NICE and SIGN, frequently underpins the 'evidence base' sections in each of the Part II chapters), though some are considered in particular detail in particular chapters (e.g. **new ways of working in primary care mental health** is considered in detail in Chapters 4 and 5; the **new mental health laws** are considered in detail in Chapters 7 and 12; and **new services**, such as assertive outreach and crisis resolution/home treatment, are considered in detail in Chapters 6 and 7). Those drivers not discussed elsewhere are worthy of some brief discussion here.

Box 3.3   Newness as the theme for change in mental health nursing (adapted from DH, 2006)

- **New expectations:** service users and carers expect standards of care to be high and choice to be an option
- **New ways of working:** mental health professions are reviewing their roles and responsibilities in the overall experience of care
- **New nursing roles**: such as nurse consultants, modern matrons and nurse prescribing
- **New services:** the development of services such as assertive outreach and crisis resolution/home treatment
- **New guidance:** emanating from bodies such as the English National Institute for Health & Clinical Excellence (NICE) and the Scottish Intercollegiate Guidelines Network (SIGN)
- **New laws:** not only mental health legislation but legislation relating to disability discrimination, mental capacity and human rights
- **New focus:** recovery; one that is positive and built on hope

---

New expectations: choice and personalised care

Personalised care has its roots in the government's **personalisation of public services** agenda. Choice is an essential feature of this agenda since personalisation is about tailoring services to the needs and preferences of citizens, and empowering citizens to shape their own lives and the services they receive (HM Government, 2007). Personalised care has made some inroads into social care through initiatives such as **direct payments** and **individual budgets**. Direct payments are cash payments made directly to people with health and social care needs (or to their carers) so that they can buy the care services they choose; individual budgets are similar to direct payments except that the recipient doesn't have the worry of managing money directly since a budget is held on their behalf by the commissioning authority. Research from some pilot projects in social care (Glendinning et al., 2009) suggests that individual budgets can have positive outcomes for service users and carers. *New Horizons* (the new strategy for mental health mentioned earlier) makes it clear that personalised care will be central to future mental health service provision, especially in terms of the interventions offered to carers and service users and the mechanisms surrounding access to those interventions.

New kinds of worker

In Table 3.4, we identified a number of non-regulated mental health workers, some of whom have emerged as a direct result of the modernisation agenda in mental healthcare: **assistant practitioners**, **IAPT psychological wellbeing practitioners**, **IAPT high-intensity workers** and the **primary care graduate mental health worker** (PCGMHW). The latter three of these four new workers are unique to mental health; assistant practitioners are not, being available in a range of healthcare disciplines including, for example, nursing, midwifery, occupational therapy and surgery.

Across the UK, assistant practitioners have, to some extent, been used to plug local gaps in those disciplines where it has sometimes been difficult to recruit. Like healthcare support workers and nursing assistants, they are unlicensed and unregulated but, unlike these workers, a qualification (normally a Foundation Degree) is required. Across England their adoption has been varied, with some NHS regions being keener to adopt assistant practitioners than others (Spilsbury et al., 2009). There are specific **mental health assistant practitioners** but there are some tensions surrounding their roles (as there are with the other new mental health workers), especially since these new workers raise questions over the roles and functions of mental health nurses (Warne & McAndrew, 2004).

The PCGMHW programme is an a English initiative, proposed in the NHS Plan (DH, 2000), that arose as a result of concerns over whether the primary care standards of the National Service Framework for Mental Health (DH, 1999a) could be achieved by the existing workforce. The logic behind its establishment was that there were a large number of graduates in disciplines such as psychology who were unable to find relevant work and the creation of these new posts would essentially kill two birds with one stone. There were concerns, however, that the PCGMHWs would use their posts as stepping stones to more prestigious careers as clinical psychologists rather than as a career in itself (NIMHE, 2003a). Though PCGMHWs are still being trained in some parts of England, their roles and posts are increasingly being subsumed into the IAPT programme.

The IAPT programme, again an English initiative, emerged from the *Layard Report* on common mental health problems (CEPMHPG, 2006). Training for two types of therapist is available with the IAPT programme: **psychological wellbeing practitioner** (formerly known as a low intensity worker) and **high intensity worker**. Because these roles are specifically associated with primary care, they are discussed in more detail in the policy section of Chapter 4.

New roles arising from new legislation

The various sets of mental health legislation that exist across the four countries of the UK specify that certain statutory duties (mostly relating to the formal detention of people with mental health problems) must fall on certain mental health professionals. Prior to the introduction of the Mental Health Act 2007 (which amended the Mental Health Act 1983 in England and Wales) and the Mental Health (Care and Treatment) (Scotland) Act 2003, the situation was pretty consistent across the whole of the UK. The person making applications for detention was always a social worker (known as the 'approved social worker' or ASW) and the person in charge on the service user's care was always a doctor, usually a psychiatrist (known as the 'responsible medical officer' or RMO). The current position is much more varied, however, in part down to the fact that *New Ways of Working* was primarily an English initiative and in part down the fact that, at the time of writing, Northern Ireland's legislation (the Mental Health (Northern Ireland) Order 1986) hasn't yet been reviewed, though a review is scheduled sometime in the future (NI Executive, 2009). Thus in England and Wales the **responsible clinician** (the term used in the legislation) can be a mental health professional other than a doctor (though in most cases, it will be a doctor), whereas in Scotland and Northern Ireland, the 'responsible medical officer' (again, the term used in the legislation) must be a doctor. In England and Wales the legislation now refers to the **approved mental health professional**, which includes nurses, occupational therapists and psychologists as well as social workers. In Northern Ireland this role remains available only to social workers as it does in Scotland, though the term used in the Scottish legislation is 'mental health officer'.

In England and Wales a new role of **best interests assessor** (BIA) was created by amendments to the Mental Capacity Act 2005. These amendments (2008 in England; 2009 in Wales) have introduced new **deprivation of liberty safeguards** which specify that people over 18 in hospital and care home settings without the mental capacity to give informed consent (e.g. someone with dementia) can only have their liberty deprived (e.g. through using sedation to admit them to hospital against their will or through locking doors and monitoring their movements) if it is in their best interests and necessary to protect them from harm. It is the BIA which determines if such actions are in the person's best interests. Social workers, mental health nurses, clinical psychologists and occupational therapists in England and Wales with two years' post-qualification experience are eligible, with additional training, to become BIAs. Psychiatrists, however, are not eligible because they are expected to take on a related role within the Mental Capacity Act, that of **mental health assessor**.

New nursing roles

The modernisation agenda has also brought about the new nursing roles of **nurse consultant**, **advanced practitioner**, **modern matron** and **nurse prescriber**. The impetus for nurse consultants and advanced practitioners (sometimes called nurse practitioners) came about largely because of the restrictions the *European Working Time Directive* placed on junior doctors' working hours.

Nurse consultants and advanced practitioners
Nurse consultants were announced in 1998 and formalised the following year in *Making a Difference* (DH, 1999b), the government's strategy for nursing. Nurse consultants have four core functions: (1) expert practice; (2) practice development, leadership and consultancy; (3) education, training and development; and (4) research and evaluation (DH, 1999c). In mental health, a nurse consultant might have a number of responsibilities, including running a specialist clinic (e.g. a self-harm clinic, or a nurse-led memory clinic), leading a specialist team (e.g. a substance misuse team), teaching (both in-house and at local universities) and collaborating in research projects.

Advanced practitioners are a grade below nurse consultants (see Table 3.5). Like nurse consultants they are highly qualified and have a core function of

TABLE 3.5   The NHS career framework for nursing

Grade[a]	Typical qualifications	Typical job titles
9 More senior staff	Masters degree (often in business or management, MBA); occasionally a doctorate	Director of Nursing; Associate Director of Nursing
8 Consultant practitioners	Masters degree or, preferably, a doctorate, whether by research (PhD) or professional (e.g. DNurs)	Nurse Consultant in Mental Health, Nurse Consultant in Self-Harm, Nurse Consultant in Substance Misuse, etc.
7 Advanced practitioners	Masters degree	Advanced Practitioner in Mental Health; Team Leader; Clinical Nurse Specialist; Ward Manager; Modern Matron *IAPT High-Intensity Worker*
6 Senior practitioners	Degree or postgraduate qualification such as a PG Certificate or PG Diploma	Community Psychiatric Nurse; Senior Staff Nurse; Assistant Ward Manager *Trainee IAPT High Intensity Worker; Senior Primary Care Graduate Mental Health Worker*
5 Practitioners *Minimum level for registered nurses*	Diploma[b] or degree	Staff Nurse, Mental Health *IAPT Psychological Wellbeing Practitioner; Primary Care Graduate Mental Health Worker*
4 Assistant practitioners	Foundation degree	Mental Health Assistant Practitioner *Trainee IAPT Psychological Wellbeing Practitioner; Trainee Primary Care Graduate Mental Health Worker*
3 Senior health care assistants	Scottish/National Vocational Qualifications Level 3	Senior Nursing/Healthcare Assistant
2 Support workers	Scottish/National Vocational Qualifications Level 2	Nursing/Healthcare Assistant
1 Initial entry level jobs	Little if any formal education or previous knowledge or experience	Nurse Cadet

[a]Aligned to the NHS pay bandings.
[b]Will be phased out in nursing by 2013.

expert practice; however, they are not necessarily involved in the remaining three core functions (leadership, education and research), although many are.

Table 3.5 outlines the NHS career framework for nursing. This framework not only illustrates where nurse consultants and advanced practitioners sit in the hierarchy, it also outlines where some of the other mental health workers we have discussed sit. Hopefully, one of the things you will have noticed about Table 3.5 is that career progression in nursing is now firmly based on the acquisition of additional knowledge and skills, often in the context of formal learning in a university setting. This is an important point since it brings into play a number of factors we have already discussed including the value of **lifelong learning** (discussed in the previous chapter) and the status of nursing as a **profession** (discussed earlier in this chapter). It should also reassure you that nursing is a good career choice since there are clear opportunities for advancement.

Modern Matrons

Modern Matrons were introduced across the NHS (including mental health services) in 2001 as a result of public and media concerns over a lack of strong clinical leadership in the NHS. Their primary roles are: (1) to provide leadership in relation to clinical care; (2) to ensure that administrative and support services (e.g. cleaning and meals) are delivered to the highest standards; and (3) to provide a visible, accessible and authoritative presence for patients in ward settings (DH, 2004). Their introduction has not been without controversy: for an initiative coming from a progressive government concerned with equality, the title 'matron' is a rather anachronistic, sexist one (men can be Modern Matrons after all), and the focus on cleaning and food delivery reflects, ironically, nursing from a bygone age rather than something you would expect to emerge from a programme of *modernisation* (Watson & Shields, 2009). The role also places undue emphasis on institutional care at a time when healthcare – mental healthcare in particular – is supposedly becoming much more primary care-centred.

Independent prescribers

From 2006, all nurses (including mental health nurses) who had passed a recognised nurse-prescribing course became **independent prescribers** of medicines, able to prescribe any licensed medication for any medical condition so long as it was within their sphere of competence (Jones, 2009). To access a recognised nurse-prescribing course, the NMC laid down some minimum standards in the same year. Nurses need to: (1) have three years post-registration clinical experience; (2) be able to study at degree level; (3) have the support of a designated medical practitioner for a minimum of 12 days supervised practice learning; and (4) have support from an employer (NMC, 2006). Jones & Jones (2005) identify three main benefits of nurse prescribing in mental health: (1) increased accessibility and better medication management (since service users tend to have higher levels of contact with nurses than other mental health professionals); (2) new forms of combination therapy (such as providing joint pharmacological and psychological therapies in depression); and (3) increased workforce capacity in that doctors would not need to be consulted or called-out regarding medication as often. There are criticisms of the role, however, in particular that it medicalises nursing (Cutliffe & Campbell, 2002), turning nurses into no more than 'mini-doctors'. Still, the evidence suggests that the public (those that really matter?) have a generally positive attitude towards nurse prescribing (Berry et al., 2006).

Inter- and multidisciplinary working

A theme running throughout the *New Ways of Working* programme is that of inter- or multidisciplinary working (sometimes referred to as inter- or multiprofessional working). *Multi* means 'many', and *inter* 'between'. Because multidisciplinary can mean both many disciplines working *alone* or many disciplines working *together*, **interdisciplinary** is a preferred term since it implies that there is communication between the many disciplines – that the disciplines are working together. As we have seen, the various mental health professions (disciplines) have their own distinct identities. Nevertheless, so long as we accept that there needs to be some common and fundamental standards that all mental health professionals adhere to, having a distinct professional identity is not necessarily detrimental to service users. To a large extent, these common and fundamental standards are the *Ten Essential Shared Capabilities* that we looked at in the previous chapter; moreover since the essential shared capabilities represent a common 'language' of mental health practice, they can only enhance interdisciplinary communication and interdisciplinary working.

Closely allied with the notion of interdisciplinary working is the notion of **skill mix** – having the most appropriately qualified staff in a service while being cognisant of the cost-effectiveness of that service. Implemented carefully, skill mix can deal with skills shortages and contain costs while improving the quality of care; implemented badly, it can lead to overstretched or bored staff, cynicism over cost-cutting and reductions in the quality of care. Consider the skill mix and degree of interdisciplinary working in the two teams in Table 3.6.

Interprofessional education (IPE), where different health and social care practitioners are educated together, is another concept closely linked with interdisciplinary working and one that is supported by the modernisation agenda (DH, 2001). IPE is not universally supported, however,

TABLE 3.6 Traditional vs. modern ways of working (adapted from CSIP/NIMHE, 2007)

	Team A (traditional)	Team B (modern)
Leadership	The assumption is that leadership is provided only by a psychiatrist	Leadership depends on who is the most able and competent irrespective of profession Leadership may be rotated or shared
Team working and attitude	The team is organised in a hierarchy. The consultant psychiatrist delegates work to others but at the same time shoulders all of the responsibility	Work and responsibility are distributed among the team based on individual members' capabilities Team members are responsible for their own decision making but also their own accountability
Service user focus	Care is delivered along profession-specific lines. Care is often seen by service users as fragmented	Care is delivered on a clear service user pathway by the most capable profession
Innovation and efficiency	Service users see a variety of professionals in an uncoordinated manner. They may end up seeing different professionals in the same week. Some professionals have long waiting lists	There is a levelling of caseload. All team members carry a similar caseload based on capability and capacity. Consultants (be they be psychiatrists, psychologists or nurses) carry caseloads with similar levels of complexity; more junior staff deal with less complex cases
Intelligent use of information	They get on with the job of providing a service but it's burdened by an ever-increasing demand. There are often tensions between team members	This team has a transparent and open caseload management system in place Supervision and audit are built into working practices

being seen by some as a transient educational fad rather than a sound, evidence-based initiative (Craddock et al., 2006). Because of the entry and exit (registration) points for the various mental health professions (see Table 3.3), IPE in mental health tends to be more common within post-graduate education and in-service training than it is in undergraduate education.

Organisational Complexities and the Limitations of this Book

The populations of the four UK nations vary on a huge range of factors – age, ethnicity, gender, intellectual capacity, genetics, disease type and sexuality to name but a few. Organising health services for such diverse populations is not easy since there is the potential to organise services according to any of the factors by which humans vary. The chapters in Part II of this book reflect some of the more common organisational frameworks employed in mental health. Services might be organised according to **age** (Chapters 8 and 9 are concerned with children and young people; Chapter 10 with older people), **condition** (Chapters 4, 5 and 6 focus, respectively, on depression, anxiety and psychosis), **behaviour** (Chapter 11 focuses on substance misuse; Chapter 12 on criminality) and **level of care** (Chapters 4 and 5 have a largely primary care focus; Chapter 7 focuses on secondary – acute – care). Critics might argue that there is no consistency in our approach to mental health service organisation but this reflects the reality of service provision across the whole of the UK. There is a major downside, however. When looking at the most common organisational frameworks, the needs of smaller population groups often get lost in the more general services that are provided for the majority. In addition, service provision can get complicated for those whose mental health problems are coupled with some other factor or behaviour such as substance misuse problems, a learning disability, or physical illness or disability.

As such – for reasons of space (and because this is, after all, an *introductory* text) – we have not given as much attention as we would have liked to black and minority ethnic (BME) mental health, maternal mental health, lesbian, gay, bisexual and transgender (LGBT) mental health, mental health services for people with a learning disability and the mental health of refugees and asylum seekers. Nevertheless, we believe that there is sufficient information in this book as a whole to provide you with some direction regarding the smaller, yet important, population groups. For those of you interested in these population groups, some key policy documents and resources can be found in Table 3.7. Consulting some of the resources listed at the end of this chapter (such as the websites of the Centre for Mental Health and the four UK health departments) and elsewhere in this book should also help you find relevant materials.

Conclusion

In this chapter you will have seen how, over the last decade or so, a variety of factors – including government policy, local, national and European demands, service user dissatisfaction and a focus on human rights – have converged to help UK mental health services, and the people who work in those services, change so that service provision is geared more towards recovery than towards containment or control. In the process, we have explored the similarities and differences between the different types of mental health worker and we have looked at some of the new roles that have emerged for (mental health) nurses

TABLE 3.7 Mental health resources for some minority groups

Minority area	Policy documents	Web resources
BME mental health	*Delivering Race Equality in Mental Health Care* report (DH, 2005) *Inside Outside* report (NIMHE, 2003b)	National BME Mental Health Network: www.bmementalhealth.org.uk Chinese Mental Health Association: www.cmha.org.uk
Maternal mental health	NICE (2007) guidance on antenatal and postnatal mental health Royal College of Midwives' guidance (RCM, 2009) Scottish Government report on the impact of maternal mental health on child development (Marryat & Martin, 2010)	
LGBT mental health	MIND report on the mental health and wellbeing of LBGT people (King & McKeown, 2003)	PACE: www.pacehealth.org.uk The rainbow Project (Northern Ireland): www.rainbow-project.org
Learning disability and mental health	Foundation for People with Learning Disabilities' *Green Light for Mental Health* initiative and toolkit (FPLD, 2004) *Good Practice in Learning Disability Nursing* (DH, 2007)	Foundation for People with Learning Disabilities: www.learningdisabilities.org.uk
Mental health of asylum seekers and refugees	Commission for Patient and Public Involvement in Health's report on asylum seekers and refugees (Palmer & Ward, 2005)	Health for asylum seekers and refugees portal (HARP) mental health and wellbeing resource: www.mentalhealth.harpweb.org Scottish Refugee Council: www.scottishrefugeecouncil.org.uk

BME = Black and minority ethnic.

as well as considering the opportunities that exist for the different types of mental health worker to work together.

If there is to be one clear message that emerges from this chapter it is that the balance of power in mental health is shifting – away from the providers of mental health services and towards those who are supposed to be the beneficiaries of such services, the service users. To provide care that is truly focused on the needs of those who use mental health services, mental health nurses need, at the very least, to be adaptable to change. At best, mental health nurses should be at the forefront of this 'new paradigm' because it not only provides significant developmental opportunities for individual mental health nurses as well as the profession as a whole, it more importantly paves the way for a new way of working in mental health that restores rights, dignity and hope to the very significant number of people who need support, guidance and, above all, care from us.

Further Reading and Resources

Key texts

Cheetham G & Chivers G (2005). *Professions, Competence and Informal Learning.* Cheltenham: Edward Elgar Publishing.
  For those interested in reading a little more about the nature of professions.

Care Services Improvement Partnership/National Institute for Mental Health in England (2007). *New Ways of Working for Everyone: A Best Practice Implementation Guide.* London: Department of Health.
  As it says, a 'best practice implementation guide' for New Ways of Working.

Department of Health (2006). *From Values to Action: the Chief Nursing Officer's Review of Mental Health Nursing.* London: Department of Health.

Scottish Executive (2006). *Rights, Relationships and Recovery: The Report of the National Review of Mental Health Nursing in Scotland.* Edinburgh: Scottish Executive.
  Reports of the reviews of mental health nursing in, respectively, England and Scotland.

Sewell H (2008). *Working with Ethnicity, Race and Culture in Mental Health: A Handbook for Practitioners.* London: Jessica Kingsley.
  Recent, practical textbook on ethnicity designed specifically for mental health practitioners.

Web resources

New Ways of Working archive: www.newwaysofworking.org.uk
  Archive of the NIMHE National Workforce Programme which finished its work in March 2009.

Information from the four UK health departments: Department of Health (England), www.dh.gov.uk; Scottish Health on the Web, www.show.scot.nhs.uk; Health of Wales Information Service, www.wales.nhs.uk; and Department of Health, Social Services & Public Safety (Northern Ireland), www.dhsspsni.gov.uk
  Gateways for health-related information for each of the four countries of the UK.

The Centre for Mental Health (formerly the Sainsbury Centre for Mental Health): www.centreformentalhealth.org.uk
  Website of a leading UK mental health charity that has been extremely influential in British mental health policy over the last decade.

NHS Careers: www.nhscareers.nhs.uk
Website providing details of all of the different professional and occupational groups working throughout the NHS (and in health care in general).

Regulatory bodies for the professions: nursing, www.nmc-uk.org; medicine, www.gmc-uk.org; health professions, www.hpc-uk.org
Websites for the three main healthcare regulators where you can find standards relating to, for example, education and professional conduct. There is also 'regulator of the regulators', the Council for Healthcare Regulatory Excellence, www.chre.org.uk

References

Berry D, Courtenay M & Bersellini E (2006). Attitudes towards, and information needs in relation to, supplementary nurse prescribing in the UK: an empirical study. *Journal of Clinical Nursing*, **15**, 22–28.

CEPMHPG (Centre for Economic Performance's Mental Health Policy Group) (2006). *The Depression Report: A New Deal for Depression and Anxiety Disorders* [The Layard Report]. London: London School of Economics. Available from: cep.lse.ac.uk [accessed 12 January 2010].

Cheetham G & Chivers G (2005). *Professions, Competence and Informal Learning*. Cheltenham: Edward Elgar Publishing.

Craddock D, O'Halloran C, Borthwick A & McPherson K (2006). Interprofessional education in health and social care: fashion or informed practice? *Learning in Health and Social Care*, **5**(4B), 220–242.

CSIP/NIMHE (Care Services Improvement Partnership/National Institute for Mental Health in England) (2007). *New Ways of Working for Everyone: A Best Practice Implementation Guide*. London: DH.

Cutliffe J & Campbell P (2002). Nurse prescribing could lead nurses away from core concepts that underpin nursing. *Mental Health Practice*, **5**(5), 14–17.

Cutcliffe JR & McKenna HP (2006). Generic nurses: the nemesis of psychiatric/mental health nursing? In JR Cutcliffe & M Ward (eds), *Key Debates in Psychiatric/Mental Health Nursing*. London: Churchill Livingstone.

DH (Department of Health) (1999a). *National Service Framework for Mental Health: Modern Standards and Service Models*. London: HMSO.

DH (Department of Health) (1999b). *Making a Difference: Strengthening the Nursing, Midwifery and Health Visiting Contribution to Health and Healthcare*. London: HMSO.

DH (Department of Health) (1999c). Nurse, midwife and health visitor consultants: establishing posts and making appointments. *Health Service Circular1999/217*. London: HMSO.

DH (Department of Health) (2000). *The NHS Plan: A Plan for Investment, a Plan for Reform*. London: HMSO.

DH (Department of Health) (2001). *Investment and Reform for NHS Staff – Taking Forward the NHS Plan*. London: DH.

DH (Department of Health) (2004). *Modern Matrons in the NHS: A Progress Report.* London: HMSO.

DH (Department of Health) (2005). *Delivering Race Equality in Mental Health Care: A Summary.* London: DH.

DH (Department of Health) (2006). *From Values to Action: The Chief Nursing Officer's Review of Mental Health Nursing.* London: DH.

DH (Department of Health) (2007). *Good Practice in Learning Disability Nursing.* London: DH.

DH (Department of Health) (2009a). *Transforming Community Services: Enabling New Patterns of Provision.* London: DH.

DH (Department of Health) (2009b). *Implementation of the Right to Choice and Information Set Out in the NHS Constitution.* London: DH.

DHSSPS (Department of Health, Social Services and Public Safety) (2005). *A Strategic Framework for Adult Mental Health Services.* Belfast: DHSSPS. Available from: www.rmhldni.gov.uk [accessed 14 February 2010].

Downie RS (1990). Professions and professionalism. *Journal of Philosophy of Education*, **24**(2), 147–159.

FPLD (Foundation for People with Learning Disabilities) (2004). *Green Light for Mental Health* [framework and toolkit]. Available from: www.learningdisabilities.org.uk [accessed 15 May 2010].

Freidson E (1970). *Profession of Medicine: A Study of the Sociology of Applied Knowledge.* New York: Dodd Mead & Co.

Garside P (2003). Are we suffering from change fatigue? *Quality and Safety in Health Care*, **13**, 89–90.

Glasby J & Lester H (2004). Cases for change in mental health: partnership working in mental health services. *Journal of Interprofessional Care*, **18**(1), 7–16.

Glendinning C, Arskey H, Jones K, Moran N, Netten A & Rabiee P (2009). *The Individual Budgets Pilot Projects: Impact and Outcomes for Carers.* York: Social Policy Research Unit.

Hall JN (1996). Working effectively with clinical psychologists. *Advances in Psychiatric Treatment*, **2**, 219–225.

HM Government (2007). *Building on Progress: Public Services. HM Government Policy Review.* London: Prime Minister's Strategy Unit.

HM Government (2009). *New Horizons: A Shared Vision for Mental Health.* London: DH. Available from: www.newhorizons.dh.gov.uk [accessed 14 February 2010].

Holmes CA (2006). The slow death of psychiatric nursing: what next? *Journal of Psychiatric and Mental Health Nursing*, **13**(4), 401–415.

Jones A (2009). *Nurse Prescribing in Mental Health.* Oxford: Wiley-Blackwell.

Jones A & Jones M (2005). Mental health nurse prescribing: issues for the UK. *Journal of Psychiatric and Mental Health Nursing*, **12**, 527–535.

King M & McKeown E (2003). *Mental Health and Social Wellbeing of Gay Men, Lesbians and Bisexuals in England and Wales: A Summary of Findings.* London: MIND.

Kingdon DG (1992). Interprofessional collaboration in mental health. *Journal of Interprofessional Care*, **6**(2), 141–147.

Marryat L & Martin C (2010). *Growing Up in Scotland: Maternal Mental Health and Its Impact on Child Behaviour and Development.* Edinburgh: The Scottish Government.

McGonagle I, Jackson C & Baguley I (2009). Mental health policy to practice; too much loose change? *Journal of Research in Nursing,* **14**(6), 493–502.

MIND (2004). *Ward Watch: Mind's Campaign to Improve Hospital Conditions for Mental Health Patients.* London: MIND.

NHS Modernisation Agency/RCPsych/NIMHE (NHS Modernisation Agency/Royal College of Psychiatrists/National Institute for Mental Health in England) (2004). *Guidance on New Ways of Working for Psychiatrists in a Multi-disciplinary and Multi-agency Context: Interim Report.* London: DH.

NES/SRN (NHS Education for Scotland/Scottish Recovery Network) (2007). *Realising Recovery A National Framework for Learning and Training in Recovery Focused Practice.* Glasgow: SRN/Edinburgh: NES. Available from: www.nes.scot.nhs.uk [accessed 7 February 2010].

NI (Northern Ireland) Executive (2009). McGimpsey announces single bill approach for mental health [press release 10 September 2009]. Available from: www.northernireland. gov.uk [accessed 7 February 2010].

NICE (National Institute for Health and Clinical Excellence) (2007). *Antenatal and Postnatal Mental Health: Clinical Management and Service Guidance [NICE Clinical Guidance 45].* London: NICE.

NIMHE (National Institute for Mental Health in England) (2003a). *Fast-Forwarding Primary Care. Mental Health Graduate Primary Care Mental Health Workers: Best Practice Guidance.* London: NIMHE.

NIMHE (National Institute for Mental Health in England) (2003b). *Inside Outside: Improving Mental Health Services for Black and Minority Ethnic Communities in England.* London: NIMHE.

NMC (Nursing and Midwifery Council) (2006). *Standards of Proficiency for Nurse and Midwife Prescribers.* London: NMC.

Norman IJ & Peck E (1999). Working together in adult community mental health services: an inter-professional dialogue. *Journal of Mental Health,* **8**(3), 217–230.

Palmer D & Ward K (2005). *'Unheard Voices': Listening to the Views of Asylum Seekers and Refugees.* London: Commission for Patient and Public Involvement in Health.

RCM (Royal College of Midwives) (2009). *Maternal Mental Health Guidance for Midwives.* London: RCM.

SCMH (Sainsbury Centre for Mental Health) (1998). *Acute Problems: A Survey of the Quality of Care in Acute Psychiatric Wards.* London: SCMH.

Scottish Office (1997). *A Framework for Mental Health Services in Scotland.* Available from: www.show.scot.nhs.uk [accessed 9 September 2009].

Scottish Executive (2006). *Rights, Relationships and Recovery: The Report of the National Review of Mental Health Nursing in Scotland.* Edinburgh: Scottish Executive.

Social Exclusion Task Force (2006). *Reaching Out: An Action Plan on Social Exclusion.* London: Social Exclusion Task Force.

Spilsbury K, Stuttard L, Adamson J, Atkin K, Borglin G, McCaughan D, McKenna H, Wakefield A & Carr-Hill R (2009). Mapping the introduction of Assistant Practitioner roles in Acute NHS (Hospital) Trusts in England. *Journal of Nursing Management*, **17**, 615–626.

Stuhlmiller C (2005). Rethinking mental health nursing education in Australia: a case for direct entry. *International Journal of Mental Health Nursing*, **14**, 156–160.

Van Tosh L, Ralph RO & Campbell J (2000). The rise of consumerism. *Psychiatric Rehabilitation Skills*, **4**(3), 383–409.

Vollmer HM & Mills DL (1966). *Professionalization*. Englewood Cliffs, NJ: Prentice-Hall.

Wallcraft J (2003). *The Mental Health Service User Movement in England* [Policy Paper 2]. London: SCMH. Available from: www.scmh.org.uk [accessed 11 January 2010].

Warne T & McAndrew S (2004). The mental health assistant practitioner: an oxymoron? *Journal of Psychiatric and Mental Health Nursing*, **11**, 179–184.

Watson R & Shields L (2009). Cruel Britannia: a personal critique of nursing in the United Kingdom. *Contemporary Nurse*, **32**(1–2), 42–54.

Welsh Assembly Government (2005). *Raising the Standard: The Revised Adult Mental Health National Service Framework and an Action Plan for Wales*. Cardiff: Welsh Assembly Government.

WHO/ILO (World Health Organisation/International Labor Organisation) (2002). *Mental Health and Work: Impact, Issues and Good Practices*. Geneva: WHO/ILO.

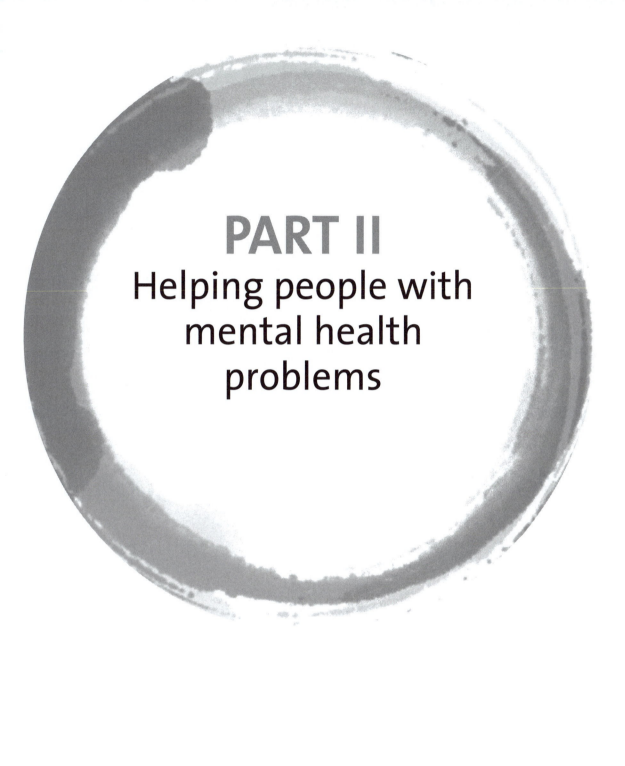

PART II
Helping people with mental health problems

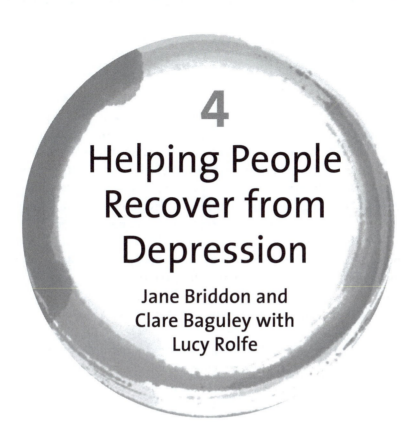

4

Helping People Recover from Depression

Jane Briddon and Clare Baguley with Lucy Rolfe

What will I learn in this chapter?

This chapter aims to provide you with an understanding of the knowledge and skills required for promoting effective, recovery-focused interventions for people experiencing problems with depression in primary care settings.

After reading this chapter, you will be able to:

- appreciate the policy framework underpinning the provision of services for people experiencing mild to moderate depression;
- identify the key symptoms and diagnostic features of depression within the context of a biopsychosocial model of depression;
- outline a structured model of assessment that incorporates a collaborative approach, shared problem formulation, SMART goal setting and joint decision making;
- recognise the principles of evidence-based practice for depression and the skills required to apply these principles in order to widen access to services and increase choice.

Introduction

Depression is a term used to describe the problems people experience when they are low in mood. It is a condition that cuts across age, gender and social group. Globally, there is increasing concern about the occurrence of depression and its effects on health: the World Health Organisation estimates that by 2020 depression will be the second largest cause of disability worldwide across the age range and for both men and women (Moussavi et al., 2007).

In the UK, depression affects around 3% of adults aged between 16 and 74, a figure that grows to over 11% when 'mixed depression and anxiety' is reported as the problem (Singleton et al., 2001). Due to its high prevalence, depression is (along with anxiety) often referred to as a **common mental health problem**. The fact that such problems are termed 'common' does not mean, however, that these conditions are any less serious than other mental health problems.

As with all mental health problems it can be useful to think of depression as having degrees of severity which exist along a continuum (see Figure 4.1, which is a redrawing of Figure 1.1 from Chapter 1). The severity of depression is determined by a range of factors, including its duration, the individual's ability to cope and the impact it has on the individual's relationships, self care, work and general quality of life.

The vast majority of people experiencing depression will have only a mild to moderate form (though it is important to recognise that even mild depression

Mental health	Mild depression	Moderate depression	Severe depression
The normal day-to-day mood fluctuations of life	Low risk and optimism about the future Temporary impact on quality of life and self care	Low to moderate risk with fluctuating hopelessness Potentially significant impact on quality of life and self care	Depressive illness Persistent high risk and hopelessness Enduring impact on quality of life and self care Recurrent relapse

FIGURE 4.1   The continuum of depression

can be disabling). Around 40% of people with depression do not seek help, the reasons being as varied as 'not thinking anyone could help', depression being something that people should be able to cope with and, perhaps most significantly, the **stigma** associated with mental health problems (NCCMH, 2009). Nevertheless, most of those with mild to moderate depression who seek help are assessed and helped entirely within **primary care** settings (Goldberg & Huxley, 1992; DH, 1999; NCCMH, 2009). Those with depression at the severe end of the continuum tend to have acute mental health needs (which may involve active thoughts of suicide) and, as such, these individuals may need to be cared for in an inpatient setting. Since these individuals are considered more fully in Chapter 7, this chapter will focus mainly on helping those with mild to moderate depression in a primary care setting.

Demographics

Some people are more vulnerable to depression than others, with a person's vulnerability likely to be down to a complex interplay of **biological** factors (e.g. gender, brain chemistry), **psychological** issues (e.g. stress, ability to cope) and **environmental** circumstances (e.g. housing status, poverty). As you will soon discover, this 'biopsychosocial' perspective is a useful one for understanding depression and one we will revisit throughout this chapter.

In terms of **gender**, prevalence rates for depression are generally 1.5 to 2.5 times higher in women than in men (NCCMH, 2009), although there are over three times as many suicides amongst men (especially younger men) than women (ONS, 2010). **Gay men** and **lesbians** are more likely to be psychologically distressed and are more likely to consult mental health professionals than their heterosexual counterparts (King et al., 2003). In terms of **age**, depression is thought to be more prevalent in the 35–54 age group than in younger or older age groups (Singleton et al., 2001).[1]

Regarding **black and minority ethnic** (BME) communities, there is some evidence that depression is more common in African Caribbean women than in white women (Shaw et al., 1999) and some evidence that physical rather than psychological presentations of depression are more likely among Asians than whites (Commander et al., 1997). In a review of the

---

[1] At this point it's worth mentioning that we will only consider depression in **adults of working age** in this chapter; depression in children and young people and in older people is discussed in Chapters 8, 9 and 10.

literature on suicide and self-harm, Bhui & McKenzie (2006) report that South Asian women (especially younger women) have higher rates of suicide than other ethnic groups while South Asian men have lower rates, and that East African men have high rates. Bhui & McKenzie also report that there may be higher rates of suicide in Irish men and women and in Scottish men. There are also issues regarding **access** to mental health services with BME groups. The *Inside Outside* (NIMHE, 2003) and *Delivering Race Equality* (DH, 2005) reports highlight continuing inequality in access to appropriate mental health care for people from BME communities in that such access often disregards primary or community care-based alternatives to hospital. In African Caribbean communities, schizophrenia (see Chapter 6) is more likely to be over-diagnosed, while depression and anxiety are more likely to be underdiagnosed. BME communities are also less likely to be accepted for psychological therapies than their white counterparts (Cahill et al., 2006).

Social factors also seem to influence depression rates: depression is more common in the unemployed, those living alone, those who are divorced or separated, those living in local authority or housing association accommodation, those with a lower socioeconomic status and/or material disadvantage and those with no formal educational qualifications (Singleton et al., 2001; Fryers et al., 2003, 2005). Social factors such as isolation, racist attacks and dissatisfaction with housing may also contribute to depression in **refugee** groups; indeed, in traumatised refugees and asylum seekers, poor social support appears to be a stronger predictor of depression in the long term than the severity of the initial trauma (Gorst-Unsworth & Goldenberg, 1998).

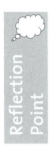

Risk factors in depression

Think about someone you know. Perhaps they are from a different ethnic or cultural background. Or they are older or younger than you, male rather than female, single rather than partnered, gay rather than straight.

What factors do you think might increase the risk of depression in that person? Try to think in terms of biological, psychological and, especially, social, economic and environmental factors.

Policy Context

A watershed in the policy framework for those with common mental health problems in England was the publication, over a decade ago, of the *National*

Service Framework for Mental Health (NSF; DH, 1999). The NSF identified as a priority those with common mental health problems (along with those with severe mental illness) and endorsed (in standards 2 and 3) primary care as the natural setting for helping and supporting this particular group of people. The wider *NHS Plan* (DH, 2000) further reinforced this position with the establishment of a new type of mental health worker, the **primary care graduate mental health worker** (PCGMHW; see Chapter 3 for further discussion), as did the introduction of a new GP contract in 2004. The new GP contract allowed primary care trusts (PCTs) to offer additional funding streams to GPs who took on 'enhanced services' – services that dealt with key areas of nationally identified clinical need – of which depression was one. PCTs would benefit from the provision of enhanced services for depression through a reduction in demand for (more expensive) secondary care services; those with depression would benefit with more convenient services and additional choice (NIMHE, 2004).

In 2006, the Centre for Economic Performance at the prestigious London School of Economics published the **Layard Report**, or to give it its formal title, *The Depression Report: A New Deal for Depression and Anxiety Disorders* (CEPMHPG, 2006). At the heart of the Layard Report was the observation that crippling anxiety and depression not only generated personal costs for a significant proportion of the population but had major social and economic implications for the country as a whole. The report supported the provision of 'talking therapies', stating that the cost of providing such therapies would be recouped within two years in savings made on incapacity benefit and lost taxes from the million-plus people who were unable to work because of mental health problems. The Layard Report was written within the context of a significant amount of research evidence, built up over the last few decades, that demonstrated that psychological therapies – cognitive behaviour therapy (CBT) in particular – could ameliorate common mental health problems like anxiety and depression so enabling people affected by these problems to live full and rewarding lives. The stumbling block, however, was *access* to these talking therapies. Even though the primary care demands of the NSF had been in operation for more than five years, many areas had waiting lists of nine months or more for these therapies; some had no waiting list simply because they had no therapists.

Out of the Layard Report came the current policy initiative on common mental health problems in England: *Improving Access to Psychological Therapies* (it's often known by its abbreviation, **IAPT**). Following a pilot in two 'demonstration' sites in Doncaster, Yorkshire and Newham, Greater London – both involving CBT – the IAPT initiative was extended in 2008 to over 30 sites in England. As Salkovskis (2008) put it, 'this is not an exercise in redistributing resources but rather the creation of an entirely new high quality way of delivering evidence-based psychological therapies to the maximum number of people possible, and doing so in their local area' (p. 1). In each of the IAPT sites, training for therapists is linked to an academic or training institution (such as a university) and is offered at two levels: **psychological wellbeing practitioner** (formally known as a low-intensity worker) and **high-intensity practitioner** (these roles were discussed in Chapter 3). In late 2009, the government committed itself to further developing the IAPT initiative, expanding the range of therapies to include not only CBT but other National Institute for Health and Clinical Excellence (NICE) approved therapies such as interpersonal therapy, couples therapy, brief dynamic therapy, counselling and collaborative care (Burnham, 2009).

Outside England, the Scottish Government has recently produced *The Matrix*, which is a guide to planning and delivering evidence-based psychological therapies within Scotland (Scottish Government/NES, 2008). *The Matrix* has significant overlaps with the English IAPT initiative but its focus is perhaps a little wider than England in that it encompasses not only anxiety and depression but also mental health issues in children and young people (see Chapters 9 and 10) and longer-term conditions in adult mental health (see Chapter 6). At the time of writing, there is no robust policy or strategy specific to anxiety and depression in Wales or Northern Ireland though elements are included in the overarching reviews of mental health services that are ongoing in the two countries – the Bamford Review in Northern Ireland (see DHSSPS, 2009) and the Williams Review in Wales (see Williams, 2008). In addition, *Book Prescription Wales*, a form of **bibliotherapy** whereby self-help books on a variety of topics including stress, anxiety, panic and depression are 'prescribed' free of charge to people with common mental health problems, has been supported by the Welsh Assembly since 2004 though its effectiveness is unknown (Porter, 2006).

In late 2009, the replacement for the English NSF (which had run its ten-year course) was announced. *New Horizons* (HM Government, 2009) is a cross-government initiative that has the twin aims of improving the mental health and wellbeing of the population and the quality and accessibility of services for people with poor mental health. As far as common mental health problems are concerned, the focus within *New Horizons* is on mental health promotion to prevent such problems occurring, and on early intervention and social support (including employment opportunities) for those who go on to develop such problems.

Stepped care

Further developments in the policy for depression came about with the publication of the NICE guidelines on the treatment and management of depression (DH, 2004; NCCMH, 2009; NICE, 2009). Based on an expert review of current evidence and best practice regarding the interventions available for depression, the NICE guidelines have been instrumental in the implementation of a framework for the delivery of primary mental health care services in England and Wales known as **stepped** care. Stepped care is a model of service delivery whereby the less intrusive, most readily accessible, evidence-based treatments are offered before more complex interventions (Bower & Gilbody, 2005a).

The stepped care model is a care pathway involving five levels of care (Figure 4.2). Steps 1 to 3 are delivered in primary care settings; while Steps 4 and 5 are delivered in secondary care settings. The steps are organised principally on the basis of the interventions on offer. As such, there has been some debate over the specific skills and competencies required to deliver the interventions at each of the levels and the types of workers best placed to undertake

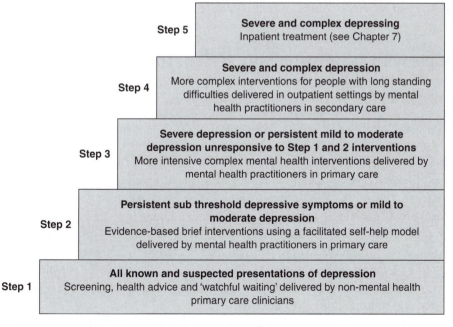

Step 5 — **Severe and complex depressing** Inpatient treatment (see Chapter 7)

Step 4 — **Severe and complex depression** More complex interventions for people with long standing difficulties delivered in outpatient settings by mental health practitioners in secondary care

Step 3 — **Severe depression or persistent mild to moderate depression unresponsive to Step 1 and 2 interventions** More intensive complex mental health interventions delivered by mental health practitioners in primary care

Step 2 — **Persistent sub threshold depressive symptoms or mild to moderate depression** Evidence-based brief interventions using a facilitated self-help model delivered by mental health practitioners in primary care

Step 1 — **All known and suspected presentations of depression** Screening, health advice and 'watchful waiting' delivered by non-mental health primary care clinicians

FIGURE 4.2   The stepped care model for depression (adapted from NICE, 2009)

the work at each level. People with more complex and severe depression may require the help of mental health practitioners who are part of a multidisciplinary team (e.g. mental health nurses, social workers, occupational therapists and psychiatrists) since such a team may be best placed to respond flexibly and promptly to the complex needs (and possible risks) associated with more severe depression.

A range of practitioners are available to meet the needs of those at steps 2 to 3, including established practitioners such as mental health nurses, occupational therapists and social workers (though additional expertise in primary mental health care is required) as well as new workers such as the PCGMHWs and IAPT therapists mentioned earlier. While the problems encountered at the lower steps were envisaged to be less severe, working with the brief time limits and high-volume case loads of primary care and using a variety of modes of delivery demands a particular skill set. Moreover, the descriptor 'mild to moderate' depression pertaining to steps 2 and 3 does not necessarily reflect the complexity and severity of the problems encountered within primary mental health care (Clark et al., 2009).

It is also worth mentioning that although stepped care is embedded into the NICE guidance on depression (NICE, 2009), it is not embraced in the more recent Scottish guidance on depression (SIGN, 2010) nor is the evidence for its effectiveness unequivocal (Bower & Gilbody, 2005b).

How People with Depression May Present to Services

Symptoms of depression

Depression is a disorder that presents with depressed mood, loss of interest or pleasure in life, low self-worth, feelings of guilt, disturbed sleep or appetite, a lack of energy and poor concentration (WHO, 2010). As we mentioned earlier, these sorts of symptoms can vary in terms of severity from mild to moderate to severe. At the severest end of the continuum, a person may be formally diagnosed as suffering from depressive illness (or 'clinical depression'). In these circumstances, diagnosis is normally undertaken by a psychiatrist who will use one of the two diagnostic systems referred to in Chapter 1 – DSM-IV or ICD-10 – to elicit and categorise a person's symptoms. These diagnostic systems require the person to be experiencing a number of symptoms for a particular duration of time (see Box 4.1).

Whilst diagnosis is an important tool for defining a problem and for guiding medical decisions regarding treatment, for mental health nurses trying to

> **Box 4.1   Core symptoms of depression (adapted from DSM-IVR; APA, 2000)**
>
> - Feels sad; empty and/or tearful
> - Loss of interest/pleasure in activities
> - Decrease/increase in appetite; weight loss or gain >5% in month
> - Insomnia or hypersomnia
> - Psychomotor agitation or retardation
> - Fatigue or loss of energy
> - Feelings of worthlessness or guilt
> - Poor concentration or indecision
> - Recurrent thoughts of death or wanting to be away from it all, with or without suicidality

understand the impact of depression on the individual at the mild to moderate end of the continuum, the reductionism of the diagnostic process is less helpful. Instead, the most helpful way for nurses to conceptualise depression is to think of it as comprising three clusters of interrelated symptoms – **autonomic**, **behavioural** and **cognitive** symptoms – together with an **environmental** component, which further gives a context to the depression. These four aspects are collectively known as the **ABC-E** model of depression.

Conceptualising depression: the ABC-E model of emotion

The ABC-E model of emotion is a biopsychosocial model of mental health care that embeds a person's emotional wellbeing into the general context of their lives. It was adapted from the ABC model of emotion – a model developed at the University of Manchester and underpinned by the cognitive and behavioural models of emotion of Lang (1971) and Beck (1976) – in order to enhance the provision of facilitated self-help for those with common mental health problems (Briddon et al., 2008).

The **autonomic (A)** aspects relate to the **physical effects** of the problem; the **behavioural (B)** aspects are best understood as the **things people do to cope with how they are feeling**; the **cognitive (C)** aspects relate to **thoughts or images** which, more often than not, are negatively 'skewed'. The **environmental** aspects (**E**) refer to those social and environmental

TABLE 4.1   Features of depression mapped according to the ABC-E model

Autonomic (A)	Behavioural (B)	Cognitive (C)	Environment (E)
Disturbed sleep	Withdrawal from activity	Sadness	Positive environmental
Disturbed appetite	Avoidance of people	Hopelessness	factors
Poor memory	Unhelpful coping	Self-criticism	Negative environmental
Poor concentration	strategies	Low self-worth	factors
Lack of energy		Rumination	Socio-political factors
Reduced libido		Poor problem solving	

factors that can have an impact on how someone is feeling. Table 4.1 outlines how depression can be understood within the framework of the ABC–E model.

Figure 4.3 outlines how the various aspects of the model interact to create what is known as the 'vicious cycle of depression'. Without intervention, the various aspects can amplify one another and may result in an increase in the overall severity of the depression, perhaps leading to thoughts of self harm and suicide. For example, disrupted sleep, amplified by noisy neighbours, may lead to the misuse of sleeping tablets; which may, in turn, lead to thoughts of being a 'failure' at not being able to cope without medication. Another practical feature of the model (as you will soon discover) is that it provides a useful intervention framework.

Social factors in depression

In May 2007 the National Director for Mental Health in England, Louis Appleby, declared that social factors, including **employment**, **housing** and **social networks**, were equally as important in the treatment of mental health problems as were the biological and psychological treatments that people had traditionally received (Appleby, 2007).

As a biopsychosocial model, the ABC–E model is one that acknowledges the interrelationships between emotion and the environment, and the role of positive and negative social and socio-political factors in a person's experience of depression. Earlier, in the introduction, we outlined how the demographics of depression are affected by various social factors. The influence of social class, gender and ethnicity, in particular, on mental health is widely understood (Pilgrim & Rogers, 2005; Rogers & Pilgrim, 2003). Indeed, seminal work on depression in women by Brown & Harris (1978) illustrates that we have been aware of the influence of some social factors for decades. In addition, socio-economic deprivation, negative life events,

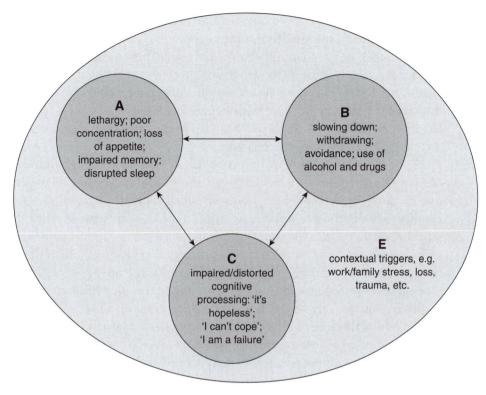

FIGURE 4.3   The maintenance cycle of depression within the ABC-E model

financial problems and not accessing health services are all predictors of depression in the general population (Ostler et al., 2001; Skapinakis et al., 2006; Viinamaki et al., 2006).

It is, as such, difficult to conceive of a model of mental health and ill health that excludes social factors. And the best person to inform us about these social factors is the service user: as Tew (2005) argues, the **lived experience** of the person with mental health problems and their '**situated knowledge**' (the knowledge they have of their own situations) are extremely important in establishing a dialogue for care.

Resilience and social capital

Not all environmental factors are risk factors for depression; some are **protective** and these protective factors can help promote **resilience**. Resilience refers to the 'positive adaptation during or following exposure to adversities that have the potential to harm development' (Masten, 2007, p. 923). This definition contains two key constructs: **adversity**, which relates to negative life circumstances, and **positive adaptation**, which relates to 'social competence' (Luthar & Ciccheti, 2000). We have seen how negative life circumstances are clearly related to depression but by exploring the contextual factors associated with positive adaptation it may be possible to enhance the capacity for resilience in those with depression. Examples of such contextual factors include having supportive friendships or supportive social structures such as faith groups, societies or clubs.

Although most of the work on resilience has focused on individuals, Masten (2007) argues that resilience can also be seen as a systems concept in that it can be applied to the systems in which individuals function, such as families, schools and workplaces. This has some overlap with another theoretical construct – that of **social capital**. Social capital relates to the social and community networks that are bound together by trust and reciprocity (Putnam, 2000). Social capital theory argues that these networks can be assets – or capital – just as money and property can be. People with extensive networks are more likely to be 'housed, healthy, hired and happy' (Woolcock, 2001). Whilst there is more work to be done in understanding how social capital theory may inform mental health practice, it is increasingly being recognised as an important foundation to the development of sustainable, healthy, economically vibrant and cohesive communities (Winter, 2000) and, as such, has significant implications for models of mental health care. Indeed, DeSilva et al. (2005), in a systematic review of the epidemiological literature, found higher levels of individual social capital (which reflects participation in high quality social relationships) to be associated with a lower risk of common mental health problems. Webber and Huxley (2007) similarly report that greater access to social resources within social networks is associated with lower levels of common mental health problems like depression and Wallcraft (2002) reported that mental health service users identified, among other factors, good relationships, enjoyable activities, and satisfying work as crucial to their recovery.

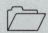 ## Case scenario: Lucy

When Lucy was 17 and studying for her A-levels, she started to experience low mood. At first she didn't recognise it as this; she just noticed that she no longer felt like going out or speaking to her friends. She also found it increasingly difficult to relate to people and hold conversations, and she gradually began to isolate herself from others more and more.

Over the next few months, Lucy sank deeper and deeper into depression and lost the ability to cope. On one particular day, no different from any other, the depression became unbearable. She became extremely distressed and couldn't bear to live like this any longer, so she attempted to overdose. Importantly, Lucy says that this was not a 'cry for help' (as so many professionals would later try to convince her it was).

Lucy also started to experience high levels of anxiety and would often have panic attacks. She couldn't concentrate on anything and would sleep for most of the day, waking up exhausted and restless. She was prescribed an antidepressant by her GP (after being made to promise that she wouldn't try to overdose), but after taking it for two weeks she found that it intensified her suicidal thoughts. The suicidal thoughts she experienced were overwhelming and it was only because of her family that she did not attempt to overdose again (although she did turn to self harming on a number of occasions as a way of coping). She completely lost her appetite and stopped eating and looking after herself. To try to calm herself down, she smoked around 20 cigarettes a day. She had a constant stream of thoughts running through her mind, telling her that she was worthless and a waste of space. At times, she felt very angry and tearful but for no clear reason. Her hands would shake because of the anxiety she was experiencing, so even when she tried to socialise and be 'normal', she was always fearful of being found out.

What A, B, C and E elements can you identify in this scenario?

Assessing Individuals with Depression

The purpose of assessment in common mental health problems is not to diagnose but to elicit an understanding of the person's problem from *their* perspective. The best way of doing this is to use a **structured assessment** that enables collaboration with the person. The ABC-E model is a useful tool, not only for assessment, but also for framing the problem and in subsequent care planning. Thus, as you will discover, the ABC-E model can help: (1) the person **disentangle the problem** and consider how the component parts impact on one another; (2) **map out the problem** in order to bring about joint decision making; and (3) **break the cycle of depression** by drawing on a variety of interventions and resources, including the person's existing resources.

Core values, skills and capabilities

In Chapter 2 we outlined a number of core values, skills and capabilities that underpin all mental health nursing practice. Without these core values, skills and capabilities, you will not be able to engage or help the person with depression. As such, these values, skills and capabilities are worth revisiting briefly.

Firstly, there are the **core values**, perhaps best summed up by the 'three Rs' of the Scottish mental health nursing review: **rights**, **relationships** and **recovery** (Scottish Executive, 2006). Embracing values such as these means that the assumptions you make about people who ask for help will be positive: that they genuinely want help, are telling the truth and trying to cope. Being positive enhances the therapeutic alliance, instils hope and recognises that people with depression have the potential for recovery.

Then there are the **core conditions** of **unconditional positive regard**, **accurate empathy** and **genuineness** (see Rogers, 1980), together with additional facilitators such as **collaboration**, **trust** and **rapport** (Beck et al., 1979). Remember that without the core conditions, rapport is unlikely to occur. On top of this are essential non-verbal skills such as **posture**, **eye contact** and **active listening** and essential verbal skills such as **questioning**, **paraphrasing** and **reflection**.

Finally, there are the essential **capabilities** (NIMHE/SCMH, 2004) – the 'sum of the parts' of all the appropriate values, attitudes and interpersonal and clinical skills you need to be an effective mental health practitioner.

Reflection Point

Values, skills and capabilities in primary care

We all use primary care services. Indeed, many of us may well have sought help for a mental health problem at a primary care level, by seeing a GP or counsellor for example. To enhance the quality and effectiveness of your own practice, it is useful to think about the positive and negative experiences you may have had as a user of primary care services, whether the contact you had related to a physical or mental health issue.

When thinking about these experiences, ask yourself two questions:

- What values, skills and capabilities were demonstrated by the healthcare professionals who provided a positive experience?
- What values, skills and capabilities were lacking in the healthcare professionals who provided a negative experience?

Person-centred interviewing

Person-centred interviewing[2] (Mead & Bower, 2000) or person-centred assessment is integral to the ABC-E model. It is an alternative to the medically based interviewing that has traditionally been the norm in primary care. Person-centred interviewing assumes that interventions are best guided by the overt problem that the person seeks help for and that the person ('patient') and clinician each bring knowledge and expertise to the problem so that recovery can be achieved through **collaboration** and an active **partnership**.

Person-centred interviewing also emphasises the importance of using the language the individual uses to describe their mental health problem, moving away from clinical jargon and terminology that only has meaning within diagnostic frameworks. This is crucial to the development of appropriate goals for recovery and a subsequent intervention strategy. Box 4.2 summarises the process of person-centred interviewing.

Box 4.2   The process of person-centred interviewing

1 Introduction and orientation
   - Confidentiality
2 Gathering information
   - The 4 Ws: what, where, when, with whom
   - ABC aspects
   - E (environmental) aspects
     - Triggers to the problem
     - Impact
   - Any other important information
   - Risk assessment
3 Formulation
   - Verbal problem statement
   - Diagrammatic problem summary

---

[2]While Mead & Bower refer to 'patient-centredness', we prefer the term **person-centred** over patient-centred as it fits better with a recovery-based approach to mental health care. However, don't confuse person-centredness (a philosophy of practice) with 'person-centred counselling' (a particular counselling approach).

Introduction and orientation

The interview begins with an introduction that involves the nurse providing **their name**, together with an explanation as to the **nature of their role** (this is especially helpful since the general public often have stereotypical views of what nurses do). **Checking** that the personal details (date of birth, address, etc.) of the referral match the details of the person sat in front of you is an important guard against potentially embarrassing or damaging errors, and also provides an opportunity to ascertain how the person would like to be **addressed** (first name? abbreviated name? Mr? Mrs?). You should then explain approximately how long the interview and any subsequent assessment will take.

Outlining the parameters of **confidentiality** is particularly important early on in the interview. You need to make sure that you are aware of any organisational or professional guidelines regarding confidentiality (e.g. those in your professional code of conduct), the circumstance in which you can (indeed, should) break confidentiality and any necessary steps you would need to take. Box 4.3 outlines a typical statement that you might use in relation to confidentiality.

Box 4.3   A typical confidentiality statement

'What we will talk about today is confidential but there are limits to confidentiality. For example, if you were to tell me that you were at risk of harm or somebody else was at risk, I would need to do something about that such as speak to your GP, but if that was necessary I would tell you what I was going to do ...'

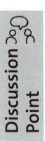

Discussion Point

Confidentiality

In each of the scenarios below think about whether confidentiality would need to be breached. If so, think about the resources available to the practitioner and the skills she or he would need to minimize distress to the service user. All of the scenarios relate to an assessment interview for someone thought to have mild to moderate depression.

- A 38-year-old woman mentions that the trigger to her problems was her uncle (who she sees occasionally at family events) raping her when she was 10 years old.

- An 18-year-old Asian girl tells you that she has been cutting herself secretly because she fears her parents are planning an arranged marriage which she hasn't consented to.
- A father of two young boys, aged 4 and 6, tells you his life has been shattered since his wife divorced him a year ago and moved away (more than 100 miles) with her new partner and the boys. He adds that his life is not worth living if he can't see his boys regularly.

Gathering information

The process for gathering information about the person's problem needs to be systematic and thorough and the model we advocate has a number of elements. We normally begin with a series of broad questions known as 'the 4 Ws'. These broad questions are not necessarily asked literally; instead they act more like a framework for questioning. Table 4.2 illustrates this framework for questioning.

TABLE 4.2 The 4 Ws as a framework for questioning

The 4 Ws	Principal questions	Subsidiary questions
What is the problem?	How would you describe the problem in a nutshell?	*Frequency*: How often is it happening?
		Severity: On a scale of 0–10, if 0 is no problem at all and 10 is very severe, how would you rate the severity of your problem?
		Duration: How long have you experienced this problem? When it is triggered how long does it last for?
Where does the problem occur?	What specific places or situations does the problem occur in?	
When does the problem happen?	What times of the day or year is the problem better or worse?	
With whom is the problem better or worse?	What people make it better or worse? (e.g. family; friends; work colleagues)	*Modifying factors:* Are there any other factors (such as alcohol or drugs) that make it better or worse?

After the 4 Ws, we follow on by asking about the ABC and E aspects of the model. The **autonomic (A)** aspects relate to the **physical effects** of the problem, e.g. headaches, dry mouth, tiredness etc. This area is especially important since a large number of people with depression present initially with somatic symptoms such as general aches and pains (Tyree & Gandhi, 2005). The **behavioural (B)** aspects are best understood as the **things people do to cope with how they are feeling**, e.g. avoiding opening the post, staying in bed, drinking more alcohol and so on. The **cognitive (C)** aspects relate to **negative automatic thoughts**, e.g. 'I'm useless', 'I'm bad', 'I can't cope'. What distinguishes these thoughts from other thoughts is that they are unsolicited; they don't have to be deliberately thought about for them to be brought to mind, they simply 'pop up' in a person's mind. Some people may describe negative automatic **images** as well as, or rather than, automatic thoughts.

There are two important dimensions to the **environmental (E)** aspects of the model: **triggers** and **impact**. Asking what trigger(s) may have initially activated the depression is helpful in understanding the context of the person's difficulties. In many cases, dealing with the triggers may be the focus of any interventions that are subsequently agreed. Often, a one-off life event is the trigger. It is important to bear in mind, however, these life events are not always negative (such as a relationship ending or a job loss); they can sometimes include events such as having a baby or moving in with a partner. Sometimes there might be no readily identifiable triggers or a trigger may seem quite innocuous on first hearing. Further questioning, however, might reveal that there are, indeed, triggers but the person hadn't connected them to the problem or that the somewhat innocuous trigger was the one that turned out to be 'the straw that broke the camel's back'. Developing an understanding of the more repetitive, day-to-day triggers that serve to maintain the problem rather than 'cause' it also helps build a picture of the problem. These may include ongoing life issues such as debt or money worries, illness of a relative or friend, or 'arguments in the home'.

Asking the person how the problem **impacts** on key areas of their life provides another layer of contextual (E) information. Investigating specific domains such as the person's **work/employment**, their **home life**, **social life** and **leisure pursuits**, their **private life** including (where relevant) **faith-based activities** and their **relationships** with others will add depth to a shared understanding of the problem's impact.

A summary of the sorts of questions that can be asked for each of the aspects of the ABC–E model are contained in Table 4.3.

Once the individual elements of the ABC–E model have been explored, there needs to be an opportunity to check that you have not missed any other important information. Ascertaining the person's **expectations** of the assessment and what they hope might be the outcome can help with shared decision making later on. You might ask for example: 'Did you come here with

TABLE 4.3 Typical questions for each aspect of the ABC-E model.

Aspect	Typical questions
A (autonomic)	It's not unusual to experience a physical change when you are feeling depressed … have you noticed any physical symptoms/ sensations?
B (behavioural)	Are there things you have stopped doing since you've been feeling depressed? Or are there things you are doing more of since feeling this way, for example drinking or using drugs?
C (cognitive)	What particular thoughts or images run through your mind when you're feeling low? Do you have images or mental pictures that come into your mind at those times?
E (environmental)	
Triggers	What do you think might have triggered this problem?
Impact	What aspects of your life have changed as a result of this problem?

any thoughts on what the outcome might be from our meeting today?' or 'Do you have any thoughts on what might help with this problem?' There is also an opportunity to ask if there any other 'symptoms' (ABC) linked to the problem that haven't been elicited or any other environmental (E) factors that are impacting on the person that haven't been captured in the assessment so far. For example, you could ask: 'Is there anything we haven't discussed, such as other physical symptoms or additional problems that you think would be helpful for me to know about?' Questions about **resilience** can also be raised here, especially within the context of past and present **coping** strategies. You might ask about coping strategies that were helpful previously but are no longer as effective, or strategies that prevent the problem getting worse but do not actually resolve it. A good question to ask here is: 'What are you doing now to cope with the problem and what have you tried in the past?' When planning and agreeing on interventions to help the person (we will look at interventions later in the chapter), it may be appropriate to try to integrate any current coping strategies into any interventions that you and the person agree upon. Even if past and present strategies didn't seem to help, the skills that the person has deployed in their attempts at coping should be acknowledged and utilised where appropriate. This approach not only recognises the expertise and skills of the person, it also emphasises the importance of working collaboratively in order to achieve recovery.

Risk assessment

The principal risks in depression are those of **self-harm** and **suicide**. Note that self-harm and suicide are not necessarily connected: while an individual episode of self-harm *might* be an attempt to end life, it might also be an attempt to communicate with others, to influence or to secure help or care from others, or a way of obtaining relief from a difficult and otherwise over-whelming situation or emotional state (Hjelmeland et al., 2002).

A number of factors increase the risk of self-harm. As with depression, many of these are social factors; people who are **single** or **divorced**, **live alone**, are **single parents** or who **lack social support** are particularly vul-nerable (Meltzer et al., 2002). Other life experiences that can trigger or increase the risk of self-harm include substance misuse, physical health prob-lems, additional mental health problems (especially phobia and psychosis), victimisation, sexual abuse, and relationship problems (NCCMH, 2004).

Risk assessment is as important in primary care as it is in an acute care setting. It is important to bear in mind that, regardless of the severity of the problem, asking people about self-harm *does not* increase the risk by 'putting ideas into their head'. Indeed, many people receiving support report the opposite to be true, describing feelings of relief that they are at last able to talk about their thoughts.

Most services offering support to people with depression will have a struc-tured risk protocol and you should incorporate this into your assessment. If not, you may find the simple protocol illustrated in Figure 4.4 useful.

Self-harm protocols often include questions about **protective** factors – those that help prevent someone self-harming. A simple question such as 'Is there anything or anyone that would prevent you from doing it?' may help the person access a seam of resilience which they may have struggled to locate had the question not been asked. Similar simple protocols can be designed to assess risk to, or risk from, other people, which may have relevance for people living in adverse circumstances such as the threat of domestic violence.

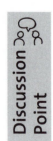

Risk assessment

Remember the scenarios from the earlier confidentiality discussion point? Have a look at them again and try to come up with a series of questions that you might ask (a simple protocol) in order to assess risk (to self or others) in each scenario.

- A 38-year-old woman mentions that the trigger to her problems was her uncle (who she sees occasionally at family events) raping her when she was 10 years old.

- An 18-year-old Asian girl tells you that she has been cutting herself secretly because she fears her parents are planning an arranged marriage which she hasn't consented to.
- A father of two young boys, aged 4 and 6, tells you his life has been shattered since his wife divorced him a year ago and moved away (more than 100 miles) with her new partner and the boys. He adds that his life is not worth living if he can't see his boys regularly.

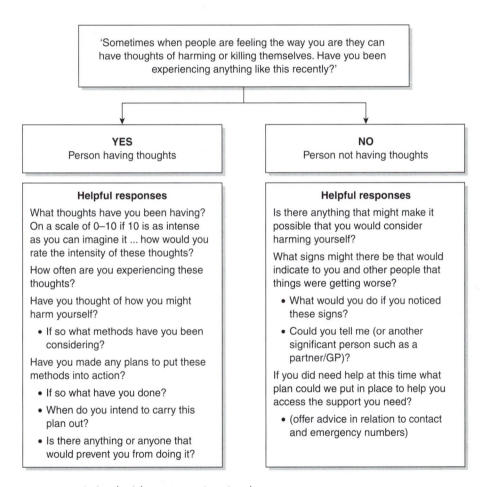

FIGURE 4.4 A simple risk assessment protocol

If a risk assessment indicates an **immediate risk** it is crucial that you are familiar with the team protocol for reporting this risk to the appropriate

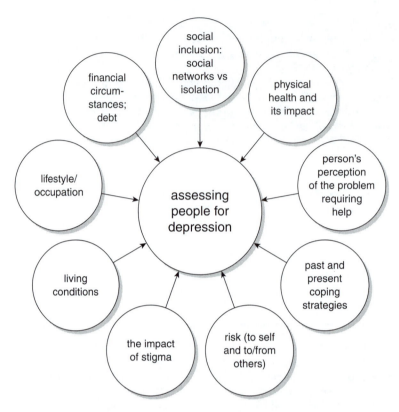

FIGURE 4.5   Things to consider when assessing people for depression

clinician (to a team manager or GP, for example). Having a list of emergency telephone numbers and contacts for out of hours services is vital in good risk management. Where there is no immediate risk but where risk is evident, it is important to respond to this within a reasonable time scale. Similarly where risk has not been identified it is useful to agree how you will monitor risk in the future. Keeping relevant practitioners (such as the person's GP) informed of the risk assessment outcome, whether there is risk present or not, is vital to good practice.

Figure 4.5 is a summary diagram of some of the things you need to think about when assessing people for depression. It's important to note that the elements listed in the diagram are not exhaustive and that – unlike the ABC-E model – the diagram is not in itself a formal model for assessment. Instead, it is merely an *aide memoire* to learning and similar diagrams are included in all of the chapters in Part II of this book. Consider also the reflection point below.

Mapping onto the ABC-E model

How might you map the elements of the diagram in Figure 4.5 onto the elements of the ABC-E model?

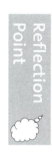

Reflection Point

Funnelling

The product of the structured assessment is a **formulation** (see the next section). To drill down to the formulation, a questioning style known as **funnelling** is useful. As the name suggests, funnelling starts with a general open question, following which, in order to clinch detail, the questions become more focused.

Figure 4.6 outlines the funnelling process, providing an example relating to physical symptoms. Funnelling isn't a single specific process. It can be (should be) applied throughout the assessment – when asking about the 4Ws, ABC elements, triggers, impact and risk. Likewise, the skills of summarising and paraphrasing should also be applied throughout the assessment to ensure that the information obtained is accurate and that it reflects the person's perspective.

Formulation

Formulation is a summary of a service user's problems that provides a framework for understanding the problem and taking action. It is an important step between assessment and taking shared action to tackle the problem(s) identified.[3] Our conceptualisation of formulation has two elements: (1) a **problem statement** (which can be verbal or, preferably, written); and (2) a **diagrammatic problem summary**. The problem statement is a synopsis of the assessment, containing brief summaries of each of the 4Ws, the ABC elements, trigger(s), impact and risk. An example of a problem statement is contained in Box 4.4.

---

[3] As you may recall when we discussed the nursing process in Chapter 1, formulation (specific problem identification) is the step between assessment and planning.

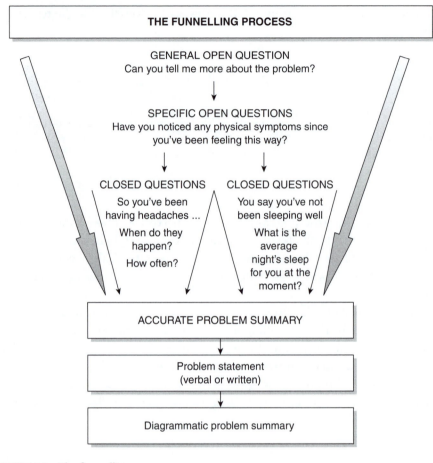

FIGURE 4.6 The funnelling process

Box 4.4   An example of a problem statement

Michael has been feeling 'low' for 6 months (*what*) since he was made redundant from a firm he had worked for since leaving school 10 years ago (*trigger*). He feels low all of the time (*when*), but it seems worse when he lies in bed first thing in the morning (*where*).

After feeding and walking his dog in the morning, he is returning to bed and stays there until late afternoon (*B*); he struggles to get off to sleep most nights, and feels tired much of the time; he suffers with tension headaches and has at least one a week

(*A*); he also has thoughts running through his head that his 'life is going nowhere' and he is a 'failure' (*C*). He is avoiding answering the phone (*B*) because friends are always ringing asking him to go out socialising. Michael is drinking three cans of strong lager each evening in order to relax (*B*; *coping mechanism*).

   The only person that makes him feel better is his sister, whom he feels he can trust and confide in; he also feels better when he walks his dog (*with whom do you feel better*). He has debt problems (*impact*) which are worse now he is out of work (*impact*). Michael doesn't experience suicidal thoughts but occasionally wishes he didn't wake up in the morning. He cannot imagine a situation that would make it more likely he would kill himself as he knows it would devastate his sister (*risk*).

The problem statement allows the person to correct any misunderstanding or misrepresentation of their problem before moving to map the problem visually onto the ABC-E model. The benefit of the ABC-E map is that it can help disentangle a problem by providing a very simple format that encapsulates the information the person seeking help has shared with you. It also helps demonstrate the vicious cycle of depression we talked about earlier and the impact that each component of the model might have on the others. It also helps the person understand how the problem developed and how it is maintained, and in so doing can help 'normalise' the problem, instilling hope and the potential for change. As you will discover when we come to discuss interventions, the ABC-E map can also help in the selection of appropriate interventions. Figure 4.7 provides an example of an ABC-E map based on the problem statement in Box 4.4.

Goal setting

Having mapped the problem onto the ABC-E model, perhaps at the same time considering interventions that may be effective in breaking the cycle of depression, you should collaboratively agree **goals** with the person you are helping. Goals are statements about changes that the person wants to achieve and, as such, they should be **person-centred** and linked to the information contained in the ABC-E map. Goals can be a way of measuring progress and checking on the appropriateness of the interventions chosen (if progress is stilted, is it time to look at different interventions?), and they are an intrinsic part of discharge planning.

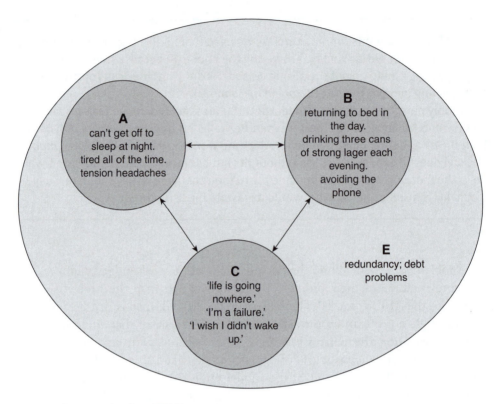

FIGURE 4.7 An example of an ABC-E map

Goal setting isn't necessarily easy. Rather than setting goals collaboratively, novice nurses often set goals according to their level of expertise (forgetting that the service user has expertise through experience!); consequently, goals are often practitioner-led, unwieldy, unrealistic and unclear. Strategies to enhance goal setting include 'turning the problem round' in order to identify goals, e.g. asking questions such as 'if you could change things, how would you like them to be?', 'what would you like back in your life?' and 'what would you be doing differently?' If there is more than one goal, the list should be prioritised by asking which is the most important, has the most benefits or is easiest to achieve, or by categorising them according to whether they are short-, medium- or long-term goals. Using the acronym 'SMART' can help you and the person seeking help build robust goals. *SMART goals* are those that are **Specific**, **Measurable**, **Achievable**, **Realistic** and **Timely** (Fennell, 1999). Box 4.5. sets out some examples of SMART goals for Michael, for whom a simple *broad goal* would be 'I just want to feel better'.

Box 4.5 SMART goals (after Fennell, 1999)

SMART goals are:

- **S**pecific: Can you explain what you want to achieve with this goal in words of one syllable?
- **M**easurable: Can you 'measure' progress with this goal? How will you know you've achieved it?
- **A**chievable: All things considered, is this goal within your reach?
- **R**ealistic: Bearing in mind factors such as resources and support, is the goal reasonable?
- **T**imely: What timescale are you working too? Can the goal be achieved within this time?

Examples of SMART goals

- To have more structure to my day by going to bed no later than 11.00pm and getting up at 9.00am each week day.
- To get back in touch with friends and in particular telephoning a close friend one evening after I've walked the dog.
- To improve my 'get up and go' by returning to the kick boxing class once a week with my friend Tom.
- To cut down my drinking by half over the next two weeks.

Shared decision making

To achieve the SMART goals, decisions will need to be made about appropriate interventions. As you will see in the next section, there are a variety of interventions available to help people with depression. The decision on which interventions to use should be a **shared** decision between the practitioner and the person seeking help, one that is person-centred and draws upon the collaborative expertise of both.

Decisions should be made on the basis of: (1) the **expressed need and goals** of the person seeking help; (2) the **formulation**; (3) an assessment of **risk**; (4) the **availability** of services and resources; (5) the **likelihood of advice being followed**; and, last but not least, (6) the **evidence base**.

Evidence-Based Interventions for Depression

In England and Wales, the NICE guidance on depression (NICE, 2009) forms the basis of best practice in the evidence-based care of people with depression. Northern Ireland endorsed the previous NICE guidance on depression (NICE,

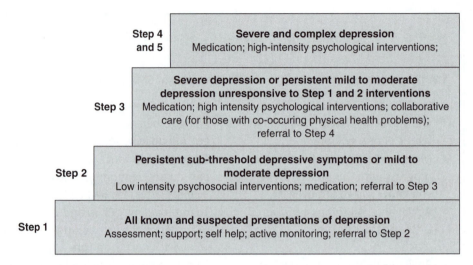

FIGURE 4.8   Evidence-based interventions within the stepped care model (adapted from NICE, 2009)

2007) but has yet to do so with the 2009 guidance.[4] Scotland has its own national guidance (SIGN, 2010). While there are substantial overlaps regarding the interventions recommended by both NICE and SIGN, the biggest difference between the two sets of guidance is that the NICE guidance embeds its recommended interventions within a framework of stepped care whereas the SIGN guidance does not. Nevertheless, we will use the stepped model of care to organise our discussion of the interventions for people with depression (see Figure 4.8).

Earlier we mentioned that one particularly useful feature of the ABC-E model was that it could also act as an intervention framework. As we discuss the various interventions for depression, we will also explain how each might map on to the four elements of the model.

Low- vs. High-intensity interventions

Figure 4.8 distinguishes between low- and high-intensity interventions. More often than not, this distinction refers to the duration and depth of the intervention rather than the specific kind of intervention used. Both low- and high-intensity interventions encompass a range of psychological

---

[4]Not because Northern Ireland necessarily disagrees with the guidance but because there will be an inevitable delay between the guidance being published (in late 2009 as it happens) and the powers that be in Northern Ireland getting round to reviewing it.

and social interventions that may be used individually or in combination with one another.

High-intensity interventions are those interventions where the involvement of the mental health practitioner is more extensive. To some extent, high-intensity interventions are akin to **psychotherapy**, though both NICE and SIGN recommend only psychotherapy founded on **cognitive behavioural principles** or on the principles of **interpersonal therapy** (NICE, 2009; SIGN, 2010).

Low-intensity interventions, on the other hand, are designed for **high volume delivery** – mainly in response to the epidemiological profile of common mental health problems (the large numbers of people in the community with depression and anxiety who do not require secondary care services). **Flexibility** and **choice** are key features of low-intensity interventions: they are less complex to deliver than formal psychotherapy, contact with service users is generally brief, and they can be delivered through a range of media (including printed materials, the telephone, computers and the Internet) and by a variety of practitioners as long as they have sufficient additional training. It is largely the new generation of workers – GPCMHWs and psychological wellbeing practitioners – who are delivering low-intensity interventions in primary care.

Since 'low-intensity psychological interventions are delivered on the explicit premise that people are the best managers of their own mental health' (IAPT, 2010, p. 6), they are intrinsically linked to the notion of **self-help**.

Self-help

Self-help can be used on its own or as a useful adjunct to interventions delivered at higher levels of care. It may provide a solution in itself or be part of a wider solution, for example while 'holding' for high-intensity work. Self-help materials are available in a variety of media: as computerised packages (either online or in CD/DVD-ROM format), as video or audio recordings, or in written form such as leaflets, manuals and books (collectively, 'bibliotherapy'). By definition, self-help means that people may well take the initiative and seek out these materials without professional help; Gellatly et al. (2007), however, have shown that supported (guided) interventions are more effective than unsupported interventions. This implies that there is a skill to facilitating self-help and that those facilitating it need to be appropriately trained.

Most guided self-help is underpinned by cognitive, behavioural or problem solving principles. Indeed, both the NICE (2009) and SIGN (2010) depression guidance recommend only guided self-help based on such principles. One specific form of guided self-help, singled out for recommendation by both the NICE and SIGN guidance, is computerised CBT (cCBT), although only *Beating the Blues* (one of many cCBT packages) has robust evidence of effectiveness in mild-to-moderate depression (NICE, 2006; NCCMH, 2009).

Since there are endless self-help resources available, it is important that any materials recommended or made available are of an acceptable quality. Signs of good-quality materials are summarised in Table 4.4.

TABLE 4.4 Quality in self-help materials

Quality dimension	Details
Evidence-based	The materials are underpinned by an appropriate model Reference is made to reputable sources Claims regarding effectiveness are realistic or reinforced by formal evaluation
Feasible	The content encourages users to reflect on their experiences The content helps users formulate their difficulties The content gives realistic and safe suggestions about self-management
Acceptable	The materials are tailored to the needs of specific audiences (children, older people, BME communities, etc.) The materials draw on the experiences of other people Service users have been consulted in the construction of materials
Accessible	The mode of delivery means it is accessible to a significant proportion of the target population The materials are communicated clearly (e.g. using diagrams to explain complicated ideas and providing summaries at regular intervals to help understanding) The materials are available in a range of languages and can be delivered in a range of settings
Cost effective	The materials are reasonably priced and affordable

Problem solving

Problem solving is a brief, structured psychological intervention that helps individuals actively find realistic solutions to key problems. A number of problem solving models exist[5] but a commonly used one is the **seven-step model** involving: (1) **identification** of the problem; (2) **exploration** of the problem; (3) the setting of **goals**; (4) identification of **possible courses of action**; (5) **selecting a course of action**; (6) **taking action**; (7) **evaluation** of the

---

[5]You may recall from Chapter 1 that the nursing process is also based on problem solving principles.

action. Problem solving can be delivered as a standalone intervention or as an adjunct to other interventions. A number of randomised controlled trials indicate that problem solving is as effective as antidepressants in reducing symptoms of depression (Dowrick et al., 2000; Mynors-Wallis et al., 2000; Kendrick et al., 2005) and it is recommended in the SIGN guidance (2010). Problem solving is a useful intervention for the E elements of the ABC-E model.

Physical exercise and interventions targeted at physical symptoms

A number of low intensity interventions attempt to break the cycle of depression by working on the physical aspects of depression, or the A of the ABC-E model. These interventions work well when built into a 'behavioural activation' schedule (see later). They include: **sleep hygiene** (techniques designed to help improve sleep); **dietary advice**, which considers the impact that a poor or limited diet might have on mood, energy levels and overall physical health; **relaxation techniques**, designed to reduce stress; and **physical exercise**, on the principle that exercise appears to improve energy levels and mood (MHF, 2007). Of these interventions, physical exercise has the best evidence being recommended – in the format of a structured programme – in both the NICE (2009) and SIGN (2010) guidance.

Social interventions

While negative thinking is associated with depression, it is important to bear in mind that, sometimes, a person's negative thoughts may be an accurate reflection of their circumstances (they may, for example, be in a violent relationship, in poor housing, have little hope of employment, little money or face harassment from 'problem' neighbours). Using 'social' problem solving (and obviously targeting the E of the ABC-E model), social interventions can be a pragmatic and effective way of breaking the cycle of depression. Social interventions include: **signposting** to supportive groups and organisations such as Welfare Rights, Citizens' Advice or SureStart; **networking** to help develop the person's activities, circle of friends and social contacts; and **bridge building**, whereby local facilities and organisations (sports, educational, arts, etc.) are explored in order to tap into new opportunities for social contact. Note that you will not be able to deliver social interventions without drawing on services provided by community groups and third sector organisations – services that may actually be more acceptable to, and more accessible for, service users than services from statutory providers like health and social care.

Interestingly, social interventions are implicit in the government's strategy for mental health, *New Horizons*, which expects all government departments – housing, environment, education, employment, etc. – to play a role in supporting mental health and wellbeing.

Medication

For many people with depression, medication is an important part of their recovery. However, the 2009 NICE guidance recommends antidepressant medication be used in conjunction with psychological interventions and it does not recommend medication as a first line treatment in mild to moderate depression. The Scottish guidance (SIGN, 2010) is notable in that its specific focus is on *alternatives* to medication.

Medication is discussed in more detail in Chapter 7, but it is worth mentioning at this point that, on average, 40% of people diagnosed with mood disorders do not take the medication prescribed (Lingam & Scott, 2002). There are a variety of reasons why people do not take antidepressant medication in primary care, including: **fears that the medications are harmful**, addictive or will not help with the depression; **dissatisfaction with the prescriber**; the **stigma** associated with mental illness; and **lack of sufficient information** (Tamburrino et al., 2009). Understanding these reasons can help the practitioner explore the issue of medication in a person-centred way, and help the individual make informed choices. To do this, the practitioner must be able to give accurate information and advice about prescribed medications and their alternatives.

Discussion Point

St John's wort

A person seeking help for mild depression asks you about St John's wort (*Hypericum*). They have been reading a lot of positive things about it on the Internet and want some advice. The current NICE and SIGN guidance on depression states that practitioners should not advise its use because of uncertainty about appropriate doses, persistence of effect, variation in the nature of preparations and potentially serious interactions with other drugs, especially the contraceptive pill.

What would you advise? What are your reasons for the advice you would give?

Medication is predominantly a **physical** intervention. As such, it falls within the remit of the A element of the model, and whether or not there is a need for further intervention (such as medication management) can be established by asking appropriate questions such as 'How does the person feel about taking the medication?', 'Are they taking it as prescribed?', 'Are they experiencing any side-effects?' Where there is a lack of knowledge, an appropriate additional intervention may be the supply of accurate information and advice (through **psychoeducation**; see Chapter 6) or, alternatively, the practitioner may want to relate concerns regarding medication management to the prescribing GP.

Cognitive behavioural interventions

Some of the cognitive behavioural techniques that are particularly useful in depression, whether used alone or in combination and which are recommended by both the NICE (2009) and SIGN (2010) guidelines, are discussed next. As we mentioned earlier, cognitive behavioural approaches are designed to break the B and C elements of the depression cycle.

Cognitive interventions

The principal cognitive interventions are those derived from Beck's cognitive therapy (which we explored in Chapter 1), in particular **cognitive themes** and **cognitive restructuring**.

In depression, the cognitive theme is one of **loss and rejection** (in anxiety, it is a perception of fear or danger) and drawing the person's attention to this can help them identify 'depressive' thoughts and so think about any subsequent interventions.

Cognitive restructuring gives the individual the opportunity to challenge the negative cycle of thoughts inherent in depression by rigorously considering the evidence that both supports and disputes it. In evaluating the evidence they can then make the decision as to whether the original thoughts reflect an accurate or a 'skewed' perspective. This process is not the same as 'positive thinking'; it asks the person to weigh up the facts and adjust their thinking to represent the fuller picture. **Thought diaries** are the tool for capturing thoughts and subsequently challenging them (there is more on thought diaries in the next chapter). **Behavioural experiments** (see below) can be used to test out 'predictions' and potentially add more weight to a new, more balanced thought. **Self-challenge** is what people may go on to do when they recognise 'patterns' to their thinking and, through cognitive restructuring, have developed the skills to challenge thoughts without necessarily having to use a thought diary.

Behavioural interventions

The principal **behavioural** therapies useful in depression are **behavioural activation** and **behavioural experiments**.

Behavioural activation (BA) is a technique designed to counter the tendency to do little or ruminate when low in mood. It initially involves the completion of a 'baseline' timetable of an individual's day-to-day activity in which each activity is rated on a scale of 0–10 for pleasure and achievement. Once this baseline is captured and reviewed, a planned schedule of activity is written into a blank timetable. This schedule includes a balance of routine tasks as well as those activities previously rated highly for pleasure and achievement. BA is often the most useful place to start when working with depression as significant gains can be made without needing to focus directly on the person's cognition (Jacobson et al., 1996). It is an effective strategy for mild to moderate depression, being recommended in both the NICE (2009) and SIGN (2010) guidelines. (Behavioural activation is also discussed in Chapter 6 in the context of helping people recover from psychosis.)

Behavioural experiments are a helpful strategy for strengthening or challenging new perspectives. They are called 'experiments' because any new or modified ways of thinking that might emerge from techniques such as cognitive restructuring are tested out in real situations. For example, if a person believes that they will fail at some particular task, the experiment will be to undertake that task and check the outcome against their preconceived belief. Behavioural experiments are discussed in more detail in the next chapter.

Discharge planning and relapse prevention

On first beginning to work therapeutically with the person seeking help, it is important that you discuss the **boundaries** of the relationship, which includes preparation for future discharge. Within a biopsychosocial approach, the therapeutic relationship is not seen as a 'cure' but as a stepping stone towards a fuller recovery. Once the therapeutic relationship ends, the person should be able to apply what they have learnt to their day-to-day lives by drawing on the support of broader networks and resources. In order to help people achieve this, it is useful to agree post-discharge goals and to develop a relapse prevention or 'staying well' plan. Agreeing goals will help the person build on any gains made while the relapse prevention plan can be used to identify signs of potential relapse and so help prevent a return of the downward spiral of depression. **Emergency plans** – formal written plans outlining what the individual should do if things take a real turn for the worse – also form an integral part of any comprehensive relapse prevention plan since a significant number of people with depression will have a recurrence in the future (Kennedy et al., 2003).

The questions listed in Box 4.6 are useful in building a relapse prevention plan; standardised relapse prevention plans also exist (see, for example, Williams, 2008).

Box 4.6   Questions that help with the construction of relapse prevention plans

- What have you learnt from our working together? What has been useful? (ideas, techniques, etc.).
- How can you build on what you have learnt? (Is there an action plan? Will you practise what you've learnt? Will you apply it to other settings such as work or college?)
- What might make it difficult to do this?
- How will you overcome these difficulties?
- What might lead to a recurrence of the problem (future stresses, personal vulnerabilities, etc.)?
- What would be the warning signs that a setback is occurring?
- If you have a setback what would you do (plan A; plan B)?

Conclusion

In this chapter we have explored ways of helping the significant number of people in primary care who experience depression. In particular, we have looked at how a specific conceptual model – the ABC-E model – might be of use throughout the therapeutic process, from assessment through to the planning of interventions. We have also considered the range of evidence-based interventions that are available for helping people with depression, including those self-help interventions where the nurse or other mental health practitioner will act as a guide, coach or facilitator.

Above all, we have emphasised the person-centredness of the whole help-ing process and the necessary values, skills and capabilities that a mental health nurse needs in order to engender a collaborative therapeutic alliance. We end with this quote from a service user with experience of depression:

I think that something as simple as listening to the person can make a world of difference. I think that giving people a choice about treatment helps to make them feel empowered and in control of their own wellness, rather than just offering medication. From my own personal experience and from meeting a wide range of service users, just giving someone the space and time to be real and open can help them to feel much less isolated. We should be empowering those with the lived experience of depression to help others, because after all, they are the experts.

Further Reading and Resources

Key texts

Bennet-Levy J, et al. (eds) (2010). *Oxford Guide to Low Intensity CBT Interventions*. Oxford: Oxford University Press.
The first comprehensive textbook outlining the low-intensity CBT method. Written by leading experts in the field, this is an essential text for those working with common mental disorders.

Beck AT (1979). *Cognitive Therapy and the Emotional Disorders*. New York: International Universities Press.
The founder of cognitive therapy provides an introduction to cognitive therapy and the emotional disorders.

Gilbert P (1997). *Overcoming Depression: A Self-Help Guide Using Cognitive Behavioural Techniques*. London: Robinson.
A self-help text which is thorough in its description of depression while also providing a guide to useful cognitive behavioural interventions. Helpful not only to service users but practitioners who wish to develop their knowledge further.

Greenberger D & Padesky CA (1995). *Mind Over Mood*. New York: Guilford Press.
More than 15 years old but still one of the most well-known self-help books around. Clearly written and includes useful worksheets that can help service users develop practical skills to overcome mental health problems.

Lovell K & Richards DA (2008). *A Recovery Programme for Depression*. London: Rethink. Available from: www.mentalhealthshop.org.
A booklet to accompanying Rethink's recovery programme for depression containing worksheets, exercises and CBT techniques to help people manage their own recovery.

Williams C (2009). *Overcoming Depression and Low Mood: A Five Areas Approach*, 3rd edition. London: Arnold.

A self-help manual, which introduces the 'five areas approach', an approach based on cognitive behavioural principles. Clearly written and includes useful worksheets (see also web resources below).

Key policy documents

Centre for Economic Performance's Mental Health Policy Group (2006). *The Depression Report: A New Deal for Depression and Anxiety Disorders [The Layard Report].* London: London School of Economics.

National Institute for Clinical Excellence (2009). *Depression: The Treatment and Management of Depression in Adults (partial update of NICE Clinical Guideline 23).* London: NICE. Available from www.nice.org.uk/CG90

Social Exclusion Unit (2004). *Mental Health and Social Exclusion: Social Exclusion Unit Report.* London: Office of the Deputy Prime Minister.

Scottish Intercollegiate Guidelines Network (2010). *Non-pharmaceutical Management of Depression in Adults: A National Guideline.* Edinburgh: SIGN.

Web resources

Depression Alliance: www.depressionalliance.org
Website of a national charity providing information and support to help those with depression.

The Improving Access to Psychological Therapies (IAPT) initiative: www.iapt.nhs.uk
Gateway website to the NHS England IAPT programme.

Beating the Blues: www.beatingtheblues.co.uk
Website of 'the only computerised CBT treatment for depression recommended for use in the NHS'.

The 'Five Areas Approach': www.livinglifetothefull.com and www.fiveareas.com/resourcearea
Two sites supporting users of Williams' 'Overcoming Depression' self-help manual. Both sites provide downloadable resources that are accessible and practical.

References

APA (American Psychiatric Association) (2000). *Diagnostic and Statistical Manual of Mental Disorders, 4th Edition* (Text Revised) (DSM–IVR). Washington: APA.

Appleby L (2007). *Breaking Down Barriers. Clinical Case for Change: Report by Louis Appleby, National Director for Mental Health.* London: DH.

Beck AT (1976). *Cognitive Therapy and the Emotional Disorders.* New York: International Universities Press.

Beck AT, Rush AJ, Shaw BF & Emery G (1979). *Cognitive Therapy of Depression.* New York: The Guilford Press.

Bhui K & McKenzie K (2006). *Suicide Prevention for BME Groups in England: Report from the BME Suicide Prevention Project*. London: Centre for Health Improvement and Minority Ethnic Services.

Bower P & Gilbody SM (2005a). Managing common mental health disorders in primary care: conceptual models and evidence base. *British Medical Journal*, **330**, 839–842.

Bower P & Gilbody SM (2005b). Stepped care in psychological therapies: access, effectiveness and efficiency. *British Journal of Psychiatry*, **186**, 11–17.

Briddon JE, Baguley C & Webber M (2008). The ABC-E model of emotion: a bio-psychosocial model for primary mental health care. *Journal of Mental Health Training, Education and Practice*, **3**(1), 12–21.

Brown G & Harris T (1978). *The Social Origins of Depression: A Study of Psychiatric Disorder in Women*. London: Tavistock Publications.

Burnham A (2009). Speech by the Rt Hon Andy Burnham, Secretary of State for Health, 26 November 2009, New Savoy Partnership Conference: Psychological Therapies in the NHS. Available from: www.dh.gov.uk [accessed 12 February 2010].

Cahill J, Potter S & Mullin T (2006). First contact session outcomes in primary care psychological therapy and counselling services. *Counselling and Psychotherapy Research*, **6**(1), 41–49.

CEPMHPG (Centre for Economic Performance's Mental Health Policy Group) (2006). *The Depression Report: A New Deal for Depression and Anxiety Disorders [The Layard Report]*. London: London School of Economics. Available from: cep.lse.ac.uk [accessed 12 January 2010].

Clark DM, Layard R, Smithies R, Richards DA, Suckling R & Wright B (2009). Improving Access to Psychological Therapy: initial evaluation of two UK demonstration sites. *Behaviour, Research and Therapy*, **47**(11), 910–920.

Commander MJ, Sashidharan SP, Odell SM & Surtees PG (1997). Access to mental health care in an inner-city health district. I: Pathways into and within specialist psychiatric services. *British Journal of Psychiatry*, **176**, 407–411.

De Silva MJ, McKenzie K, Harpham T & Huttly, SR (2005). Social capital and mental illness: a systematic review. *Journal of Epidemiology and Community Health*, **59**, 619–627.

DH (Department of Health) (1999). *National Service Framework for Mental Health: Modern Standards and Service Models*. London: DH.

DH (Department of Health) (2000). *The NHS Plan: A Plan for Investment; A Plan for Reform*. London: DH.

DH (Department of Health) (2004). *Organising and Delivering Psychological Therapies*. London: DH.

DH (Department of Health) (2005). *Delivering Race Equality in Mental Health Care: An Action Plan for Reform Inside and Outside Services and the Government's Response to the Independent Inquiry into the Death of David Bennett*. London: DH.

DHSSPS (Department of Health, Social Security and Public Safety) (2009). *Delivering the Bamford Vision: The Response of the Northern Ireland Executive to the Bamford Review of Mental Health and Learning Disability. Action Plan 2009–2011*. Belfast: DHSSPS. Available from: www.dhsspsni.gov.uk [accessed 2 November 2009].

Dowrick C, Dunn G, Ayuso-Mateos JL, Dalgard OS, Page H, Lehtinen V, Casey P, Wilkinson C, Vazquez-Barquero JL & Wilkinson G (2000). Problem solving treatment and group psychoeducation for depression: multicentre randomised controlled trial. *British Medical Journal*, **321**, 1450.

Fennell M (1999). *Overcoming Low Self Esteem*. London: Robinson.

Fryers T, Melzer D, Jenkins R (2003). Social inequalities and the common mental disorders. *Social Psychiatry and Psychiatric Epidemiology*, **38**, 229–237.

Fryers T, Melzer D, Jenkins R & Brugha T (2005). The distribution of the common mental disorders: social inequalities in Europe. *Clinical Practice and Epidemiology in Mental Health*, **1**(14). Available from www.cpmentalhealth.com [accessed 12 February 2010].

Gellatly J, Bower P, Hennessy S, Richards D, Gilbody S & Lovell K (2007). What makes self-help interventions effective in the management of depressive symptoms? Meta-analysis and meta-regression. *Psychological Medicine*, **37**(9), 1217–1228.

Goldberg D & Huxley P (1992). *Common Mental Disorders: A Bio-Social Model*. London: Routledge.

Gorst-Unsworth C & Goldenberg E (1998). Psychological sequelae of torture and organised violence suffered by refugees from Iraq: trauma-related factors compared with social factors in exile. *British Journal of Psychiatry*, **172**, 90–94.

Hjelmeland H, Hawton K, Nordvik H, Bille-Brahe U, De Leo D, Fekete S, Grad O, Haring C, Kerkhof JF, Lönnqvist J, Michel K, Renberg ES, Schmidtke A, Van Heeringen K & Wasserman D (2002). Why people engage in parasuicide: a cross-cultural study of intentions. *Suicide and Life-Threatening Behavior*, **32**(4), 380–393.

HM Government (2009). *New Horizons: A Shared Vision for Mental Health*. London: Department of Health. Available from: www.newhorizons.dh.gov.uk [accessed 14 February 2010].

IAPT (Improving Access to Psychological Therapies) (2010). *Good Practice Guidance on the Use of Self-Help Materials within IAPT Services*. Available from www.iapt.nhs.uk [accessed 23 April 2010].

Jacobson NS, Dobson KS, Truax PA, Addis ME, Koerner K, Gollan JK, Gortner E & Prince SE (1996). A component analysis of cognitive-behavioral treatment for depression. *Journal of Consulting and Clinical Psychology*, **64**(2), 295–304.

Kendrick T, Simons L, Mynors-Wallis L, Gray A, Lathlean J, Pickering R, Harris S, Rivero-Arias O, Gerard K & Thompson C (2005). A trial of problem-solving by community mental health nurses for anxiety, depression and life difficulties among general practice patients. The CPN-GP study. *Health Technology Assessment*, **9**(37), 1–104.

Kennedy N, Abbott R & Paykel ES (2003). Remission and recurrence of depression in the maintenance era: long-term outcome in a Cambridge cohort. *Psychological Medicine*, **33**, 827–838.

King M, McKeown E, Warner J, Ramsay A & Davison O (2003). Mental health and quality of life of gay men and lesbians in England and Wales: controlled, cross-sectional study. *British Journal of Psychiatry*, **183**, 552–558.

Lang P (1971). The application of the psychophysiological methods to the study of psychotherapy. In AE Bergin & SL Garfield (eds), *Handbook of Psychotherapy and Behaviour Change*. New York: Wiley.

Lingam R & Scott J (2002). Treatment non-adherence in affective disorders. *Acta Psychiatrica Scandinavica*, **105**(3), 164–172.

Luthar SS & Ciccheti D (2000). The construct of resilience: implications for interventions and social policies. *Development and Psychopathology*, **12**, 857–885.

Masten AS (2007). Resilience in developing systems: progress and promise as the fourth wave rises. *Development and Psychopathology*, **19**, 921–930.

Mead N & Bower P (2000). Patient centredness: a conceptual framework and review of the empirical literature. *Social Science and Medicine*, **51**, 1087–1110.

Meltzer H, Lader D, Corbin T, Singleton N, Jenkins R & Brugha T (2002). *Non-fatal Suicidal Behaviour Among Adults Aged 16 to 74 in Great Britain*. London: TSO.

MHF (Mental Health Foundation) (2007). *Up and Running? Exercise Therapy and the Treatment of Mild or Moderate Depression in Primary Care*. London: MHF.

Moussavi S, Chatterji S, Verdes E, Tandon A, Patel V & Ustun B (2007). Depression, chronic diseases, and decrements in health: results from the World Health Surveys. *The Lancet*, **370**, 851–858.

Mynors-Wallis LM, Gath DH, Day A & Baker F (2000). Randomised controlled trial of problem solving treatment, antidepressant medication, and combined treatment for major depression in primary care. *British Medical Journal*, **320**, 26–30.

NCCMH (National Collaborating Centre for Mental Health) (2004). *Self-Harm: The Short-Term Physical and Psychological Management and Secondary Prevention of Self-Harm in Primary and Secondary Care*. London: NICE.

NCCMH (National Collaborating Centre for Mental Health) (2009). *Depression: The Treatment and Management of Depression in Adults (partial update of NICE Clinical Guideline 23)*. London: British Psychological Society/Royal College of Psychiatrists.

NICE (National Institute for Health and Clinical Excellence) (2006). *Computerised Cognitive Behaviour Therapy for Depression and Anxiety [review of Technology Appraisal 51]*. London: NICE.

NICE (National Institute for Health and Clinical Excellence) (2007). *Depression (Amended): Management of Depression in Primary and Secondary Care*. London: NICE.

NICE (National Institute for Health and Clinical Excellence) (2009). *Depression: The Treatment and Management of Depression in Adults (partial update of NICE Clinical Guideline 23)*. London: NICE.

NIMHE (National Institute for Mental Health in England) (2003). *Inside Outside: Improving Mental Health Services for Black and Minority Ethnic Communities in England*. London: NIMHE.

NIMHE/SCMH (National Institute for Mental Health England/Sainsbury Centre for Mental Health) (2004). *The Ten Essential Shared Capabilities: A Framework for the Whole of the Mental Health Workforce*. London: DH.

NIMHE (National Institute for Mental Health in England) (2004). *Enhanced Services Specification for Depression under the New GP Contract: A Commissioning Guidebook*. Hyde, Cheshire: NIMHE North West.

ONS (Office for National Statistics) (2010). Suicide rates in the United Kingdom 1991–2008. Newport: ONS. Available from www.ons.gov.uk [accessed 21 February 2010].

Ostler K, Thompson C, Kinmonth A-L K, Peveler RC, Stevens L & Stevens A (2001). Influence of socio-economic deprivation on the prevalence and outcome of depression in primary care: The Hampshire Depression Project. *British Journal of Psychiatry*, **178**, 12–17.

Pilgrim D & Rogers A (2005). *A Sociology of Mental Health and Illness,* 3rd edition. Maidenhead: Open University Press.

Porter A (2006). *An Evaluation of Book Prescription Wales: Final Project Report.* Swansea: AWARD. Available from: www.awardresearch.org.uk [accessed 12 February 2010].

Putnam RD (2000). *Bowling Alone: The Collapse and Revival of American Community.* New York: Simon & Schuster.

Rogers CR (1980). *A Way of Being.* New York: Houghton Mifflin.

Rogers A & Pilgrim D (2003). *Mental Health and Inequality.* Basingstoke: Palgrave Macmillan.

Salkovskis P (2008). Editorial. *Behavioural and Cognitive Psychotherapy*, **36**, 1–2.

Scottish Executive (2006). *Rights, Relationships and Recovery: The Report of the National Review of Mental Health Nursing in Scotland.* Edinburgh: Scottish Executive. Available from: www.scotland.gov.uk [accessed 15 February 2010].

Scottish Government/NES (NHS Education for Scotland) (2008). '*The Matrix': A Guide to Delivering Evidence Based Psychological Therapies in Scotland.* Edinburgh: Scottish Government/NES. Available from: www.nes.scot.nhs.uk [accessed 12 February 2010].

SIGN (Scottish Intercollegiate Guidelines Network) (2010). *Non-pharmaceutical Management of Depression in Adults: A National Guideline* Edinburgh: SIGN.

Shaw CM, Creed F, Tomenson B, Riste L & Cruickshank JK (1999). Prevalence of anxiety and depressive illness and help seeking behaviour in African Caribbeans and white Europeans: two phase general population survey. *British Medical Journal*, **318**, 302–306.

Singleton N, Bumpstead R, O'Brien M, Lee A, & Meltzer H (2001). *Psychiatric Morbidity Among Adults Living in Private Households, 2000.* London: TSO.

Skapinakis P, Weich S, Lewis G, Singleton N & Araya R (2006). Socio-economic position and common mental disorders: longitudinal study in the general population in the UK. *British Journal of Psychiatry*, **189**, 109–117.

Tamburrino MB, Nagel, RW, Chahal, MK & Lynch DJ (2009). Antidepressant medication adherence: a study of primary care patients. *The Primary Care Companion to the Journal of Clinical Psychiatry*, **11**(5), 205–211.

Tew J (2005). Social perspectives: towards a framework for practice. In J Tew (ed.), *Social Perspectives in Mental Health: Developing Social Models to Understand and Work with Mental Distress.* London: Jessica Kingsley.

Tyree A & Gandhi P (2005). The importance of somatic symptoms in depression in primary care. *The Primary Care Companion to the Journal of Clinical Psychiatry*, **7**(4), 167–176.

Viinamaki H, Tanskanen A, Honkalampi K, Koivumaa-Honkanen H, Antikainen R, Haatainen K & Hintikka J (2006). Recovery from depression: a two-year follow-up study of general population subjects. *International Journal of Social Psychiatry*, **52**, 19–28.

Wallcraft J (2002). 'Turning Towards Recovery?' A Study of Personal Narratives of Mental Health Crisis and Breakdown. Unpublished PhD thesis. London: London South Bank University.

Webber M & Huxley P (2007). Measuring access to social capital: the validity and reliability of the Resource Generator-UK and its association with common mental disorder. *Social Science and Medicine*, **65**(3), 481–492.

WHO (World Health Organisation) (2010). *Depression*. Geneva: WHO. Available from: www.who.int [accessed 12 February 2010].

Williams MAH (2008). *Iechyd Meddwl Cymru: A Well Being and Mental Health Service Fit for Wales*. Cardiff: Welsh Assembly Government. Available from: www.wales.nhs.uk [accessed 12 February 2010].

Winter I (2000). *Towards a Theorised Understanding of Family Life and Social Capital* (Working Paper No. 21). Melbourne: Australian Institute for Family Studies.

Woolcock M. (2001). The place of social capital in understanding social and economic outcomes. *Isuma: Canadian Journal of Policy Research*, **2**(1), 1–17.

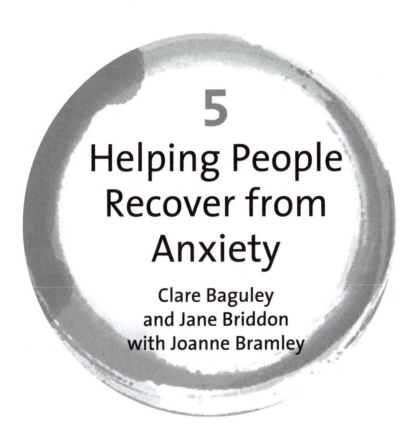

5
Helping People Recover from Anxiety

Clare Baguley
and Jane Briddon
with Joanne Bramley

What will I learn in this chapter?

This chapter aims to provide you with an understanding of the knowledge and skills required for promoting effective, recovery-focused interventions for people experiencing problems with anxiety in community and primary care settings.

After reading this chapter, you will be able to:

- identify the key symptoms and diagnostic features of the different types of anxiety, appreciating in particular the impact anxiety has on individuals;
- appreciate the role of the cognitive behavioural model in understanding anxiety disorders;
- outline a structured approach to assessing anxiety that incorporates collaborative approaches to problem formulation and goal setting;
- recognise the principles of evidence-based care for anxiety, and the skills required to deliver a range of evidence-based interventions.

Introduction

Anxiety is normal and something that every one of us experiences at some point in our lives. Indeed, it is important for our survival that we have the capacity to become anxious because the heightened physiological arousal that underpins anxiety also raises our performance when we are faced with new or unfamiliar demands or dangers. Anxiety can become problematic, however, if it is persistent, if it occurs without plausible explanation, or if it is accompanied by overwhelming feelings of dread, apprehension or impending disaster. In such cases, anxiety can interfere with our ability to meet the demands of daily life, including those related to work, home and relationships. Some people are so affected by anxiety that they withdraw completely – a situation that can have a devastating effect on their quality of life and sense of wellbeing (DH, 2004).

As we mentioned in the previous chapter, anxiety is (along with depression) often referred to as a **common mental health problem**. It is important to recognise, however, that this does not mean that anxiety does not have potentially serious and disabling effects.

Prevalence and demographics

According to the Office for National Statistics (ONS, 2001), common mental health problems across Great Britain (England, Scotland and Wales) affect around 1 in 6 (17%) of the population. Of these, roughly half experience mixed anxiety and depression, the remaining half experiencing either depression or one of the anxiety disorders. The most common anxiety disorder is **generalised anxiety disorder** (4.4% prevalence). To put things into perspective (and to appreciate why the term 'common' is used), almost 2.3 million people in England alone have an anxiety disorder (McCrone et al., 2008).

Anxiety disorders tend to be more common in women than in men (though panic disorder has equal rates). They are most prevalent in the 40–55 age range, with rates peaking for men in the middle of this range (45–49) and women at the top end (50–55). Social risk factors are similar to those for depression and include being divorced or separated and living alone or as a lone parent.

The economic costs of anxiety are significant: in terms of work days lost, effects on the economy and health care usage, figures from 2007 estimate the costs to be in the region of £9 billion (McCrone et al., 2008).

Policy Context

In relation to policy, anxiety disorders are rarely discussed in isolation from depression, the two being handled together under the label of **common mental health problems** (or common mental disorders). As such, most of the policy context for anxiety has already been covered in the respective section in the previous chapter and you are advised to refer to that section for direction. In particular, to see how policy varies across the UK, you should revisit the discussion about the Layard Report (CEPMHPG, 2006) and IAPT initiatives in England, *The Matrix* in Scotland (Scottish Government/NES, 2008), the Williams Review (Williams, 2008) in Wales and the Bamford Review (DHSSPS, 2009) in Northern Ireland.

In 2004 the National Institute for Health and Clinical Excellence (NICE) published guidance on the management and treatment of anxiety disorders in primary, secondary and community settings. This provided the first clear analysis of the evidence base for the treatment of anxiety and the ways in which services should aim to provide access to timely and effective interventions. The detail of this guidance – which was updated in 2007 – is outlined more fully later.

How People with Anxiety May Present to Services

In psychiatry, the broad umbrella term 'anxiety' is divided into different sub-diagnoses largely differentiated by the types of fearful thoughts that the person experiences and the effect these have on their behaviour. These categories are defined in the psychiatric manuals that we mentioned in Chapter 1 – DSM-IVR (APA, 2000) and ICD-10 (WHO, 2007) – and are used mainly by psychiatrists to diagnose anxiety when it is severe enough to be referred to mental health services. The different types of anxiety disorder are listed in Box 5.1.

Box 5.1   Main types of anxiety disorder (from ICD-10/ DSM-IV)

- Panic disorder (with or without agoraphobia)
- Social anxiety

(Continued)

(Continued)

- Health anxiety
- Generalised anxiety disorder
- Obsessive–compulsive disorder
- Post–traumatic stress disorder
- Specific phobias

As we mentioned in the previous chapter, formal diagnoses like these are important for guiding medical decisions regarding treatment. Since you will be working with some mental health professionals who will use these diagnoses, you should know the basics of them; as mental health nurses trying to understand the impact of anxiety on the individual, however, the reductionism of the diagnostic process isn't always helpful. Instead, as with we saw with depression, the most helpful way to conceptualise anxiety may be to think of it in terms of its **autonomic**, **behavioural** and **cognitive** aspects.

Understanding anxiety: the ABC-E model

Whilst the symptoms of each of the anxiety disorders have a slightly different clinical presentation, the core elements are the same. These core elements relate to the ways in which the person's body is affected, the ways in which they think and the ways in which they behave. It can be helpful to conceptualise this in terms of the ABC-E model that we introduced in the previous chapter: the **physical symptoms** of arousal as a result of involuntary activation of the sympathetic nervous system are the **autonomic** (**A**) aspects; the **actions** the person takes to try to manage the perceived danger are the **behavioural** (**B**) aspects; and the dominant **thoughts** of perceived threat or danger are the **cognitive** (**C**) aspects.

Anxiety can be triggered by a wide range of objects or situations, real or imagined. These may be **external** to the person (**environmental, E**) triggers such as social situations, relationship difficulties or work stress), or they may be **internal** (unpleasant bodily sensations or frightening thoughts or images, for example). Once anxiety has been triggered, interactions between the A, B and C aspects of the model conspire to maintain it. The central feature of anxiety is **fear**; not only fear of the triggering object or situation, but also fear that the effects of the anxiety disorder will result in physical, social or psychological harm.

In a moment, we will consider how each of the aspects of the ABC-E model impact on one another to create a 'vicious cycle of anxiety' – a cycle that can be very difficult to break without an understanding of what is happening – but firstly, consider the reflection point below.

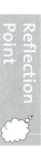

How you experience anxiety

Think about a time when you have felt anxious, worried or panicky. Perhaps it was when you first started school, college or work, or a time when things soured in a relationship.

How did you feel? What thoughts went through your head? What did you do? Try to categorise your answers according to whether they would fit into the A, B, C or E aspects of the model.

The A of anxiety: how our bodies react when we are anxious

To keep us safe, we are physically 'hardwired' to recognise and respond to threat, a mechanism known as **fight or flight**. This instinctive survival mechanism prepares the body for immediate action and is managed by the **sympathetic nervous system** (technically, the sympathetic branch of the autonomic nervous system). When we are faced with a real or perceived threat (a 'stressor'), the sympathetic nervous system automatically and instantaneously mobilises the body's resources to respond to the threat. The stress hormones **adrenalin** and **cortisol**, secreted by the adrenal glands, provide a burst of energy, increase blood flow to the major muscles such as the heart, increase breathing, heighten alertness and perception, and divert blood and energy away from less immediately vital systems such as digestion.

This emergency system works very well when the threat is real and our body needs to respond immediately, such as having to jump out of the way of an oncoming car when crossing the road or fighting back at an attacker. Unfortunately, the system works equally as well in response to a **perceived** threat. Take social anxiety for example. A very common trigger for this type of anxiety is the fear of being on show to a large group of people or having to perform publicly. The threat here is not that there is any real danger to you from the crowds; it is more about the **thought** that you might be embarrassed or make a fool of yourself, perhaps by sweating profusely, by fainting or by being sick. That these worries are related to some of the physical symptoms of anxiety (sweating; light-headedness; dry mouth; butterflies in the

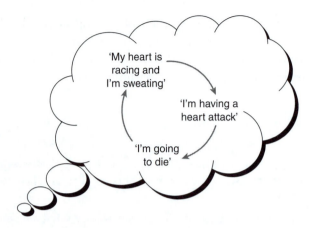

FIGURE 5.1   Catastrophic interpretation of anxiety

stomach) explains why people with social anxiety can get locked in a negative cycle of avoidance.

Panic attacks

A panic attack is a sudden and acute attack of anxiety during which a person experiences physical symptoms or sensations which they appraise and then attribute a catastrophic meaning to. For example, a racing heart may be interpreted as 'I'm having a heart attack', breathlessness as 'I'm going to collapse', visual disturbances as 'I'm going blind', and fingers tingling as 'I'm having a stroke'.

These catastrophic thoughts rapidly set up a feedback loop: the sympathetic nervous system responds to these thoughts as additional threats, producing yet more stress hormones which, in turn, increases the severity of the symptoms, provoking even more frightening thoughts (see Figure 5.1).

Another example involves the changes in breathing that occur in anxiety. Changes in breathing patterns can produce unpleasant and frightening effects. Breath holding is common amongst people when they are anxious and can be indicated by involuntary yawning or sighing. At the other end of the spectrum, over-breathing or **hyperventilation** can occur during a panic attack. During hyperventilation, breathing becomes rapid and shallow causing the person to feel light-headed and dizzy.

Severe or persistent hyperventilation can lead to the alarming muscle-cramping symptoms of **tetany**. This happens because excessive amounts of carbon dioxide are exhaled, so increasing the pH of the blood and reducing calcium plasma levels (a condition known as **alkalosis**). When caused by hyperventilation, tetany is not dangerous but it can be very frightening and is easily misinterpreted as a stroke or a fit by people who do not understand what is happening. While we will discuss interventions in more detail later on in this chapter, it is useful at this point to offer a simple first aid tip for hyperventilation (Box 5.2).

Box 5.2   A simple first aid technique for hyperventilation

Get the person to re-breathe their exhaled air. They can do this by holding a paper bag over their nose and mouth and continuing to breathe. This helps correct the body's carbon dioxide levels, so helping breathing to return to normal.

The C[1] of anxiety: how our thinking is affected when we are anxious

Our intellectual processes – the way we absorb information from our environment, the thoughts we have, and the way we attribute meaning to things – are collectively known as **cognition**. Anxious cognitions are characterised by thoughts of **risk** and **threat**. We all have anxious cognitions at times; for example, we might be scared of walking into a dark tunnel in case we get trapped, or we might get up in the night to check that the door has been locked to prevent a burglar getting in. While these types of thoughts tend to go away fairly quickly, they can sometimes become persistent, intrusive and difficult to control. We may, as such, change our behaviour in ways that we think help (in that they reduce anxiety) but that are actually quite unhelpful in the longer term – avoidance being a good example. To understand anxious thinking, it as useful to think of it as a continuum (Figure 5.2).

Catastrophic thinking
Normal anxious thinking varies across the continuum according to what we are doing, our level of confidence and our experience of similar situations. When a person becomes anxious to the point that it might be considered an

---

[1]With the ABC-E model, you might be wondering where behaviour (the B) is. It does indeed appear in a short while; it's just that, as far as anxiety is concerned, it is more logical to talk about cognitions (the C) first.

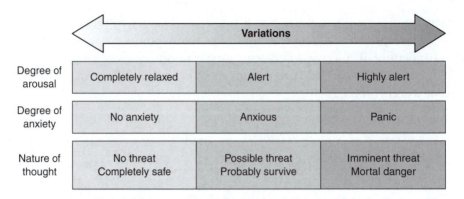

FIGURE 5.2   The continuum of anxious thinking

anxiety disorder, their ability to move along the continuum becomes impaired in that they become restricted to the higher end of the continuum which is characterised by a loss of flexibility and a lack of objectivity in thinking. The person may interpret their symptoms and the stimuli around them as an imminent sign of danger, i.e. the situation or event is **catastrophically mis-interpreted**. Different anxiety disorders have their own catastrophic themes, summarized in Table 5.1 below.

Images and processing of self as a social object

Images or 'mental pictures' can be as powerful – if not more powerful – than other types of cognition for people with anxiety. For a person experiencing social anxiety, images typically focus on how they believe they appear to

TABLE 5.1   Catastrophic themes for the various anxiety disorders

Type of anxiety disorder	Main fear
Panic disorder	Imminent catastrophe whether physical, social or psychological in nature *I'm going to die; I'm losing my mind*
Social anxiety	Negative social evaluation by others *I'm going to collapse and make a fool of myself*
Health anxiety	(Serious) physical illness *I've got cancer*
Obsessive–compulsive disorder	Responsibility for preventing harm to self or to others *If I don't do this (check), something bad will happen*
Specific phobias	Harm or danger from a specific object or situation *Being in the same room as a spider means it will attack me and do me serious harm*

others. They may, as such, have a mental picture of themselves with an enlarged, red, sweaty face – an image that in no way reflects how they appear in reality. This is known as the **processing of self as a social object**. These mental images are extremely powerful and fuel behaviours which maintain anxious beliefs about the degree of risk inherent in social situations.

Appraising risk

There are some situations or events where we all experience fear to a lesser or greater degree. So why do some people face their fears and meet head-on these situations or events while others avoid them at all costs? Salkovskis (1996) thinks it is down to the way in which we appraise risk. He claims that we make decisions about risk by unconsciously carrying out a complex calculation using **the risk equation** (Box 5.3).

Box 5.3   The risk equation

$$\text{Degree of perceived risk} \quad = \quad \frac{\text{Likelihood of threat} \quad \times \quad \text{'Awfulness' of threat}}{\text{Personal resources to survive} \quad + \quad \text{Environmental rescue factors}}$$

The risk equation provides a very helpful way of understanding how a person can be extremely anxious and unwilling to challenge their fear even when the likelihood of a threat occurring is low. For example, it is very common for people to be afraid of flying despite the fact that, statistically, the risk of a plane crashing is low. By applying the risk equation this can be explained by the 'awfulness' of crashing being high together with the possibility of surviving or being rescued by others being low. This raises the degree of perceived risk and results in a high degree of anxiety for the person who thinks in this way. Those less afraid of flying may still perceive the threat to have high 'awfulness' but they may think the likelihood of a crash happening to be minute and/or they might think the chances of surviving a crash or being rescued are reasonable. In a similar vein, the perception of risk may increase in new parents because the loss of their child will rank extremely high in terms of 'awfulness' and they may also feel that they don't have the personal resources (experience and knowledge) to deal with any threats (illness, accidents, etc.) to their children.

Since our own perception and interpretation of another person's fears can be inaccurate, we must be careful to avoid making assumptions. For example, a person saying that he or she is 'afraid of dying' is not as straightforward as it might seem. For some, it holds less fear because of their beliefs about what happens to them after death; for others, the fear might not necessarily be about them but about the welfare of the loved ones they will leave behind.

Cognitive processes that reinforce anxiety

As well as having thoughts and images about threat and danger, anxious people also develop instinctive patterns of spotting and seeking out information that reinforce the way they are feeling. Three main cognitive processes are behind these instinctive patterns. **Hypervigilance** is where the person becomes habitually alert to anything that may signal a threat and so becomes hypersensitive to any unexpected or sudden noises or movements. **Selective attention** happens when a person who is anxious about an aspect of their environment notices only those things that fit in with their fear – even if those things are not logically relevant. For example, a person who is anxious about being attacked on the street may constantly scan their environment for what they consider to be warning signs in people's behaviour such as 'being looked at'. The effect of selective attention is that the person collects increasing amounts of evidence to convince them that their fears are true. **Thought suppression** is where people try to cope with their fears and worries by trying not to think about them. The problem with thought suppression is that the more they try not to think about something that is worrying them, the more those worries start to intrude, that is pop into the person's mind when they least expect it (a particular problem in both obsessive–compulsive disorder and post-traumatic stress disorder). These intrusions can be frightening and they can make the person feel they are 'going mad' or that they are out of control. They can also lead to avoidance and other such behaviours that help maintain the anxiety, as we shall see in the next section.

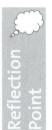

Reflection Point

Suppressing thoughts

Here is a simple exercise to help you understand the self-defeating power of thought suppression.

- Sit on your own and try very hard *not* to think about a pink elephant sat in a tree. What happens? Is it easy or hard to do?
- Now ... if you were told that every time you thought about a pink elephant sat in tree you would be fined £10 what would happen? Would it make it easier or harder still?

This simple exercise shows how when you believe it is very important not to think about something it will intrude into your thinking more and more.

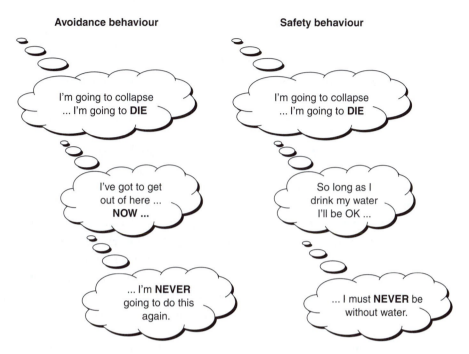

Avoidance behaviour

I'm going to collapse ... I'm going to **DIE**

I've got to get out of here ... **NOW ...**

... I'm **NEVER** going to do this again.

Safety behaviour

I'm going to collapse ... I'm going to **DIE**

So long as I drink my water I'll be OK ...

... I must **NEVER** be without water.

FIGURE 5.3 Avoidance vs. safety behaviours

The B of anxiety: what people do when they are anxious

As we have seen, when a person is fearful or anxious, their initial response is governed by the sympathetic nervous system – a system that mobilizes the body to either run away from the threat or fight it. When anxiety becomes habitual and entrenched people will engage in two particular types of behaviour to try to manage their anxiety levels: **avoidance behaviours** and **safety behaviours**. Crucially, while these behaviours are employed in a bid to control the threat and reduce the anxiety, they actually work against the person by maintaining the sense of threat and by preventing a realistic appraisal of beliefs about the feared situation or object. An illustrative example of how avoidance and safety behaviours can be employed in the same situation is contained in Figure 5.3.

Avoidance behaviours

Avoidance – where all possible steps are taken to avoid having to face a feared object or situation – is a very common response in anxiety disorders. Avoidance invariably means leaving the situation or not going near it in the first place (see the left-hand side of Figure 5.3). We all engage in avoidance to some extent, especially in difficult times or in anxiety-provoking situations. For example, many of us would not choose to go into a tank of snakes and avoidance here can hardly be called dysfunctional (unless, of course, we worked as a herpetologist[2] at a zoo!). However when a feared situation is a normal and healthy part of everyday life – such as touching other people, going to the shops or using public toilets – the use of avoidance behaviours can be disabling. One further and important consequence of avoidance is that we never find out if our fears are true. For example, would we really have a heart attack if we carried on exercising in a hot room when we felt breathless? Or if we did collapse in public would everyone really stand around and laugh at us?

In some circumstances, avoidance can spread to areas of our lives that resemble or remind us of the original trigger. This can be the case in post-traumatic stress disorder (PTSD) where a person who has had a traumatic or near-death experience can find themselves avoiding any reminders of the event (such as driving on the same stretch of road or even talking or thinking about the incident) with the disabling consequence that large areas of the person's daily life become shut off. Avoidance can also bring people into conflict with those who do not understand their reasons for refusing to do something. People with anxiety are often **ambivalent** about tackling avoid-ant behaviours because, from their perspective, there can be significant risks in changing such behaviours. Consequently, personal relationships can become strained as friends and partners seek to help by offering advice or, perhaps, compensating for the avoidant behaviour by taking over responsibil-ity for the day-to-day activities the person with anxiety is unable to do. As the avoidant behaviour becomes reinforced, the person with anxiety may become more demanding, which may result in an increasing burden on and additional stress for those close to them. This pattern also occurs in profes-sional relationships: a mental health practitioner might become frustrated at a person's apparent inability to change, and so resort to labelling the person as 'unmotivated' or 'difficult'. Since it is very important to be alert to the dangers of falling into this trap and to know how to respond, we will be looking at strategies for dealing with ambivalence later on.

Safety behaviours
Sometimes a person simply cannot avoid a situation they are fearful of and they may be forced to confront it – having to go to the shops for food or taking

---

[2]Someone who studies reptiles!

a child to school, for example. In these circumstances, **safety behaviours** may be adopted to help the person manage the situation.

Safety behaviours, which are also very common in anxiety disorders, are actions or strategies that are intended to minimise the likelihood of the feared event happening, but which actually make the problem worse. They often serve to maintain the sense of threat and, crucially, as with avoidance, they can stop the person from noticing evidence that their fears may not be true. The impact of engaging in safety behaviours is that the safety behaviour becomes the 'rescue' factor and the reason why the feared event did not happen or the person survived. For example, if someone believes that taking sips of water when they feel panicky stops them from collapsing, they will see sipping water as the reason why they didn't collapse (see the right-hand side of Figure 5.3). They are, as such, unlikely to challenge whether this really is the case, that is, put themselves in the position of thinking 'I may well be anxious if I don't have water with me, but will I actually collapse?'

As with avoidance behaviours, we all engage in safety behaviours to some degree. Some safety behaviours, such as carrying a mobile phone when driving the car, are logical and practical; others, such as touching wood for luck or saluting a magpie to avoid bad things happening, are less rational but emotionally powerful or culturally reinforced all the same. For the person with an anxiety disorder, however, these safety behaviours can be unhelpful to say the least; at the worst, they can be very disabling, as we shall see when we talk about the rituals and checking behaviour of obsessive–compulsive disorder (OCD).

There are many different types of safety behaviour that people use to cope. Table 5.2 shows some common ones associated with the different types of anxiety disorder.

TABLE 5.2 Examples of safety behaviours

Anxiety type	Safety behaviour	Example
Panic disorder	Bodily monitoring and avoidance	Checking heart rate and looking for escape routes
Social anxiety	Rehearsal and self–monitoring	Practising conversations and mentally monitoring performance
Health anxiety	Checking and reassurance seeking	Continually checking lumps and habitually seeing doctor
Obsessive–compulsive disorder	Rituals and checking	Touching an object many times and mentally counting
Post-traumatic stress disorder	Avoidance of reminders of the trauma	Not talking, and avoiding thinking, about the incident

Reassurance seeking is a particular type of safety behaviour that occurs most frequently in people with **health anxiety**, though it may be seen in other anxiety disorders. Since the ability to give and receive reassurance when things are tough and/or we need a confidence boost to meet a challenge is part of the normal course of life, seeking reassurance is hardly an abnormal activity. For a person with an anxiety disorder, however, reassurance seeking can be unhelpful because it becomes a way of avoiding having to deal with the fear. While reassurance seeking will give short-term relief from anxiety, the downside is that it very quickly loses its power so that the person becomes stuck in a loop of repeated reassurance seeking. For example, a person who fears they will have a heart attack may phone their partner for verbal reassurance when their heart rate increases. Initially, this seemingly innocuous behaviour may provide the necessary relief. However, it may become their only way of coping, causing tension and potential burnout for the reassurance giver. More importantly, it may prevent more rational reflections, such as how a telephone call to a partner might actually prevent a heart attack! Because of the physical symptoms inherent in anxiety, many GPs will arrange physical investigations (both as good practice and as a means of reassurance) for those who complain of specific physical symptoms. These investigations often give the person a clean bill of health, yet they may continue to return to the doctor for reassurance or they may seek opinion from elsewhere (including online) which may result in conflicting information which serves only to increase their fear.

Reassurance is as easy to give as it is to seek. Health professionals may be particularly vulnerable to reassurance seeking behaviour as their roles inherently require that they help people to both be better and feel better. Bear in mind that where time and availability is limited, giving reassurance can act as a quick fix but without proper attention to the underlying anxiety, it may serve only to maintain the problem.

Checking is a common behaviour that can be very useful. For example, it can help us make sure that we have completed a task accurately or help us improve the safety of ourselves and those around us (most formal health and safety procedures have a degree of checking built into them). When a person is overly anxious, however, checking behaviour can become excessive. This is the case in OCD where the demand to act (the compulsion) on specific occupying thoughts (the obsessions) can lead to checking behaviours that prevent people from getting on with other tasks of daily living.

As with reassurance seeking, checking provides relief from anxiety in the short term but very quickly loses its power, and so the person repeatedly checks. A person with **health anxiety**, for example, may constantly check their body for signs and symptoms, or monitor their blood pressure and feel around their body for 'abnormalities' or 'changes'. Again, while this is something we all do (indeed, the breast and testicular care campaigns actively encourage us to do just this), the effect of checking too often is that normally occurring variation in our bodies can end up being misinterpreted as the signs and symptoms of illness.

Rituals are elaborate and stereotypical ways of ensuring that something bad doesn't happen. Again, we all engage in rituals at times (indeed some, such as touching wood to make sure something we have said doesn't happen, are culturally reinforced) but, in conditions like OCD, these can become exaggerated and habitual to the point of causing disability.

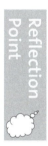

Avoidance and safety behaviours

As with the earlier reflection point, think about the times you have felt anxious, worried or panicky.

How did you behave in these circumstances? What actions did you take? Did you use any avoidance or safety behaviours? And did they have the desired effect (i.e. was there a reduction in your anxiety)?

Reflection Point

The E of anxiety: the effect of the environment

Anxiety is a very individual experience that arises partly from our individual physiologies and the individual ways in which we view and think about the world, and partly from the way in which we have been shaped by our current and past environments. Our environments provide the foundation upon which we learn to judge risk, cope with anxiety, behave with others and develop coping strategies for dealing with stress. For example, a child with a parent who is afraid of spiders will assimilate into their own world-view (through observing the parent's reaction to spiders) the perception that 'spiders are dangerous', unless they are exposed to the alternative viewpoints of other significant adults. Our environments also provide many of the triggers for anxiety (see Box 5.4).

Box 5.4   Common environmental triggers for anxiety

- Relationship and family problems
- Excessive work demands
- Loss of occupation and role
- Sudden trauma or loss
- Illness or death
- Bullying and alienation

Past experiences and environments can also have an impact on an individual's vulnerability to anxiety and the degree to which they are **resilient** (we discussed resilience in more detail in the previous chapter). If a specific way of coping helped someone successfully emerge from an anxious situation in the past, that coping strategy – whether personal (using problem solving skills, for example) or social (seeking the support of friends, for example) – may well be useful in the present or in the future when we are faced with the sorts of challenges listed in Box 5.4. On the other hand, if our past experiences haven't prepared us for a particular challenge (because, for example, it is a rare event like a disaster or an event that we are encountering for the first time in our lives, like a relationship break up), then we may well experience anxiety. Moreover, if we cannot find the personal and social resources needed to cope or if those resources are ultimately maladaptive (as with avoidance and safety behaviours), we may find the anxiety maintained and amplified through the vicious cycle of anxiety so much so that anxiety becomes problematic and an **anxiety disorder** develops. Figure 5.4 illustrates this vicious cycle within the framework of the ABC-E model of emotion.

 Case scenario: Joanna

Joanna grew up as a self-conscious girl who struggled to feel comfortable around people. She would often feel panicky and burst into tears, usually if it had anything to do with a social event. She'd feel hot and flustered, sick and shaky and get palpitations. At times, she felt as if she had been punched in the stomach. Her mouth would feel so dry she'd struggle to

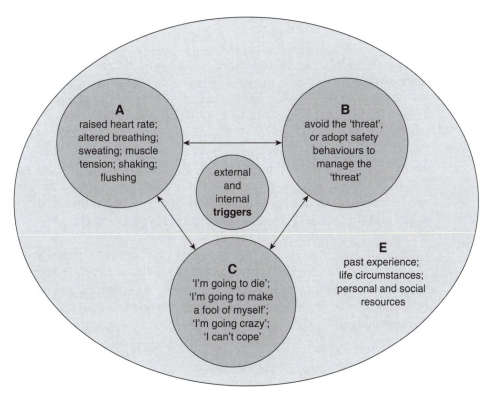

FIGURE 5.4   The maintenance cycle of anxiety within the ABC-E model

speak. Her face and neck would turn a vivid shade of red (so much so that she felt like she was on fire), her cheeks would sting and blotches would appear on her neck. Her head would feel as though it had a tight band of steel around it.

These symptoms were so overwhelming that she found it impossible to focus on anything else other than how awful she was feeling. She felt powerless to control these symptoms and was worried that they would cause her real harm. Worst of all was the embarrassment she felt because her symptoms were so visible, symptoms that she felt would appear to others as a sign of weakness and that people would laugh at her. She didn't feel normal like everyone else; she felt a failure and believed she was odd. All she wanted was to be just like everyone else.

(Continued)

(Continued)

Because she was so self-conscious, Joanna started to find it more and more difficult to mix with people. If she couldn't avoid a social function then she would see if she could take someone with her for support. She'd arrive as late as she could and be the first to leave. She'd always sit or stand near a door so that she could 'escape' into the fresh air if she became 'trapped'. She wouldn't eat anything because she found it difficult to eat in front of others and because she never had any appetite anyway because of her anxiety. She wouldn't initiate any conversation because she felt too shy and she could never think of anything interesting to say as she was too preoccupied with keeping her symptoms under some sort of control.

Joanna would always wear high-necked tops so that no one would notice the red blotches on her neck. To avoid panic setting in, going out became 'like a military exercise'; for example, she spent a great deal of time (and a small fortune) on make-up that she hoped would conceal her flushed face.

What A, B, C and E elements can you identify in this scenario? Can you identify any avoidance or safety behaviours?

Assessing Individuals with Anxiety

In the previous chapter we outlined a person-centred, structured assessment and formulation process for depression, framed within the ABC-E model (Briddon et al., 2008; see Box 5.5). The same assessment and problem formulation principles can be applied to people experiencing anxiety so long as they are shored up by an understanding of the nature of anxiety and the individual effects it can have on people.

As with depression, it is essential that the practitioner possesses the right values, skills and capabilities to work with and help people with anxiety. The cornerstone for success in psychotherapeutic interventions is, after all, the **therapeutic relationship** (see Chapter 2). People experiencing anxiety need practitioners that have a calm and reassuring manner coupled with a genuinely curious and enquiring approach.

Box 5.5 The process of person-centred interviewing

1 Introduction and orientation

- Confidentiality

2 Gathering information

- The 4 Ws: what, where, when, with whom
- A-B-C aspects
- E (environmental) aspects

  - Triggers to the problem
  - Impact

- Any other important information
- Risk assessment

3 Formulation

- Verbal problem statement
- Diagrammatic problem summary

To work with a person experiencing anxiety, you need to adopt a compassionate and normalising approach, underpinned by an assumption that whatever the person is doing, or however they are behaving, **they are trying their best to cope**. Remember that by asking them to work on their fears and challenge avoidance, you are asking them to take a very big leap of faith; that either their fears are not going to happen or, if they do, that they will be able to cope. During engagement, and when delivering interventions, it is equally important not to give false reassurance. Bear in mind the risk equation: it's often not the probability of something occurring that matters; instead, it's the ability to cope and/or the degree of perceived 'awfulness'.

The structured assessment process

As with any therapeutic encounter, you should begin with an **introduction** that includes a statement of **confidentiality**. The next stage of the assessment and formulation process is to gather appropriate information. Here you should

TABLE 5.3 Typical questions for each aspect of the ABC-E model

Aspect	Typical questions
General	When was the last time that you felt anxious?
A (Autonomic)	How did your body feel? What sensations did you experience?
B (Behavioural)	What did you do to cope?
C (Cognitive)	What ran through your mind? What was the worst thing you were thinking?
E (Environmental)	What (or who) in your life makes the anxiety worse? What helps?

use a **structured questioning** framework – the 4Ws and the questions appertaining to the fours aspects (ABC-E) of the model (see Table 5.3), for example. Remember that structured questioning coupled with the **funnelling** technique is a powerful way of helping you hone in on the problem formulation. In gathering appropriate information, you might also use formal **psychometric measures** (see 'establishing a baseline' below), **observation** (perhaps observing the person in their natural environment as well as in any sessions you have with them), and tools such as **diaries** and informal **questionnaires**.

Establishing a baseline

It is important to get an initial measure of how often, frequent and severe the person's anxiety is so that you can: (1) **assess and understand its severity** and the impact it has on the person's day-to-day functioning; (2) **monitor the success of interventions** by measuring any change from the baseline; and (3) discuss any changes, and **provide feedback** to the person seeking help.

There are a number of ways of getting baseline measurements. You might use a standardised **general questionnaire**, such as the **GAD-7** (*Generalized Anxiety Disorder Assessment*; Spitzer et al., 2006) to provide a general score that indicates the severity of the anxiety. Alternatively, you might use a standardised **disorder specific measure** to provide more detailed information about the content, severity and frequency of specific symptoms. Examples include the **Y–BOCS** (*Yale–Brown Obsessive Compulsive Scale*; Goodman et al., 1989) for symptoms of OCD, and the CAPS (*Clinician Administered PTSD Scale*; Blake et al., 1995) for PTSD. Finally, you might use a non-standardised (informal) **personalised measurement scale** such as an

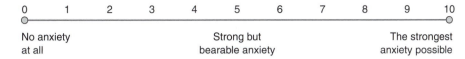

FIGURE 5.5   A self-rating anxiety scale

adapted Likert scale. These are a relatively simple and quick way of getting a rating on any aspect of the person's presentation such as strength of anxiety or belief in particular thoughts. The scale should be carefully set up by defining both ends of the scale and the points between. Figure 5.5 provides an example personalised scale.

Problem formulation

Problem formulation is the bridge between assessment and intervention. It has a number of important functions, namely: (1) to organise assessment information in a **manageable and understandable format**; (2) to **normalise and personalise** the person's experience; (3) to develop a 'map' to guide **shared decision making** and **goal setting**; and (4) to **instil hope**, with the message that 'we can work on this together'.

After the structured assessment, the problem formulation can be drawn out using the ABC-E model as a framework (but adapting it to incorporate specific features of each anxiety disorder as required). The development of the problem formulation can often act as an intervention in itself, especially if the problem formulation is mapped diagrammatically (perhaps by using the diagram in Figure 5.4). By mapping the formulation, you can make the overwhelming and frightening simple. Through an explanation of the links between emotions, thoughts, behaviour, physiology and environment, you can also help the person understand their anxiety and the way in which it is maintained so as to help them progress towards recovery.

A summary of the things you might need to consider when assessing people experiencing anxiety is contained within Figure 5.6.

Evidence-Based Interventions for Anxiety

As well as heaping misery on a significant proportion of the population, anxiety also has major social and economic costs (CEPMHPG, 2006;

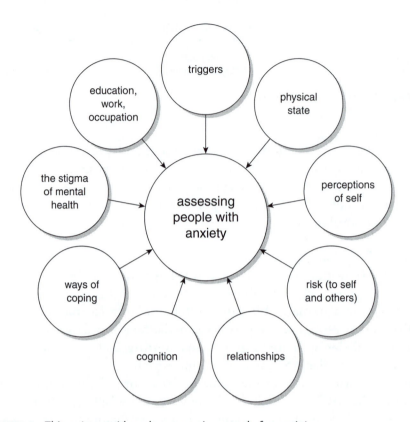

FIGURE 5.6   Things to consider when assessing people for anxiety

NICE, 2007). Moreover, anxiety disorders often go undetected (and therefore untreated) in primary care despite the fact that (as we shall see) highly
effective treatments for these conditions are available. As a result of these concerns, the National Institute for Health and Clinical Excellence (NICE) in
England published, in 2004, a set of guidelines relating to the management of
anxiety (see NICE, 2007 for the updated version). These were followed a year
later by specific guidance on OCD (NICE, 2005a) and PTSD (NICE,
2005b). Although the Scottish equivalent of NICE, the Scottish Intercollegiate
Guidelines Network (SIGN), has recently published guidance on depression
(SIGN, 2010), they have not, at the time of writing, published any guidance
on the anxiety disorders.

The recommendations from the various sets of NICE guidance relating to
anxiety are summarized in Table 5.4.

TABLE 5.4   A summary of the NICE guidance relating to anxiety

Anxiety disorder	Recommended interventions	Source
Panic disorder	*In order of length of effect, most effective first:* • CBT • an SSRI antidepressant licensed for panic disorder • self-help based on CBT principles *Not recommended: benzodiazepine medication*	Guidance on panic disorder and generalised anxiety disorder (NICE, 2007)
Generalized anxiety disorder (social anxiety, health anxiety and phobias are included here)	*In the short term:* • short-term (2–4 weeks) use of benzodiazepine medication *In the longer term, in order of length of effect, most effective first:* • CBT • an SSRI antidepressant licensed for panic disorder • self-help based on CBT principles	Guidance on panic disorder and generalised anxiety disorder (NICE, 2007)
Obsessive–compulsive disorder	*Where there is mild functional impairment:* **low intensity** (<10 sessions) psychological interventions: • facilitated self-help using CBT-based principles, particularly exposure and response prevention (ERP) • telephone CBT (including ERP) • group CBT (including ERP) *Where there is moderate functional impairment:* • an SSRI antidepressant • **high intensity** (>10 sessions) psychological treatment involving CBT (including ERP)	Guidance on OCD (NICE, 2005a)
Post-traumatic stress disorder	*Either:* • trauma-focused CBT or • eye movement desensitisation and reprocessing (EMDR) *Not recommended: drug treatments as a first line treatment.*	Guidance on PTSD (NICE, 2005b)

Cognitive behavioural interventions

Given their dominance in the treatment of anxiety, the bulk of this section will focus on those interventions that are underpinned by cognitive behavioural principles. To alleviate any distressing psychological symptoms, cognitive behavioural interventions may be combined with a medication such as an SSRI antidepressant or a benzodiazepine anxiolytic; as such, to work with people with anxiety, practitioners not only need to become skilled in these interventions, they also need to understand the effects and side-effects of any medications prescribed.

This section outlines some of the key features of the various cognitive behavioural interventions that can be used effectively with anxious people. In particular, we will look at **graded exposure**, **cognitive restructuring** and **behavioural experiments**. However, bear in mind that in a book like this, we can only provide you with some basic information to get you started. In integrating cognitive behavioural interventions into your everyday practice as a mental health nurse, you will need to further develop your knowledge and skills in this area. The further reading and resources we list at the end of this chapter can help you enhance your knowledge about cognitive behavioural approaches; to enhance your skills, however, there is no better solution than practice, though you should bear in mind your level of capability and the importance of mentorship and supervision.

Before discussing specific cognitive behavioural interventions in detail, it's worth discussing one or two prerequisites to intervening, prerequisites that are essentially interventions in their own right.

Normalising and providing psychoeducation

Having developed a shared problem formulation, the first step of any intervention for anxiety is to provide a **normalising** rationale for the anxiety. This can be achieved by discussing the continuum of anxious thinking (see Figure 5.2) and exploring any triggers if they are apparent. Box 5.6 contains some examples of how you might provide a normalising rationale for the anxiety.

Box 5.6 Examples of normalising statements

'Given what you have been dealing with, there is a logic to why you have become anxious.'

'Anyone thinking the same thoughts as you are at the moment would be experiencing anxiety too.'

In addition, the provision of understandable and accessible information through self-help and psychoeducational materials (which tie in directly with the collaboratively agreed problem formulation) is important in helping the person begin to develop a new perspective on their anxiety. If appropriate, these materials can also be shared with friends and family who often want to understand the problem and offer meaningful support.

Graded exposure

The first specific cognitive behavioural intervention we will consider is **graded exposure.** Where an anxiety disorder is maintained by avoidance – in **specific phobias** and **panic disorder with agoraphobia,** for example – this is the best first line approach. When a person is stuck in a cycle of avoidance, they will instinctively avoid the perceived threatening situation, object or event as their anxiety builds up. Getting the person to gradually confront the fear so that they begin to realise that panic symptoms will subside naturally if dealt with in the right way is how exposure is used to break the cycle of avoidance (Figure 5.7).

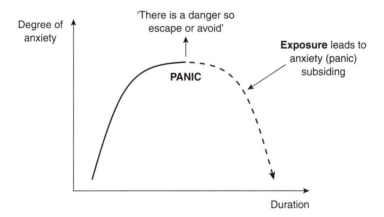

FIGURE 5.7 Avoidance vs. exposure

The core principles of exposure are that it is **gradual, regular, prolonged** and **measured**. 'Gradual' refers to the process of using small steps that are linked to goals. It can be useful to create a hierarchy of steps leading to the person's ultimate goal (Figure 5.8).

'Regular' means that the exposure is planned and practised **every day**. 'Prolonged' means that each step of the exposure hierarchy is conducted **for at least one hour** or until the anxiety symptoms have **subsided to 50%**

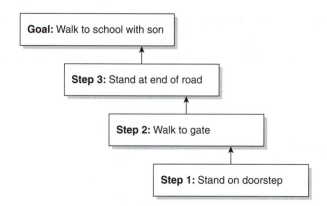

FIGURE 5.8   Hierarchy of exposure linked to a goal

or less of the original rating, and 'measured' means that some sort of **self-rating tool** (such as the one in Figure 5.5) is used to record changes in anxiety levels and provide feedback on progress. A self-rating sheet (Figure 5.9) is a useful way of recording any such measurements.

It is common for many people with anxiety to have a range of avoidance behaviours. Where this is the case, you can get the person to make a list of all

Overall goal:		
Exposure steps for this week	Anxiety rating before 0–10	Anxiety rating after 0–10
1.		
2.		
Comments:		

FIGURE 5.9   An exposure self-rating sheet

of their avoidance behaviours, getting them to prioritise the list in terms of the easiest or most important to tackle. By selecting one specific area of avoidance to work on, you can teach the person the principles of exposure, which they can then apply to other areas of avoidance as and when the opportunity arises.

Generally when working on exposure, you should ensure that progress results in positive feedback (praise). Enlisting the help and support of a family member or significant other is also useful as they can often support the person in their home environments. It's also worth planning in advance for potential **obstacles** (by asking, for example, 'what might get in the way of you doing this?') so that there is a readily available solution should these obstacles arise.

Exposure with response prevention (ERP), recommended for people with OCD, is exposure coupled with strategies to prevent the person carrying out safety or avoidance behaviours (their 'response'). For example, a person with excessive hand washing may be asked to create a hierarchy of the situations and thoughts that lead to hand washing behaviour (thinking about bins, touching a doorknob, emptying a bin, etc.) and as they are exposed to the various elements of this hierarchy so they also agree to refrain from washing their hands (the safety behaviour).

Exposure on its own is sometimes insufficient. Its success as a 'single strand' intervention is often determined by the nature of the beliefs that the person holds about the feared situation or object and the extent to which they explore and examine these beliefs.

Anxious thoughts are very powerful as they are **involuntary** and occur spontaneously, and they are often **plausible** in that they are very believable to the person holding them. As such, cognitive behavioural techniques that focus on the anxious thoughts are often a useful adjunct to a single strand intervention like exposure. **Cognitive restructuring**, which we explored in the previous chapter, is perhaps the main such technique.

Cognitive restructuring: examining and challenging anxious thoughts

Cognitive restructuring in relation to anxiety has three basic steps: (1) **recognising and capturing** the anxious thoughts; (2) **examining the evidence** for those thoughts and developing more realistic or accurate beliefs; and (3) **testing out** alternative beliefs via behavioural experiments.

Anxious thoughts can be identified through specific questioning during the assessment interview – by asking questions such as 'what runs through your mind when you are anxious?' However, the real detail of

Date and time	Situation	Anxiety rating	Thoughts
When did it happen?	Where were you? What were you doing? Who was with you?	How strong was the feeling of anxiety on a scale of 0–10?	What exactly were your thoughts? To what degree did you believe the thought(s) on a rating scale of 0–10?

FIGURE 5.10   A diary for capturing anxious thoughts

anxious thoughts is only fully accessible when the person is directly exposed to the situations that trigger the anxiety. Recreating the anxiety-provoking situation or accompanying the person to such a situation can be a very useful way of capturing the thought, though this is not always possible and inexperienced practitioners should always carry out this type of intervention under close clinical supervision. An alternative approach is to use a **thought diary** (Figure 5.10). Thought diaries have two purposes: first, they can help the person differentiate between anxious feelings, physical symptoms and thoughts; and secondly, they allow the specific details (such as the context) of the anxious thoughts to be captured as and when they occur.

The thought diary should be used between sessions. The person seeking help should be encouraged to be as precise as possible in recording their anxious thoughts by writing them down as soon as they occur while also rating them on a scale of 0–10 according to how strong the anxiety was and how much the person believed the thought. This rating is important as the more strongly held a belief, the more likely it is to be unresponsive to exposure alone and more likely it will need to be examined and tested through cognitive restructuring.

During sessions, the content of the diary can be examined so that key anxious thoughts can be identified, together with the evidence for and

Identified anxious thought	Evidence for the anxious thought	Evidence against the anxious thought	Alternative thought
What were you thinking when you were anxious? What does this mean for you? What is the worst thing about it?	What helps you support this view? What is the evidence for the thought?	What evidence is there that contradicts or does not support the thought?	What might a more realistic/balanced thought be? To what degree do you believe the new thought(s) on a rating scale of 1–10?

FIGURE 5.11   Examining anxious thoughts worksheet

against them. Once this has been done, an action plan for testing out alternative thoughts or collecting new evidence to test out the belief can be devised. This can be done with the help of an 'anxious thoughts worksheet' (Figure 5.11).

Discussion of the anxious thoughts worksheet should lead to a plausible alternative perspective–a perspective that needs to be articulated in a thought that has a high rating of believability. This alternative then needs testing out through a **behavioural experiment**.

Behavioural experiments

In the previous chapter, we saw how behavioural experiments were a useful tool to use with the negative thoughts that underpin depression. Behavioural experiments are equally as useful with anxious thoughts in that they help the person become curious about their problems rather than feel at the mercy of them.

There are four steps for undertaking a behavioural experiment: (1) **identify the thought** or belief to be tested; (2) **construct an experiment**; (3) **do the experiment**; and (4) **review the outcome**, that is consider the evidence for and against the new thought or belief. Some examples of behavioural

What is the thought/belief being tested? Rate how much you believe this on a 0–10 scale.	Describe the experiment *What?* *Where?* *When?* *With whom?*	What do you predict will happen?	Record here what <u>actually</u> happens	What have you learnt? How does it match the thought/belief being tested? Rate how much you believe this now on a 0–10 scale.

FIGURE 5.12   Behavioural experiment record sheet

experiments are: getting the person to stop trying to control their breathing; getting the person to leave the house without a 'safe' object such as emergency anxiety medication; and getting the person to observe the practitioner doing something such as simulating a faint in a public place to see what actually happens. When undertaking a behavioural experiment, it is useful to have a recording sheet (such as the one illustrated in Figure 5.12) so that the outcome can be easily reviewed.

Working with ambivalence and blocks to progress

Earlier, we mentioned that ambivalence – having mixed feelings about something – is common in people experiencing anxiety. Remember that people use coping strategies such as avoidance and safety behaviours so as to minimize perceived risk. As such, changing these behaviours may result in an unacceptable increase in (perceived) risk to the person with anxiety, with any potential benefits being relegated into the background. In these circumstances, a **cost–benefit analysis** table can be a very useful way of exploring ambivalence and finding potential levers for change. An example of a cost–benefit analysis table, undertaken with a person suffering from panic disorder with agoraphobic avoidance, can be found in Table 5.5.

TABLE 5.5 Example of a cost–benefit analysis for panic disorder with agoraphobia

Timescale	Reasons for changing	Reasons for not changing
Short term This week	I'm fed up	It'll be very difficult There's no one to help me I'll panic
Medium term 6 months	I'll feel better about myself I'll be able to go to the park with my son and he'll be happier	I'll need a lot of will power People will expect me to do more things
Long term 2 years	I'll be able to get fit I could go back to college It will affect my son if I can't take him to school	I'll feel worse if I fail.

By using a cost–benefit analysis, you can help the person understand that, while it may be overwhelming to achieve the short-term gains, the effort involved is worth it because the longer-term gains have real rewards. For most people, keeping sight of these longer-term goals is the key to dealing with ambivalence and managing any setbacks. Cost–benefit analyses can also be helpful in identifying **blocks** to progress. If these are identified, then they need to be directly discussed. For example, a statement such as 'there's no one to help me' can be discussed and problem solved with a view to finding out what sort of help is needed and what resources are actually available, from within the person's own world as well as from the professionals.

In addition, asking the person 'what would you say to someone that you cared about if they were talking to you about this as their problem?' can help them get a 'meta-perspective' on their problems, a perspective where instinctive responses emerging from their own anxiety are avoided. Anxious people can very often give excellent advice to others while ignoring it for themselves!

Some blocks are more difficult to problem solve, particularly when there are tangible short term gains to be had by staying the same – keeping control of a relationship or maintaining financial stability through disability benefits, for example. Importantly, the cost–benefit table allows the person and the professional to look at these issues together objectively. Drawing the person's attention to the longer-term benefits can help them shift perspective. However, it is important to recognise that the immediate costs can sometimes outweigh the gains. Open and honest discussion between the person seeking help and the professional can, however, lead to agreement about the way forward – whether it is a re-prioritisation of the problem or, perhaps, a plan to do nothing but review things after an agreed period of time. The strength of working on blocks in this way is that challenges are confronted within the framework of a collaborative approach to decision making. It also allows the practitioner to understand why a person is not engaging when all the signs are that they should benefit from intervention.

Discharge planning and relapse prevention

As with depression, planning for discharge should be a key consideration from the outset of any programme of help. In primary care, most interventions for anxiety aim to be time-limited; as such, the ultimate goal of any such intervention is to give the person the knowledge and skills necessary for them continue to work on their problems beyond the time limits of the therapy.

The final stage of intervention, as a prerequisite to discharge, is **relapse prevention**. This involves: a structured review of what has been learnt from the therapy; identification of what remains to be worked on post discharge; planning for this continued effort; and identification of potential setbacks. A specific session should be set aside for this work, supported by preparatory between-session work that the person seeking help will have undertaken. The questions contained in Box 5.7 provide a useful framework for this between-session work, as well as for the relapse prevention session itself.

Box 5.7   Questions that help with the construction of relapse prevention plans

- What have you learnt about your anxiety?
- What key things have been helpful in learning to manage your anxiety?
- What do you need to do next to build on what you have learnt?
- How will you go about this? (perhaps write a plan)
- What might lead to a setback? What would the 'warning' signs be?
- What do you need to do if you notice this happening? What *can* you do? What help might you need and from whom?

By working through these questions, discharge planning becomes a **collaborative** exercise – one that enables incomplete goals to be factored into the next steps of the person's recovery, and one that allows the possibility of setbacks, and how they might be managed, to be discussed in a normalising and open way. The information gleaned through this exercise can then be shared with the people most likely to make a difference in the person's path to recovery: family members and those close to them, as well as key members of the primary care team.

Conclusion

In this chapter we have shown that anxiety is a common mental health problem; it is a problem that mental health nurses (indeed, all nurses) will encounter in a variety of settings throughout their clinical practice. Although anxiety is described as a *common* mental health problem, we have shown that it can have a serious and enduring impact on a person's quality of life and their ability to function.

Regarding the assessment of people experiencing anxiety, we have outlined a structured approach to assessment and problem formulation, using the ABC-E model as a framework. We have considered anxiety predominantly from a cognitive behavioural perspective because this is the perspective that offers the most effective interventions for those experiencing anxiety and we have outlined a number of evidence-based cognitive behavioural techniques that are helpful in dealing with specific aspects of anxiety. Moreover, we have discussed the necessary core skills and qualities that mental health nurses require if they are to embed such cognitive behavioural approaches into their routine clinical practice.

Further Reading and Resources

See also the further reading and resources listed in the previous chapter.

Key texts

Bennet-Levy J, et al. (eds) (2010). *Oxford Guide to Low Intensity CBT Interventions*. Oxford: Oxford University Press.
As listed in the previous chapter.

Greenberger D & Padesky CA (1995). *Mind over Mood*. New York: Guilford Press.
  Again, as listed in the previous chapter.

Kennerley H (1997). *Overcoming Anxiety*. London: Constable Robinson.
  This simple self-help book is one of a series covering mental health topics and CBT techniques. As helpful for clinicians as for service users!

Wells A (1997). *Cognitive Therapy of Anxiety Disorders: A Practice Manual and Conceptual Guide*. Chichester: John Wiley & Sons.
  This book has been reprinted several times and remains the best all-round clinical overview of the anxiety disorders. An excellent core text for both the theoretical and practical aspects of cognitive therapy.

Willson R & Branch R (2006). *Cognitive Behavioural Therapy for Dummies*. Chichester: John Wiley & Sons.
  Yes, there really is a 'for dummies' book on CBT! Useful as an introduction, but perhaps too basic as an academic source.

Key policy documents

National Institute for Health and Clinical Excellence (2005). *Obsessive Compulsive Disorder: Core Interventions in the Treatment of Obsessive Compulsive Disorder and Body Dysmorphic Disorder*. London: NICE. Available from: www.nice.org.uk/CG31.

National Institute for Health and Clinical Excellence (2005). *Post-Traumatic Stress Disorder (PTSD): The Management of PTSD in Adults and Children in Primary and Secondary Care*. London: NICE. Available from: www.nice.org.ukcg26.

National Institute for Health and Clinical Excellence (2007). *Anxiety (amended): Management of Anxiety (Panic Disorder, with or without Agoraphobia, and Generalised Anxiety Disorder) in Adults in Primary, Secondary and Community Care*. London: NICE. Available from: www.nice.org.uk/CG22.

Web resources

Anxiety UK: www.anxietyuk.org.uk
  Website of the main charity offering support to people with anxiety.

The Improving Access to Psychological Therapies (IAPT) initiative: www.iapt.nhs.uk
  As listed in the previous chapter.

Beating the Blues: www.beatingtheblues.co.uk and Fear Fighter: www.fearfighter.com
  Websites of NICE-recommended computerised CBT treatment for panic and phobia.

The 'Five Areas Approach': www.livinglifetothefull.com and www.fiveareas.com/resourcearea
  As listed in the previous chapter.

Glasgow Steps: www.glasgowsteps.com
  The website of a Glasgow-based primary mental health care service that has useful video clips and downloadable resources for anxiety and other mental health problems.

References

APA (American Psychiatric Association) (2000). *Diagnostic and Statistical Manual of Mental Disorders, 4th Edition* (Text Revised) (DSM–IVR). Washington: APA.

Blake DD, Weathers FW, Nagy LM, Kaloupek DG, Gusman FD, Charney DS & Keane TM (1995). The development of a clinician-administered PTSD scale. *Journal of Traumatic Stress*, **8**, 75–90.

Briddon JE, Baguley C & Webber M (2008). The ABC-E model of emotion: a bio-psychosocial model for primary mental health care. *Journal of Mental Health Training, Education and Practice*, **3**(1), 12–21.

CEPMHPG (Centre for Economic Performance's Mental Health Policy Group) (2006). *The Depression Report: A New Deal for Depression and Anxiety Disorders* [The Layard Report]. London: London School of Economics. Available from: cep.lse.ac.uk [accessed 12 January 2010].

DH (Department of Health) (2004). *Organising and Delivering Psychological Therapies.* London: DH.

DHSSPS (Department of Health, Social Security and Public Safety) (2009). *Delivering the Bamford Vision: The Response of the Northern Ireland Executive to the Bamford Review of Mental Health and Learning Disability. Action Plan 2009–2011.* Belfast: DHSSPS. Available from: www.dhsspsni.gov.uk [accessed 2 November 2009].

Goodman WK, Price LH, Rasmussen SA, Mazure C, Fleischmann RL, Hill CL, Heninger GR & Charney DS (1989). The Yale–Brown Obsessive Compulsive Scale. I: Development, use, and reliability. *Archives of General Psychiatry*, **46**, 1006–1011.

McCrone P, Dhanasiri S, Patel A, Knapp M & Lawton Smith S (2008). *Paying the Price: The Cost of Mental Health Care in England to 2026.* London: Kings Fund.

NICE (National Institute for Health and Clinical Excellence) (2005a). *Obsessive Compulsive Disorder: Core Interventions in the Treatment of Obsessive Compulsive Disorder and Body Dysmorphic Disorder.* London: NICE.

NICE (National Institute for Health and Clinical Excellence) (2005b). *Post-Traumatic Stress Disorder (PTSD): The Management of PTSD in Adults and Children in Primary and Secondary Care.* London: NICE.

NICE (National Institute for Health and Clinical Excellence) (2007). *Anxiety (amended): Management of Anxiety (Panic Disorder, with or without Agoraphobia, and Generalised Anxiety Disorder) in Adults in Primary, Secondary and Community Care.* London: NICE.

ONS (Office for National Statistics) (2001). *Psychiatric Morbidity among Adults Living in Private Households, 2000.* London: ONS. Available from: www.statistics.gov.uk [accessed 15 February 2010].

Salkovskis P (ed.) (1996). *Frontiers of Cognitive Therapy: The State of the Art and Beyond.* London: Guildford Press.

Scottish Government/NES (NHS Education for Scotland)(2008). 'The Matrix': A Guide to Delivering Evidence Based Psychological Therapies in Scotland.* Edinburgh: Scottish Government/NES. Available from: www.nes.scot.nhs.uk [accessed 12 February 2010].

SIGN (Scottish Intercollegiate Guidelines Network) (2010). *Non-pharmaceutical Management of Depression in Adults: A National Guideline.* Edinburgh: SIGN.

Spitzer RL, Kroenke K, Williams JBW & Löwe B (2006). A brief measure for assessing generalized anxiety disorder: the GAD-7. *Archives of Internal Medicine,* **166**, 1092–1097.

WHO (World Health Organisation) (2007). *International Classification of Disease, 10th Revision.* Geneva: WHO. Available from www.who.int [accessed 12 February 2010].

Williams MAH (2008). *Iechyd Meddwl Cymru: A Well Being and Mental Health Service Fit for Wales.* Cardiff: Welsh Assembly Government. Available from: www.wales.nhs.uk [accessed 12 February 2010].

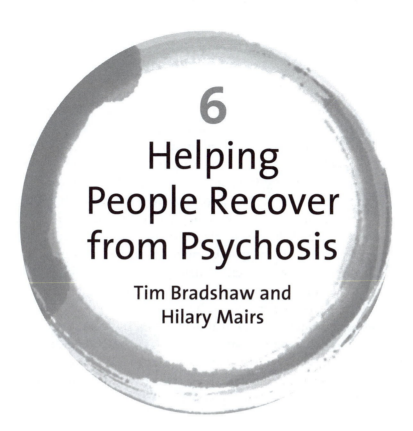

6

Helping People Recover from Psychosis

Tim Bradshaw and Hilary Mairs

What will I learn in this chapter?

The aim of this chapter is to examine optimal mental health nursing practice for people who require long-term support from mental health services because they experience psychosis as a relapsing or ongoing condition.

After reading this chapter, you will be able to:

- explain the context in which modern mental health services for people with psychosis are delivered;
- reflect on the nature and diversity of problems experienced by this group;
- describe evidence-based strategies that will enable you to work in collaboration with service users, their families and the wider community in order to reduce the distress and stigma associated with psychosis.

Introduction

A significant proportion of people with ongoing (or enduring) mental health needs who remain in long-term contact with mental health services are likely to have a case-note diagnosis of **schizophrenia**. This diagnostic category is, however, problematic and it has been argued that it lacks both scientific credibility and clinical utility (Bentall, 2004). Given the controversy surrounding the term, some commentators have suggested that schizophrenia is a redundant term that should be revised (Kingdon & Turkington, 2005). Even those who refute these challenges to the diagnosis concede that it is a heterogeneous disorder and that it may be more fruitful to research and work with individual symptom groups rather than the overall syndrome of schizophrenia. While we support the search for an alternative to the term 'schizophrenia', we are somewhat stuck for the time being as it is difficult to discuss relevant background, optimal treatment approaches and so on without referring to a body of literature that has the schizophrenia syndrome as its specific focus. So, while we prefer an approach that focuses upon individual symptoms or the arguably less stigmatising term **psychosis**, we have been forced at times to use the term schizophrenia.

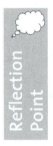

Schizophrenia

Take a moment to think what images, thoughts and feelings are conjured up for you by the word 'schizophrenia'. Where have you got these images, thoughts and feelings from? Have you been influenced by your friends and family? How do the media portray people with schizophrenia?

Onset, Cause and Course of Schizophrenia

Epidemiological data suggest that the prevalence of schizophrenia lies within the range of 1.4 to 4.6 per 1,000 and that the incidence is between 0.16 and 0.42 per 1,000 of the population (Jablensky, 2000). The incidence is higher in men and people living in urban areas (McGrath et al., 2004) and is influenced by ethnicity and social capital (Kirkbride et al., 2006, 2007). Kirkbride et al. (2006), for example, reported a higher incidence in London compared to two other less densely populated UK cities, reporting further (Kirkbride et al., 2007) that, even within London, variations exist between neighbourhoods.

A higher incidence is found in those areas with lower social capital (measured by voter turnout at local elections) and higher degrees of ethnic fragmentation (segregation of different ethnic groups within communities). Environmental factors, therefore, clearly affect levels of diagnosis; indeed, the role of environmental and social factors in the onset and course of psychosis will be reflected throughout this chapter.

Schizophrenia onset typically occurs in late adolescence/early adult life (Nadeem et al., 2004). The cause of onset is not well understood. Evidence does not point to any one single cause, but is thought to result from a complex interaction of multiple factors as conceptualised by early **stress–vulnerability** models (Zubin & Spring, 1977). Such models propose that onset is activated by an interaction between vulnerability factors and later experiences of stress. Vulnerability factors may be biological, psychological or social and may include genetic inheritance, Asian flu in pregnancy, cranial trauma during childbirth, abuse in childhood, migration and so on. Vulnerability, in turn, can be activated by life events that are stressful and/or traumatic. The degree and nature of stressors required to trigger underlying vulnerability will differ between individuals and the model suggests that people with higher risks of developing psychosis are those who are less resilient to the effects of stress.

Stress-vulnerability models have been influential in focusing attention beyond a single biological cause and, consequently, the development of non-drug treatments for psychosis. They are, however, subject to a number of limitations. One of the primary limitations of stress-vulnerability models is that while they help explain why some people develop psychosis, they do not explain why some people hear voices rather than develop strange, unusual beliefs or vice versa (Kingdon & Turkington, 2005). At the same time, we think that the emphasis on vulnerability can be a somewhat negative one and that it may be better to think of them as **stress–resilience** models. Such a move would be in line with current data that has challenged the view that schizophrenia has a chronic deteriorating course, highlighting instead a varied course that can be favourably influenced by a supportive social environment and access to a range of evidence-based pharmacological and psychosocial treatments (Malik et al., 2009).

Prejudice, Stigma and Social Exclusion

Negative opinions about mental health problems among the adult population of the UK appear to lie on a continuum with the more pronounced negative opinions being reserved for people who have a diagnosis of schizophrenia, and those who misuse alcohol and drugs (Crisp et al., 2000). For example, more than 70% of those interviewed reported that people with a diagnosis of schizophrenia were 'a danger to others' and half stated that this group would never recover. It is especially important for you to know that negative and pessimistic views about people with psychosis are also held by mental health professionals. Marwaha et al. (2009), for example, surveyed UK clinicians and found that they were pessimistic about people with psychosis being able to work in competitive employment settings. This is in spite of the fact that surveys suggest that people with psychosis want to work and there is no conclusive evidence that working precipitates relapse. However, one recent UK survey (O'Brien et al., 2002) found that 70% of people with a diagnosis of schizophrenia were unemployed and 54% had no social support, illustrating that it is not just work settings from which this group are socially excluded.

Reflection Point

Changing negative perceptions

In the previous reflection point we asked what images, thoughts and feelings the term 'schizophrenia' conjured up. Were those images, thoughts and feelings largely negative or largely positive?

If they were largely negative, do you think there is anything you could do to try to change your and other people's perceptions of people with schizophrenia?

Policy Context

For most of the twentieth century, services for people with psychosis were typically provided in large institutions geographically removed from the communities they served (Shorter, 1997). Driven by human rights concerns, developments in pharmacological treatments and the high cost of institutional care, the latter half of the twentieth century saw a shift to community mental health care and the closure of many of these institutions (DH, 1990). This change in the provision of care was not without its critics. It was argued that the community infrastructure was insufficiently developed, that money liberated from the large psychiatric hospitals would be spent by hospital management on other areas of healthcare (Leff et al., 2000) and that psychiatric nurses and other workers were inadequately prepared for their new roles

(Butterworth, 1994). In the 1990s, high profile (yet isolated) incidents such as the killing of Jonathon Zito by a man diagnosed with schizophrenia (Ritchie et al., 1994) led the then Health Minister for England, Frank Dobson, to conclude that 'community care had failed many vulnerable people' and to announce a root and branch reform of service provision for the mentally ill (BBC News, 1998). As a result, key policy documents for England were published including the *National Service Framework for Mental Health* (DH, 1999) and the NHS Plan (DH, 2000). Elsewhere in the UK, Scotland had already published its policy recommendations a year or so earlier (Scottish Office, 1997) while Wales and Northern Ireland published their recommendations a few years later (Welsh Assembly Government, 2002; DHSSPS, 2005).

The English policy documents proposed an increase in spending on mental health of £700 million. In relation to people with psychosis, they recommended increased provision of secure hospital beds and the development of a network of specialised community services across England including: (1) **assertive outreach** teams for people with complex needs; (2) **early intervention** teams for young people with first episode psychosis; and (3) **crisis resolution/ home treatment** teams. These recommendations were supported by a set of policy implementation guidelines (DH, 2001) and have been mirrored, to some extent, elsewhere in the UK. Further guidance regarding the specific services these teams should provide is summarised in the National Institute of Health and Clinical Excellence (NICE) guidance for schizophrenia (NICE, 2009). Key NICE recommendations are discussed in more detail in the evidence-based interventions part of this chapter. At this stage, however, it is worth mentioning that there has been a shift towards the inclusion of **psychosocial** treatments and the current expectation is that hope and optimism should pervade mental health services for people with psychosis rather than the pessimistic views that are still held by the general public and, sadly, some mental health practitioners. Indeed, both England (*New Horizons*; HM Government, 2009) and Scotland (*Towards a Mentally Flourishing Scotland*; Scottish Government, 2009) have recently launched new mental health strategies which, as well as building upon the progress made by their respective former strategies, incorporate this much more positive view of mental health.

Typical Presenting Problems in Those with Psychosis

The problems experienced by people with psychosis vary considerably from individual to individual and it is difficult to summarise typical presenting problems. Each individual with psychosis will present with his or her own unique combination of symptoms, the pattern and course of which is influenced by their individual circumstances (NICE, 2009). For some people with psychosis, their main problems will be solely related to the symptoms they experience, but for others it may be the side effects of the medication they are prescribed, the difficulty in finding socially inclusive activities or low self-esteem triggered by societal perceptions of psychosis. The presenting problems discussed in this section should not, therefore, be considered an exhaustive list of the problems faced by people with psychosis.

It has become customary, though somewhat simplistic, to view these symptoms as falling into the two key domains of **positive** and **negative** symptoms (Jones et al., 2004). These labels were not applied because positive symptoms are 'good' and negative symptoms are 'bad' (as lay people may understandably think), but because positive symptoms were judged 'additional' (+, plus) to the usual range of human experiences and negative symptoms reflect things that are 'taken away' (−, minus). The symptoms are summarised in Table 6.1 and are discussed in more detail in the following sections.

TABLE 6.1   Positive and negative symptoms

Positive (+) symptoms	Negative (−) symptoms
Additional to the usual range of human experience	Lessened when considering the usual range of human experience
<ul><li>delusions (unusual thoughts)</li><li>hallucinations (disturbances in perception)<ul><li>– visual</li><li>– auditory ('hearing voices')</li><li>– olfactory/gustatory (smell/taste)</li><li>– tactile ('skin crawling')</li></ul></li></ul>	<ul><li>alogia (reduction in the expression of thoughts)</li><li>affective flattening/blunting (reduction in the expression of feelings)</li><li>avolition (decreases in activity levels)</li></ul>

Positive symptoms

Positive psychotic symptoms include unusual thoughts, which are referred to as **delusions**, and disturbances in perception, called **hallucinations**. Common delusions observed in people with psychosis include **paranoid** or **persecutory delusions**, with people believing, for example, that others are plotting to harm or even kill them, and **delusions of reference** whereby people believe that special messages are being communicated from media such as television and radio (Morrison et al., 2004).

Historically, delusions were thought to be false, fixed beliefs, which were held with absolute conviction (believed 100% of the time) and which could not be challenged even in the face of overwhelming evidence to disprove them (Kingdon & Turkington, 2005). More recently, this idea has been challenged. We know, for example, that lots of people who do not have psychosis hold 'unscientific' beliefs for which there is no evidence. For example, in one survey of the UK general population, Cox & Cowling (1989) found that more than 50% of people believed in thought transference between people, 50% believed that it was possible to predict future events and more than 25% believed in ghosts.

Discussion Point

Who's delusional?

A Roman Catholic nun tells you that she believes the Virgin Mary is within her.

A woman with a history of schizophrenia tells you that she believes the Virgin Mary is within her.

Which of these two women is delusional? Is it the nun, the woman with a history of schizophrenia, both or neither? What factors influence your answers to these questions?

There is also evidence from a significant number of research studies that levels of conviction in delusions vary at different times. Hence, some people may totally believe that they are being followed when out in public and feeling anxious, but be less convinced that this is true when sat at home watching television in a relaxed atmosphere with close friends. Data further suggest that delusional beliefs are not necessarily fixed; for instance people who participate in therapies such as cognitive behavioural therapy (CBT) may be helped to reappraise their beliefs and find alternative explanations for the events around them (see, for example, Sensky et al., 2000).

Hallucinations are experiences that have the compellingly real sense of a true perception, but occur in the absence of any identifiable external source (Andreasen, 1984a). Hallucinations may occur in any sensory modality but by far the most commonly observed in people with psychosis are **auditory hallucinations**, or the **hearing of voices** (Morrison et al., 2004). The voices heard may be of either gender, familiar or unfamiliar, critical or complimentary. Typically the voices heard by people with psychosis are experienced as unpleasant and negative. Some people hear voices that provide a running commentary on their behaviour or two voices that talk to each other, usually discussing the individual concerned and often in a derogatory way (Andreasen, 1984a).

The view that hallucinations are only experienced by people with a psychosis-related diagnosis is now disputed. Voice-hearing is relatively common in members of the general population who do not come into contact with mental health services (Honig et al.,1998). Studies have found that people in hostage situations, those deprived of sleep and people who are recently bereaved may also hear voices (Kingdon & Turkington, 2005). It has been speculated that the reason why some people require support from mental health services whereas others do not relates to the beliefs held about the voices and the degree of distress they cause. For example, two people may hear a voice they attribute to a recently deceased relative: one may find it reassuring to hear guidance from a loved one; the other, in contrast, may feel they have no control over a voice that is present all of the time and subsequently find it extremely distressing.

Negative symptoms

Negative symptoms relate to behaviours that are normally present in a 'healthy' population but are reduced or absent in psychosis (Stahl & Buckley, 2007). Negative symptoms include a reduction in the expression of thoughts (referred to as **alogia** in the literature) and feelings (described as **affective flattening** or blunting), and a decrease in activity levels (**avolition**). Since negative symptoms represent something that is missing rather than something that is present, they are difficult to detect and are often missed or misunderstood by healthcare professionals (Stahl & Buckley, 2007). It has been suggested that even people who experience negative symptoms often fail to recognise them or are indifferent to the limited expression of thoughts and feelings or the reduced activity levels they experience. Indeed, some have suggested that negative symptoms cause more problems and dissatisfaction for family and friends rather than the individual themselves (Winograd-Gurvich et al., 2006). Nevertheless, there is a growing awareness that people with negative symptoms are aware of them and that they do find them distressing (Selten et al., 1993).

The impact of negative symptoms can be far-reaching. Negative symptoms have not received the same research attention that positive symptoms have and are less well understood (Stahl & Buckley, 2007). It is likely, however, that people experience negative symptoms to different degrees. It has been suggested that for some people a complete 'shut-down' of thoughts and feelings may be a necessary part of recovery after a psychotic episode, in the same way that people often take time to recuperate after a physical health problem (Watkins,

1996). However, for other people, finding it hard to communicate what they are thinking and feeling or to motivate themselves to get up and take part in routine activities can cause stress and distress (Selten et al., 1993). Limited activity levels may also be implicated in the poor physical health often seen in people with schizophrenia, an issue we will discuss shortly.

Thought disorder

Another category of symptoms that is associated with psychosis is called **thought disorder**. Thought disorder is manifested in disorganised thought and speech patterns. People with thought disorder may give responses to questions in an oblique or irrelevant way, jump between different topics in a conversation or make up new words. Table 6.2 lists some of the most common manifestations of thought disorder.

TABLE 6.2   Common manifestations of thought disorder (after Andreasen, 1979)

Type	Details	Examples
Pressure of speech	Over-talkativeness; rapid and frenzied speech	
Tangentiality	Replying to questions in an oblique, tangential or irrelevant manner	Q: 'What's your name?' A: 'Ah, well, that would be telling. It's not Mary or Joseph. Is it Jesus? You tell me.'
Knight's move thinking (derailment)	Jumping from one topic to another in a unrelated or barely related manner (cf. the way a Knight moves in chess)	'I need to go to the shop to get some milk ... Is Cowes on the Isle of Wight? Scotland is cold, you know.'
Word salad (incoherence)	Real words are strung together in an unintelligible manner	'There is nothing like office cars to help me when I'm falling with junior creators. I've got vision in my party rats.'
Neologisms	New words are used	'It's bestinkingall here.' 'Please, I need help finding my ingootuber.'
Echolalia	Repeating the speech of others or yourself	Q: 'How are you today?' A: 'I'm not so good. How are you today? How are you today? How are you today?'
Blocking	Train of speech is interrupted mid sentence (there's usually an embarrassing pause)	
Clang association (clanging)	The sounds of words rather than their meaning governs speech	'I live in Manchester with Uncle Fester and I am bester because of it.'

Associated problems

The 'true' symptoms of psychosis (positive and negative symptoms, and thought disorder) will vary considerably between individuals, as will the degree of distress and disruption related to them. At the same time, there are a number of other difficulties associated with a diagnosis of schizophrenia which mental health nurses need to take into account. These are discussed below.

Anxiety and depression

Given the content of the unusual beliefs and/or voices that people with psychosis experience, it is not surprising that everyday functioning is disrupted and, as such, levels of depression and anxiety are high in this group, as are rates of suicide (Siris, 2001). It is also important to recognise that people may become low in mood and anxious as a result of other factors, such as high levels of criticism, stigma and social exclusion. We have already highlighted how people may become distressed as a result of worrying delusional beliefs and how stigma can generate anxiety for some people. There is also a growing awareness that levels of post-traumatic stress disorder (PTSD) are high in this group (Frame & Morrison, 2001). Although the specific trauma may date back to an individual's childhood or early adult life, the trauma can be related to the experience of developing psychosis and/or the way services respond. For example, a compulsory admission to hospital under mental health legislation[1] may be traumatic event for many – if not most – people. The view that services and treatments themselves can have unintended and unwanted consequences is explored further in the discussion on physical health in the next subsection.

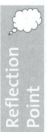

Reflection Point

Anxious thoughts

How anxious would you feel if you were absolutely convinced that there was a plot to assassinate you and you found evidence to support this belief every time you left the house?

How you would feel if you repeatedly heard a voice that told you you were useless, there was no point trying to do anything because you would fail, and that no one liked you?

---

[1] The various UK Mental Health Acts are discussed in more detail in the next chapter.

Physical health of people with schizophrenia

There is now clear evidence that people with a diagnosis of schizophrenia have a reduced life expectancy of approximately 15 years compared to others in the general population (Brown et al., 2000). Furthermore, although rates of suicide are high in people with schizophrenia (Siris, 2001) approximately two-thirds of 'excess' mortality in this group can be attributed to deaths from natural causes (Bradshaw et al., 2005). Two key factors appear to account for the poor physical health of this group: an **unhealthy lifestyle** and the **side-effects of neuro-leptic medication**. People diagnosed with schizophrenia generally eat a less healthy diet, take less exercise and are twice as likely to smoke than others in the general population. They are significantly more likely to be overweight or obese (Brown, 2006), a problem that may be due to poor diet, but is compounded by the side-effects of the medications frequently prescribed for psychosis. One study found that 91% of a group of people experiencing a first episode of psychosis who were prescribed a commonly used drug, olanzepine, had gained more that 7% of their baseline body weight one year after commencing the medication. The average weight gain was around 37 lb (2.5 stones or 17 kg; Strassnig et al., 2007). Clearly, the impact of such rapid weight gain on both physical and mental health is likely to be a negative one.

Substance use

People with a diagnosis of schizophrenia often use illicit substances and/or drink alcohol to excess (Holland, 2002), a presentation often referred to as **dual diagnosis**. As well as impacting upon their physical health, such drug and alcohol use may exacerbate mental state; indeed, for some people, substance use – cannabis especially – has been implicated in the onset of psychosis. Higher levels of substance use present a barrier to engaging people in treatment approaches, as people may forget appointments, not be able to concentrate in sessions or forget what has been discussed. Dual diagnosis is considered in more detail in Chapter 11.

Relations with family and friends: expressed emotion

The concept of **expressed emotion** originated in research into the relationship between people with schizophrenia and their families after discharge from hospital (Bebbington & Kuipers, 1994). The term is used to describe the emotional climate within the home environment. Research suggests that people in regular contact with high expressed emotion relatives (marked by high levels of **criticism**, **hostility** and/or **emotional over-involvement**) are exposed to a greater risk of relapse. Interest in the climate within the family home prompted the development of family-based treatment approaches that were originally designed to reduce levels of expressed emotion and hence prevent or delay relapse. We will discuss these treatment approaches in further detail later. Early studies into these treatment approaches suggested that they were beneficial and more recent research has suggested that there may be other positive outcomes such as reduced levels of burden on family carers (Pilling et al., 2002).

Unfortunately, expressed emotion is now often misused as a term and is sometimes applied as a negative judgement on families who may be experiencing difficulty in coping with the effects of psychosis. This is unhelpful as it can encourage barriers between mental health professionals and family members. At the same time, given the nature of psychosis, it is not surprising that relatives may become critical (of a relative who stays in bed until late afternoon, for example) or over-involved (by monitoring the medication of a relative who has taken an overdose, for example). Acknowledging that such responses are understandable can be an important first step in beginning to work collaboratively with family members.

 Case scenario: expressed emotion

As a community mental health nurse, you make a routine home visit to Chris, a 23-year-old man diagnosed with schizophrenia while at university a few years ago. He has had one or two episodes of paranoia in the past (all of them leading to hospitalisation) but his positive symptoms seem well controlled, a fact his mother – Dianne – puts down to compliance with his depot medication.

Chris displays mainly negative symptoms such as lying in bed until late in the afternoon, having little interest in any activities other than passively watching TV or playing on his games console in his room. Dianne is very supportive of Chris but she is so worried that he will relapse if he doesn't have his medication that she feels she has to constantly monitor him. Dianne's husband, Dave (who is Chris' stepfather), says Dianne interferes too much in Chris' life and she should 'let him be' and get on with her own life. You know Dianne well as she's almost always there when you visit and she nearly always speaks on Chris' behalf when you're assessing his progress. She despairs of Chris' lying in bed all day and is constantly fussing around him to 'do something'. Chris says (affectionately) that she never stops nagging him.

On arrival, you find Dianne really upset. She says she had attended a local support group for families and friends of people with mental health problems and remembers someone talking about 'high expressed emotion'. She's been reading about it on the Internet. She says it means she's a 'bad mother' and it's her fault that Chris got schizophrenia.

What can you do to reassure Dianne?

(We will revisit this scenario later.)

Assessing Individuals with Psychosis

Given the diversity of problems faced by people with psychosis, the focus of assessment is likely to be broad and take some time. Indeed assessment should continue throughout a course of treatment, as levels of symptoms, distress and disruption to functioning may change over time.

As you will recall from Chapter 2, the process of engagement and assessment should start with the development of a **therapeutic relationship** and the formation of **trust**. This may present some challenges when working with someone who has psychosis. For example, the service user may be distracted by voices they are hearing which may be telling them not to answer any questions or they may be worried that they are 'going mad' and will be taken to a locked ward if they disclose too much information. People with marked negative symptoms may find to difficult to answer questions at any great length. Consequently it may take longer to complete a thorough assessment. We find it important not to rush through assessment schedules and questioning, and to take some time to engage in conversation about non-mental health topics. From the first meeting, it is important to **instil hope**, but refrain from making unrealistic promises.

All meetings or sessions should begin with a simple explanation of the purpose of the meeting and what will happen afterwards. Remember some people may be paranoid and it is important to give a clear rationale as to why you want to find out what has been happening for them and also, why you might want to take notes, for example. The extent of **confidentiality** should be made explicit. We recommend avoiding jargon and clinical language, particularly the term schizophrenia (given its negative connotations), and listening carefully to find a common language to help you develop a shared understanding of the particular problems that have brought the person into contact with mental health services. In contrast to other mental health problems, some people with psychosis may be introduced to services because

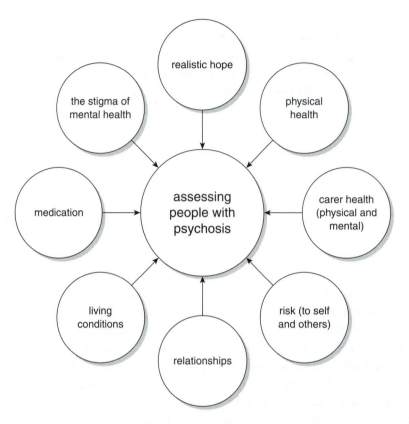

FIGURE 6.1   Things to consider when assessing people with psychosis

other people are concerned about them and their behaviour and the service user may not think that they require mental health nursing input.

The structure of each meeting should be individually tailored for each service user. As well as providing a simple explanation of the purpose of the meeting, it can be beneficial to negotiate how long the session will last, and whether the service user would like to take a break at anytime. Providing regular summaries of what you think you have heard and checking out its accuracy is particularly important with this group of service users as some of the discussion may be highly unusual or even bizarre, and it will help the service user feel listened to.

We recommend a process of assessment that begins with a global (overall) assessment of need and potential symptoms and then funnels down to explore, in further details, the *specific* needs and/or symptoms that appear to be problematic. The introduction of any assessment schedule should be preceded by a clear rationale and explanation of what will happen to the information that is elicited. Remember to show genuine curiosity and interest in the service user's experiences to avoid turning the assessment into an interrogation.

Needs assessment

People with long-term psychotic conditions frequently have multiple unmet health and social needs. Unmet needs can generate stress, which as we highlighted earlier, can have a detrimental effect on their mental state. There are a number of needs assessments available and some services have adapted schedules for their own purposes.

The **Camberwell Assessment of Need** (CAN; Phelan et al., 1995) is a global assessment of need that is widely used. It assesses 22 areas of psychosocial need, but is relatively quick to administer (taking around 25 minutes). Each item is scored on a three-point scale, which indicates whether there is no problem in that specific area, that there is a problem but resources are available to help overcome it, or that there is an unmet need that requires attention. Both the service user and a 'reliable other' can be interviewed using the CAN if it is suspected that the person may have an unrealistic view of their own needs. Where unmet needs are identified, an action plan should be drafted. This plan might indicate the need for further detailed assessment or a specific intervention to meet the need.

It is beyond the scope of this chapter to discuss further assessments for all 22 of the needs areas that the CAN deals with, so we will concentrate on the three most commonly occurring problems: **symptoms**, **medication side-effects** and **physical health**. We will refer to some validated assessment schedules, but it should be noted that these are by no means the only tools available for further assessing these areas. Other important aspects of assessment, such as **signs of relapse** and **coping strategies** for dealing with distressing symptoms, will be discussed later in the section on evidence-based interventions. **Risk** is also an important issue and warrants a brief comment here. Assessment schedules in common use in psychosis are summarised in Table 6.3 and discussed in more detail in the remainder of this section.

Assessing risk
All mental health assessments should include attention to any risks that may be present. Given the increased rates of suicide in this client group, risk of self-harm should be assessed and any identified risk monitored and managed. Risk to the safety of others, particularly in people with a forensic history, will also need to be assessed. We do not cover this in any detail here, as services usually have their own well-defined risk assessment and management

TABLE 6.3   Some commonly used assessment tools in psychosis

Type of assessment	Name of assessment	Originators
1. Global assessment of needs		
	CAN – Camberwell Assessment of Needs	Phelan et al. (1995)
2. Specific assessment tools		
Broad-based symptom scales	KGV-M – Krawiecka, Goldberg & Vaughn Symptom Scale, Modified Version	Krawiecka et al. (1977); Lancashire (1998)
	PANSS – Positive and Negative Syndrome Scale	Kay et al. (1987)
	SAPS – Scale for the Assessment of Positive Symptoms	Andreasen (1984a)
	SANS – Scale for the Assessment of Negative Symptoms	Andreasen (1984b)
Specific symptom scales	PSYRATS – Psychiatric Rating Scales for auditory hallucinations and delusional beliefs	Haddock et al. (1999)
	SENS – Subjective Experience of Negative Symptoms	Selten et al. (1993)
Medication side-effects	LUNSERS – Liverpool University Side Effects Rating Scale	Day et al. (1995)
Physical health	PHC – Physical Health Check	Phelan et al. (2004)

procedures that they expect all staff to observe. Risk (especially in relation to forensic environments) is discussed in detail in Chapter 12.

Assessing symptoms

People with long-term psychosis will experience a diverse range of symptoms, not all of which will cause distress. We recommend therefore that a broad-based assessment is used in the first instance to determine which commonly reported symptoms are experienced by each service user. Additional assessments can then be introduced to explore in further detail whether the symptom is problematic for the service user or their family/friends, how often it is experienced, how distressing it is for them and so on. Broad-based symptom assessments commonly used in practice and research settings at the present time include (see Table 6.3) the **KGV-M**, the **PANSS**, the **SAPS** and its complement, the **SANS**. Many service providers now stipulate which measures of mental state are to be used and provide training for new staff to ensure that they use these measures reliably.

Results from broad-based symptom schedules will usually indicate areas for further assessment. More detailed assessment of positive symptoms (again, see

Table 6.3) can be completed via the **PSYRATS**. The PSYRATS assesses a wide range of the phenomenological aspects of both voices and delusions including volume of voices, beliefs about origin, distress and disruption to daily living caused by symptoms. Advantages of the PSYRATS include the detailed understanding of psychotic symptoms they elicit and the fact that they can be used to monitor symptom changes during the course of treatment. The **SENS** is a detailed schedule which provides a subjective account of the level of distress and disruption experienced in relation to any negative symptoms identified.

Assessing medication side-effects

Both the newer and more traditional medications prescribed for schizophrenia have potential side-effects and it is important that these are assessed soon after medication is commenced and then monitored regularly over time. By far the most user-friendly instrument for assessing side-effects is the **LUNSERS** (again, see Table 6.3). Originally developed to assess side-effects in first-generation anti-psychotics, the LUNSERS has also been used in studies investigating side-effects in second-generation medications (Jung et al., 2005). It can be filled in by service users on their own or with help from the assessor and takes between 5 and 20 minutes to complete. It is a 51-item self-report questionnaire containing 41 questions relating to seven major groups of neuroleptic side-effects and ten 'red herring' questions relating to symptoms not known to be side-effects of neuro-leptics. Each of the 51 items is rated on a five-point frequency scale where the service user is required to indicate how often they have experienced that side-effect ranging from 0 (not at all) to 4 (very much). Having completed the LUNSERS, side-effect scores for each of the seven key areas should be calcu-lated, followed by discussion with the service user about how much discomfort or distress each side-effect causes them. Where side-effects are particularly prob-lematic, discussion with the prescribing clinician about changes to the service user's medication regimen may be required. Note that service users who score highly on the red herring questions may well have exaggerated their symptoms in general (the point of such questions is to improve the accuracy of tests like the LUNSERS after all) and, where this is the case, care should be taken when interpreting the LUNSERS results for the seven key areas.

Physical health assessment

Given the generally poor physical health of people with schizophrenia, the routine monitoring of the physical health of this client group is an important task for mental health nurses. The **PHC** is a tool that helps identify unmet physical health needs and an action plan to address these needs. The PHC assesses medical history, current treatments, lifestyle factors, physical symptoms (via a checklist), when screening checks such as cholesterol levels were last undertaken, body mass index, waist circumference, blood pressure and urinalysis. Any mental health professional can use the PHC without special training as long as they read the guidance notes supplied (these are available on the RETHINK website; see the list of Web resources at the end of this chapter). It is not intended that mental health professionals will carry out further investigations themselves but that they explore areas of unmet need with the service user and draw up an action plan to address these areas. The PHC takes a maximum of 30 minutes to complete.

 Case scenario: assessing psychosis

A GP refers Albert, a 52-year-old man, to you as a member of a Community Mental Health Team. The GP informs you that Albert is prescribed 2.5 mg of lorazepam per day and he would like you to help him to withdraw from this. During your first home visit to meet Albert you find he lives alone in a very poorly maintained and dirty ground floor flat. He has no furniture and sleeps on a pile of old clothes and blankets. He lives of a diet of pork pies and cold baked beans. There are cat faeces all over the floor of the flat.

Albert tells you that he used to be 'very ill' but is alright now. As a younger man he received inpatient mental health treatment on over 20 occasions and has made several serious suicide attempts. Eight years ago Albert stopped attending the psychiatric outpatient department and the service failed to follow him up in the community. In addition to lorazepam, he is prescribed temazepam 20 mg and haloperidol 5 mg twice a day. He often takes the temazepam in the middle of the day and then wakes in the early hours of the morning. He says his only symptoms now are hearing voices occasionally, but they do not cause him any distress.

On further inquiry you find out that he has previously been referred to social services on several occasions but, having been assessed, they decided that the way he lives is a 'lifestyle choice' and they decided not to intervene.

Your initial thoughts are that, while the positive symptoms of Albert's illness might be much less acute than when he was younger, his ability for self-care is being severely affected by negative symptoms.

What assessments might it be appropriate for you to complete with Albert to either confirm or eliminate your hypothesis?

What information do you think you might need to convey to social services as a result of your assessment?

Evidence-Based Interventions for Psychosis

The primary treatment for psychosis remains antipsychotic medication, although recent developments in psychological and psychosocial treatments now offer additional treatment choices (NICE, 2009). This is an important point since even when people are compliant with medication regimes, they often continue to experience symptoms (Kane et al., 1996) and the side-effects of some medications, such as weight gain, may be unpalatable for some people. At the same time, service users and their families are increasingly demanding access to a greater repertoire of treatments. In the following section we review the evidence for psychosocial treatment approaches with this service user group, providing details of several evidence-based interventions that we think are vital to mental health nursing practice.

Psychosocial interventions

Current evidence (e.g. NICE, 2009) suggests that the optimal psychosocial treatments for psychosis are individual **cognitive behavioural therapy** (CBT) and **family intervention** (FI).

As you will recall from Chapters 1 and 4, CBT is a psychological treatment based on the premise that thoughts, feelings and behaviour are interrelated and that changing thoughts and/or behaviour can lead to positive shifts in feelings. CBT was originally devised as a treatment for depression, but has since evolved as the treatment of choice for a range of other mental health problems, including psychosis. At the time of writing, data from more than 30 randomised controlled trials are available and meta-analysis of these trials generally concurs that CBT is effective in reducing the positive symptoms associated with schizophrenia (Wykes et al., 2008).

Family intervention is a structured approach to working with service users and their families. Models of family intervention differ in their emphasis but share a number of key features including **information sharing**, **stress management** and **goal planning**. Interventions are delivered in regular meetings with family members, either as a single family or in multiple family groups. A series of well-designed randomised controlled trials have found participation in family work to be associated with a reduced risk of relapse for the service user and some suggest that there may be benefits for other family members as well (Pilling et al., 2002).

The weight of the evidence has led to NICE (2009) recommending that all people with a diagnosis of schizophrenia be offered a programme of CBT and, for those in regular contact with family members, a course of family intervention. In making these recommendations, NICE notes that specialist training is required to facilitate FI and CBT competently, but that there is insufficient data to judge the precise level of training required. It is likely that some of the questions will be addressed in the near future and some mental health nurses may opt to undertake further training in these therapies. However, not all nurses will want to pursue this route and it is important to note that comprehensive services for people with psychosis need to offer a broader base of interventions. This is reflected in the limited external validity (generalisability) of the clinical trials that have evaluated psychosocial interventions for psychosis. For example, the studies that have evaluated CBT have often excluded people who use substances, have pronounced negative symptoms or are subject to detention under mental health legislation. Unlike these trials, mental health nurses do not exclude people with these characteristics from their caseloads and, as such, they need to be able to develop treatment plans for these service user groups.

In the family work literature, there is an acknowledgement that even when the therapy is provided by experts, many families either do not want the intervention when it is offered or they drop out of treatment (Mairs & Bradshaw, 2005a). These limitations suggest that while CBT and FI are effective in research settings, their usefulness in routine practice may be compromised. This is perhaps one reason why these evidence-based treatment approaches have not yet been widely disseminated (Tarrier, 2005). While further training is required to deliver CBT and FI in line with the NICE (2009) recommendations, both treatment approaches offer a number of components which nurses may find beneficial when working with people with psychosis and their families. We have identified four key components of psychosocial interventions which we think are relatively straightforward and do not require intensive training: (1) **information sharing** (psychoeducation); (2) **coping strategy enhancement** for distressing positive symptoms; (3) **behavioural activation** (sometimes referred to as activity scheduling) for negative symptoms and/or depression; and (4) **relapse prevention strategies**. Each of these treatment approaches is summarised below, together with details of further resources to support their application in routine practice.

Information sharing

A key skill for all professionals working with people with psychosis is the timely provision of accurate and appropriate information. Historically, the aspects of any intervention that relate to the provision of information and education to service users and their families about the diagnosis, treatment, resources, prognosis, and so on has been termed **psychoeducation** (Pekkala & Merinder, 2002). There is good evidence that the provision of such information is helpful for people experiencing a range of physical and mental health conditions. However, there are also data to suggest that there may be negative effects associated with the provision of information in psychosis. Psychoeducation has been associated with an increase in suicidal thinking (Cunningham-Owens et al., 2001) and depression (Rathod et al., 2003) in schizophrenia. This may be due to the highly stigmatising nature of the diagnosis and common myths about a uniformly poor prognosis or a link with dangerousness. Earlier, we recommended avoiding using the term schizophrenia and, further, that clinical language and jargon should be kept to a minimum. At the same time, we prefer the term **information sharing** to psychoeducation, as it does not conjure up images of teachers in classrooms imparting expert knowledge. Instead it allows for information sharing to be mutual (after all service users and families are the experts in their experience of living with psychosis), individualised and based upon what people have already been told or their existing (potentially culturally diverse) beliefs about mental health problems (Barrowclough & Tarrier, 1997).

When working with people with psychosis, information sharing can operate on a number of different levels: we might share information about psychosis (its onset, cause and so on), or supply information about treatments (including medications) or, in light of the poor physical health of this group, health education may be important.

Sharing information about psychosis

We have adopted the 'normalising' approach to information sharing in psychosis introduced by Kingdon & Turkington (1994, 2005). Underpinning the approach is a philosophy that we all are at risk of developing psychosis and, therefore, the people who do are not different from us, but have different experiences or maybe experience them to a different degree (Kingdon & Turkington, 2005). This normalisation approach has long been recognised in relation to the common mental health problems of anxiety and depression (see Chapters 4 and 5), but has only recently been accepted (at least in some circles) in psychosis. This shift has been generated by the findings regarding the incidence of psychotic phenomena in the general population highlighted earlier in this chapter. Indeed, studies now report this in samples of mental health professionals. For example, in a recent study of nurses and other mental health professionals in Scotland, 16% reported hearing voices and 21% indicated that they had experienced delusions (Fleming & Martin, 2009).

The specific content of the information shared should primarily be determined by what service users and families request, but useful topics include discussing the onset and course of psychosis within a stress–vulnerability (or resilience) framework and sharing information about 'normal' circumstances in which psychotic symptoms can occur. For example, people in stressful situations such as hostage situations often report hearing voices, as do people who are deprived of sleep. Of course, it is important not to minimise the distress that people with psychosis experience. Instead, normalisation should promote understanding of psychotic experiences, reduce worries and fears relating to 'going mad' and set the scene for later intervention.

One of the aims of information sharing is to help service users and their families make sense of the experiences that can be difficult to understand and extremely distressing. It may well be the negative symptoms associated with a diagnosis of schizophrenia that families find difficult to cope with, possibly because they attribute them to personality characteristics rather than to the illness. Helping families to understand that their relative is not being lazy, but that negative symptoms are common in psychosis, can reduce levels of criticism which, in turn, reduces stress for the service user.

Education about medication and general health

People with psychosis and their families often ask for further information about the medication that has been prescribed, or indeed alternatives that may be available. Consequently, mental health nurses need to remain up to date with research findings about which medications seemed to work best and also any associated side-effects. It is helpful that bodies like NICE summarise the research evidence pertaining to optimal pharmacological and psychosocial treatment. The NHS-approved website www.choiceandmedication.org.uk is also helpful when it comes to educating service users and their families about medication.

In light of the poor physical health and premature mortality of this group, information about healthy living, diet, exercise and so on should be offered regularly. At the same time, information about local resources, exercise facilities and services to help people stop smoking should be made widely available.

Educating the general public

We have focused above on sharing information with individual service users and their families, but we think it is important to highlight the role of all mental health professionals in challenging the myths and stereotypes that persist about all mental health problems, but seem particularly loaded and detrimental in relation to psychosis and schizophrenia. Although hampered by a powerful mass media that is often hostile to people with psychosis, the mental health charities MIND and RETHINK are determined to educate the public about mental health issues in general. In particular, their *Time to Change* campaign has been at the forefront of challenging myths and stereotypes associated with mental health, and mental health nurses would certainly benefit from exploring the website www.time-to-change.org.uk.

Coping strategies for dealing with distressing symptoms

Studies have shown that people who experience psychotic symptoms develop naturalistic coping strategies to help to reduce the associated distress (Tarrier, 1987). These may be positive and active (e.g. physical activity) or negative and passive (e.g. alcohol misuse). Examples of the types of coping strategies reported by service users in research studies are illustrated in Table 6.4. As can be seen, a wide variety of strategies have been described and they seem to be highly idiosyncratic; thus, what works for one person may make another's symptoms worse.

In a series of studies, Tarrier and colleagues investigated whether service users could be trained to use coping strategies in a systematic way and whether this use would result in a reduction in positive symptoms (Tarrier et al., 1993, 1998). The results of the research were positive, with a significant

TABLE 6.4 Examples of coping strategies used in psychosis

Type of coping strategy	Examples
Cognitive	Attention switching Attention narrowing Self-instruction
Behavioural	Increasing solitary activities Increasing social interaction Social disengagement Reality testing
Physiological	Relaxation Controlled breathing
Counter stimulation	Turning the radio on Listening to music through headphones Ear plugs

number of participants in both studies reporting a 50% or more reduction in symptoms. The main components of **coping strategy enhancement** (CSE), as Tarrier and colleagues call it, are outlined below.

Coping strategy enhancement

The first stage of CSE is to perform an assessment of the positive psychotic symptoms which the service user experiences. A target symptom is then collaboratively identified; this is normally the symptom which causes the most distress. A more detailed analysis of the target symptom is completed focusing particularly on what triggers the symptom and how the service user responds to it emotionally and behaviourally. If the person is already using coping strategies, an analysis of their effectiveness and how consistently the person applies them is completed. A **formulation** is then developed with the service user which helps to explain the development and maintenance of the symptom. A rationale for developing existing coping strategies and exploring new ones is provided (see Box 6.1 for an example); this rationale may need to include a discussion of the need to drop existing coping strategies, such as shouting back at voices if the formulation suggests this is actually making them worse.

Box 6.1   Example of a rationale for coping strategy enhancement

'Many people who experience unpleasant voices or worrying beliefs find that certain things they do can help make them less distressing, however these things vary from person to person. What I would like us to do is explore how you currently respond to your voices/beliefs and then test out other ways of responding to see if you find them helpful. How does that sound to you?'

If the service user accepts the rationale you can begin to explore with them alternative coping strategies for their symptoms, such as those outlined in Table 6.4. Once a suitable coping strategy has been identified the service user should be taught to apply the strategy within the relative safety of the interview/session before being encouraged to practise it in the real world. Goals for practising the coping strategy between sessions should be negotiated and the service user should be encouraged to keep a diary that lists occasions and situations when the target symptom occurred, how they coped with it and what level of distress they experienced on each occasion. At the next session, the effectiveness of the coping strategy should be reviewed. If the service user has found it helpful, try to establish *why* it was helpful by referring back to the formulation. This may help the service user learn important lessons such as 'high levels of noise make my symptoms worse' which can then be applied to other aspects of their lives.

CSE in the format described above is a relatively skilled and complex intervention that should be undertaken only by someone with CBT training. However, in its simplest form – that is to say helping service users explore whether changing their behaviour reduces the distress they experience as a result of symptoms – can be safely practised by even novice mental health workers. Things that we have found useful for people in the past include **listening to music on an MP3 player** to help with voices, **keeping busy** to prevent rumination about distressing beliefs and **carrying a mobile phone** to talk into should someone feel compelled to respond to their voices in public situations.

Behavioural activation

As you will recall from Chapter 4, behavioural activation (BA) is an intervention that has been found to be effective in treating depression (Dimidjian et al., 2006). Because depression shares overlapping features with negative symptoms, it has been suggested that BA (which is also referred to as **activity scheduling** in the literature) may be a useful treatment for negative symptoms. Although evidence for this approach is sparse, it is included here because: (1) there is a paucity of evidence for treatments for negative symptoms; (2) many people with psychosis experience depression and there is evidence for BA in depression; and (3) increasing activity levels is an important strategy in counteracting the poor physical health of this population.

The brief review of the treatment presented here is based upon the techniques outlined by Lejuez et al. (2001) and Richards et al. (2008), which have recently been synthesised into a manual of BA for negative symptoms (Mairs et al., 2006). In its simplest form, the treatment is comprised of four stages or steps, which are summarised in Figure 6.2.

As with all nursing interventions, a clear explanation of the treatment and what it entails should be offered to the service user.

In the **first step**, people are encouraged to keep a diary (like the one in Figure 6.3) of their current weekly routine. The aim of this is to gather a baseline of their current activity levels and also help them begin to think about what they like about their weekly routine and what they would like

Step 1	Step 2	Step 3	Step 4
			How can I start to include them in my weekly routine?
	What would I like to be doing?	Which of these activities are the easiest to include in my weekly routine?	
What am I doing now?			

FIGURE 6.2 The steps of behavioural activation

	Time of day	Mon	Tues	Wed	Thurs	Fri	Sat	Sun
Morning	6:00–8:00							
	8:00–10:00							
	10:00–12:00							
Afternoon	12:00–2:00							
	2:00–4:00							
	4:00–6:00							
Evening	6:00–8:00							
	8:00–10:00							
	10:00–12:00							

FIGURE 6.3 An example of a diary

to change about it. It is not easy to recall exactly what we have done when thinking back over a week, so we encourage service users to record what they have been doing on a daily basis if possible.

Of course, there are a number of reasons why people with negative symptoms may find it difficult to complete this task. It is therefore crucial to spend time ensuring that the rationale for the task is understood and that any obstacles to successful completion are elicited. One obvious obstacle would be if the service user could not write or was embarrassed about writing things down. Alternative approaches, such as using a tape recorder or involving a supportive friend or family member in the process, could then be suggested. We recommend completing part of the diary in session with the service user in order to model the process.

The **second step** of the process is to help the person think about the things that they would like to do, based upon what they have stopped doing since they developed psychosis. Some of these things will simply be routine jobs that need to be done, such as housework or cooking. Some will be pleasurable activities, such as going out and meeting people. Others will be important necessary activities that you are avoiding, such as paying bills. If the service user is leading a sedentary lifestyle, it may help to try to include some task that requires physical activity.

The **third step** is to make a list of these activities in a hierarchy, with the most difficult at the top of the list and some easier activities at the bottom, making sure there is a mix of routine, pleasurable and necessary activities.

The **fourth step** in BA is to use a diary sheet to plan how to start doing these things starting near the bottom of the list and working upwards. It is important when choosing activities to start small and choose the things the service user is likely to be successful at achieving/is already doing but would like to do more. It is also crucial to spell out exactly what the activity is, where it will be done, when it will be done, how it will be done, who it will be done with (if anyone) and what steps are needed to complete the activity. This is most easily achieved by setting goals that are 'SMART' (**S**pecific, **M**easurable, **A**chievable, **R**ealistic and **T**imely see Box 4.5).

Although these steps are presented in a linear way, it is unlikely that every service user will progress through the stages of the treatment in this way. Indeed, it is important to note that for some people, negative symptoms may serve as a protective function. The timing and pacing of activation should therefore be carefully tailored to each individual. It may be helpful to spend some time exploring the advantages and disadvantages of becoming more active with people who seem indifferent to changing their weekly routine. At the same time, it is important to continue to monitor positive symptoms and other aspects of mental state to ensure that increased activity does not cause a relapse.

Relapse prevention planning

Although recovery from first episode psychosis is normally good the chance of relapse within five years is around 82% (Robinson et al., 1999) and each relapse raises the possibility of future relapses and poorer outcome (McGlashan, 1988). In view of this an important aspect of working with people with psychosis is helping them to identify their own early signs of relapse and develop an action plan to prevent relapse when these occur. One of the most accessible approaches to relapse detection and prevention is the *Back in the Saddle* (BITS) approach developed by Max Birchwood at the University of Birmingham (Birchwood et al., 2000). We have based the information below on the BITS approach with some adaptations from our own clinical experience. Table 6.5 contains a summary of the stages involved in relapse prevention planning.

TABLE 6.5   Stages of relapse prevention planning (after Birchwood et al., 2000)

Stage	Details
Stage 1 Engagement	Service users need to be engaged in a **collaborative** relationship with mental health professionals. Service user perceptions of their health problems are important: Do they accept that they have a mental health problem? Do they believe that they may be able take control and prevent future relapse? Do they wish to learn more about how to do this?
Stage 2 Identification of the relapse signature	The service user's own early signs are identified in what is known as a **relapse signature**. This is done through recalling the period of time which led up to the person last becoming ill and through reviewing of a list of common early signs reported by others (perhaps by having these early signs written on cards that the service users can select). The service user is then asked to place the identified early signs in the order in which they think they appeared
Stage 3 Development of a relapse drill	An action plan is developed outlining what the service user should do if they observe early signs of relapse in the future. The **relapse prevention plan** should include details of how to access mental health services 24 hours a day, a list of helpful interventions, a list of helpful personal coping strategies and where appropriate instructions relating to medication
Stage 4 Rehearsal and monitoring	Agreement is made on how the development of early signs will be **monitored**. The service user may, for example, recognise a need to be vigilant at times known to be stressful to them. With the service user's agreement, family or friends may also be asked to monitor for specific early signs. The action plan also needs to be **rehearsed**
Stage 5 Clarification of the relapse signature and drill	The service user should be given a written copy of the relapse plan and encouraged to think about where it will be kept for easy access (on a fridge door, in a bedside cabinet, etc.) With the service user's agreement, a copy of the plan should be sent to all key stakeholders involved in their care

Regarding stage 1, we have already discussed the importance of engaging people with psychosis in a collaborative relationship when assessing their problems. Box 6.2 gives an example of how engagement can be facilitated through explaining relapse prevention work to a service user.

Box 6.2 Explaining relapse prevention to a service user

'Research shows that most people with mental health problems like yours have several weeks between early signs showing and the onset of acute symptoms and that service users and their families are good at identifying these signs. The signs themselves are very individual to each person and because of this are sometimes called a relapse signature. What I would like to do is for us to work together to help you to identify your own early signs and then decide what you could do to avoid becoming ill again should these occur. How does that sound to you?'

The aim of the next stage is to identify the service user's own early signs and to construct a relapse signature for them. It should be remembered that asking service users to recall the last time they were ill may bring back frightening, distressing or embarrassing memories for the service user and this should be completed in a sensitive and supportive way. Regarding the list of common early signs reported by others, Birchwood et al. (2000) helpfully provide (p. 98) a list of 55 early warning signs reported by service users who have taken part in research studies. The information gathered can then be used to construct a timeline which maps out events from when the service user first noticed something was wrong through to the actual episode of psychosis. In addition, significant life events, persistent worries or concerns and anything else that might have triggered or accelerated their relapse can be added to the timeline.

The action plan – stage 3 – may include medication. However, medication should be reserved for the later stages of relapse to avoid unnecessary prescribing. In the early stages of relapse, personal coping such as exercise, gaining support from others, stress management and problem solving (see Chapter 4) may be more appropriate interventions. Stage 4 is the monitoring phase, which can be done in variety of ways (service user vigilance or the keeping of a daily 'thoughts, feelings and activities' diary). It is helpful for significant others to be involved in this stage. When early signs are observed many people become very frightened of relapse and they may cease to think clearly. It is important that the action plan is rehearsed. This can be done by role play or posing problem scenarios to the service user and asking them to tell you how they would respond. Rehearsal should be as stress-free as possible and humour and a good rapport can help in achieving this.

Once everything is finalised (stage 5), it is useful to revisit the plan periodically so it is fresh in the service user's mind.

Case scenario: Chris revisited

Remember Chris from our first case scenario? Chris displays mainly negative symptoms such as lying in bed until late in the afternoon, having little interest in any activities other than passively watching TV or playing on his games console in his room. Dianne, his mother, is very supportive of Chris but she is so worried that he will relapse if he doesn't have his medication that she feels she has to constantly monitor him. Dianne's husband, Dave (who is Chris' stepfather), says Dianne interferes too much in Chris' life and she should 'let him be' and get on with her own life.

What evidence-based interventions do you think Chris might be interested in?

Conclusion

In this chapter we have provided an overview of how people who require long-term support because they experience psychosis as a relapsing or ongoing condition might be helped by mental health nurses. We have provided a brief review of governmental policies and how they have shaped the development of modern mental health services in the UK. Some of the many difficulties commonly experienced by people with psychosis have been discussed and we have tried to emphasise that these problems may not just be a consequence of the effects of the illness itself but may also result from the stigmatising effects of psychosis and the negative reactions of others.

The general principles of engaging in therapeutic relationships and undertaking assessments with people who have psychosis have been described and some of the more user-friendly assessment tools have been recommended. Finally, we have discussed the evidence base that underpins psychosocial interventions but have also highlighted some of the difficulties in practising such therapies in routine settings without additional specialist training (Mairs & Bradshaw, 2005b). In light of this we have selected four parsimonious interventions that we believe can be safely practised by mental health nurses without specialist training and that may be of significant thera-peutic benefit to many service users with psychosis and to their family and friends. We believe that interventions such as those we have described can help to empower service users, enabling them, as such, to take greater control of their lives. Ultimately, this means that people with psychosis should be able to reduce their dependence on mental health services, instead taking advan-tage of more mainstream and less stigmatising primary care health services.

Further Reading and Resources

Key texts

Turkington D, Kingdon D, Rathod S, Wilcock SKJ, Brabban A, Cromarty P, Dudley R, Gray R, Pelton J, Siddle R & Weiden P (2009). *Back to Life, Back to Normality: Cognitive Therapy, Recovery and Psychosis*. Cambridge: Cambridge University Press.
Written to help make cognitive behavioural therapy (CBT) more widely available to service users and their carers. It can be used by service users as a guided self-help manual, or as a training aid for mental health professionals who want to learn more about using CBT in psychosis.

Harris N, Williams S & Bradshaw T (eds) (2002). *Psychosocial Interventions for People with Schizophrenia*. Basingstoke: Palgrave Macmillan.
A good, general introduction to psychosocial interventions that includes information on training and supervision. Most of the contributors to this book are mental health nurses.

Smith G, Gregory K & Higgs A (2007). *An Integrated Approach to Family Work for Psychosis: A Manual for Family Workers*. London: Jessica Kingsley.
A practical guide to engaging family and friends of people with psychosis in collaborative relationships.

British Psychological Society (2000). *Recent Advances in Understanding Mental Illness and Psychotic Experiences: A Report by the British Psychological Society, Division of Clinical Psychology*. Leicester: BPS. Available from: www.bps.org.uk.
A BPS publication that contains very informative and accessible information about psychosis, including potential causes, treatments and the factors influencing its outcome.

Key policy documents

HM Government (2009). *New Horizons: A Shared Vision for Mental Health*. London: Department of Health. Available from: www.newhorizons.dh.gov.uk.
Scottish Government (2009). *Towards a Mentally Flourishing Scotland: Policy and Action Plan 2009–2011*. Edinburgh: The Scottish Government. Available from: www.scotland.gov.uk.

Welsh Assembly Government (2002). *Adult Mental Health Services: A National Service Framework for Wales.* Available from: www.wales.nhs.uk.

National Institute for Health and Clinical Excellence (2009). *Core Interventions in the Treatment and Management of Schizophrenia in Primary and Secondary Care (Update) [National Clinical Practice Guideline Number 82].* London: NICE. Available from: www. nice.org.uk/CG82.

Web resources

RETHINK: www.rethink.org.uk
> *Formerly the National Schizophrenia Fellowship, now a more generic mental health charity. The Physical Health Check and guidelines for use can be downloaded from RETHINK's website.*

Time to Change campaign: www.time-to-change.org.uk/home/
> *A joint MIND/RETHINK campaign aimed at reducing the discrimination and stigma associated with mental health.*

The Hearing Voices Network: www.hearing-voices.org
> *An organisation offering information, support and understanding to people who hear voices and those who support them.*

Choice and Medication: www.choiceandmedication.org.uk
> *Excellent website, written for a service user and carer audience, that helps service users and carers make informed choices (where possible) regarding medications used in mental health settings.*

References

Andreasen N (1979). Thought, language, and communication disorders. I. A clinical assessment, definition of terms, and evaluation of their reliability. *Archives of General Psychiatry*, **36**(12), 1315–1321.

Andreasen N (1984a). Scale for the Assessment of Positive Symptoms (SAPS). Iowa: University of Iowa.

Andreasen N (1984b). Scale for the Assessment of Negative Symptoms (SANS). Iowa: University of Iowa.

Barrowclough C & Tarrier N (1997). *Families of Schizophrenic Patients – Cognitive Behavioural Intervention.* Cheltenham: Nelson Thornes.

BBC News (1998). Health: Latest News. 'Third way' for mental health [web page]. Available from: news.bbc.co.uk/1/hi/health/latest_news/141538.stm [accessed 16 September 2009].

Bebbington P & Kuipers L (1994). The predictive utility of expressed emotion in schizophrenia: an aggregate analysis. *Psychological Medicine*, **21**, 707–718.

Bentall RP (2004). *Madness Explained: Psychosis and Human Nature.* London: Penguin.

Birchwood M, Spencer E & McGovern D (2000). Schizophrenia: early warning signs. *Advances in Psychiatric Treatment*, **6**, 93–101.

Bradshaw T, Lovell K, Bee P & Mairs H (2005). Why do adults with schizophrenia have poorer physical health than the rest of the population? *Mental Health Practice*, **9**(4), 28–30.

Brown S (2006). Schizophrenia, weight gain and atypical antipsychotics. *British Journal of Psychiatry*, **188**, 191–192.

Brown S, Inskip H & Barrowclough B (2000). Causes of the excess mortality of schizophrenia. *British Journal of Psychiatry*, **177**, 212–217.

Butterworth T (1994). Working in partnership: a collaborative approach to care. The review of mental health nursing. *Journal of Psychiatric and Mental Health Nursing*, **1**, 41–44.

Cox D & Cowling P (1989). *Are You Normal?* London: Tower Press.

Crisp AH, Gelder MG & Rix S (2000). Stigmatisation of people with mental illnesses. *British Journal of Psychiatry*, **177**, 4–7.

Cunningham-Owens DG, Carroll A, Fattah S, Clyde Z, Coffey I & Johnstone EC (2001). A randomized, controlled trial of a brief interventional package for schizophrenic out-patients. *Acta Psychiatrica Scandinavica*, **103**, 362–369.

Day JC, Wood G, Dewey M & Bentall RP (1995). A self rating scale for measuring neuroleptic side-effects: validation in a group of schizophrenic patients. *British Journal of Psychiatry*, **166**, 650–653.

DH (Department of Health) (1990). *National Health Service and Community Care Act*. London: HMSO.

DH (Department of Health) (1999). *National Service Framework for Mental Health: Modern Standards and Service Models*. London: HMSO.

DH (Department of Health) (2000). *The NHS Plan: A Plan for Investment, Plan for Reform*. London: HMSO.

DH (Department of Health) (2001). *The Mental Health Policy Implementation Guide*. London: HMSO.

DHSSPS (Department of Health, Social Services and Public Safety) (2005). *The Bamford Review of Mental Health and Learning Disability (Northern Ireland): The Review of Mental Health and Learning Disability (Northern Ireland), A Strategic Framework for Adult Mental Services*. Belfast: DHSSPS.

Dimidjian S, Hollon SD, Dobson KS, Schmaling KB, Kohlenberg RJ, Addis ME, Gallop R, McGlinchey JB, Markley DK, Gollan JK, Atkins DC, Dunner DL & Jacobson NS (2006). Randomized trial of behavioural activation, cognitive therapy and anti-depressant medication in the acute treatment of adults with major depression. *Journal of Consulting and Clinical Psychology*, **74**(4), 658–670.

Fleming MP & Martin CR (2009). A preliminary investigation into the experience of symptoms of psychosis in mental health professionals: implications for the psychiatric classification model of schizophrenia. *Journal of Psychiatric and Mental Health Nursing*, **16**(5), 473–480.

Frame L & Morrison A (2001). Causes of post-traumatic stress disorder in psychotic patients. *Archives of General Psychiatry*, **58**, 305–306.

Haddock G, McCarron J, Tarrier N & Faragher EB (1999). Scales to measure dimensions of hallucinations and delusions: the psychotic symptom rating scales (PSYRATS). *Psychological Medicine*, **29**, 879–889.

Holland M (2002). Dual diagnosis – substance misuse and schizophrenia. In N Harris, S Williams & T Bradshaw (eds), *Psychosocial Interventions for People with Schizophrenia*. Basingstoke: Palgrave Macmillan.

HM Government (2009). *New Horizons: A Shared Vision for Mental Health*. London: Department of Health. Available from: www.newhorizons.dh.gov.uk [accessed 12 January 2010].

Honig A, Romme MAJ, Ensink BJ, Escher SDM, Pennings MHA & de Vries MW (1998). Auditory hallucinations: a comparison between patients and nonpatients. *Journal of Nervous and Mental Disease*, **186**, 646–651.

Jablensky A (2000). Epidemiology of schizophrenia: the global burden of disease and disability. *European Archives of Psychiatry & Clinical Neuroscience*, **250**, 274–285.

Jones C, Cormac I, Silveira da Mota Neto JI & Campbell C (2004). Cognitive behaviour therapy for schizophrenia. *The Cochrane Database of Systematic Reviews*, Issue 4, Article CD000524. Available from: www.cochrane.org [accessed 12 December 2009].

Jung HY, Kim JH, Ahn YM, Kim SC, Hwang SS & Kim YS (2005). Liverpool University Neuroleptic Side-Effect Rating Scale (LUNSERS) as a subjective measure of drug-induced parkinsonism and akathisia. *Human Psychopharmacology*, **20**(1), 41–45.

Kane JM, Schooler NR, Marder SW, Wirshing D, Ames D, Umbricht A, Safferman R, Baker R & Ganguli R (1996). Efficacy of clozapine versus haloperidol in a long term clinical trial. *Schizophrenia Research*, **18**, 127.

Kay SR, Fiszbein A & Opler LA (1987). The Positive and Negative Syndrome Scale (PANSS) for schizophrenia. *Schizophrenia Bulletin*, **13**, 261–276.

Kingdon D & Turkington, D (1994). *Cognitive–Behavioural Therapy of Schizophrenia*. Hove: Guilford Press.

Kingdon D & Turkington D (2005). *Cognitive Therapy of Schizophrenia*. Hove: Guilford Press.

Kirkbride JB, Fearon P, Morgan C, Dazzan P, Morgan K, Tarrant J, Lloyd T, Holloway J, Hutchinson G, Leff JP, Mallett RM, Harrison GL, Murray RM & Jones PB (2006). Heterogeneity in incidence rates of schizophrenia and other psychotic syndromes: findings from the 3-Center ÆSOP study. *Archives of General Psychiatry*, **63**, 250–258.

Kirkbride JB, Morgan C, Fearon P, Dazzan P, Murray RM & Jones PB (2007). Neighbourhood-level effects on psychoses: re-examining the role of context. *Psychological Medicine*, **37**, 1413–1425.

Krawiecka M, Goldberg D & Vaughn M (1977). A standardised psychiatric assessment scale for chronic psychiatric patients. *Acta Psychiatrica Scandinavica*, **55**, 299–308.

Lancashire S (1998). *KGV-M Symptom Scale Version 6.1*. London: Institute of Psychiatry.

Leff J, Trieman N, Knapp M & Hallam A (2000). The TAPS Project: a report on 13 years of research, 1985–1998. *Psychiatric Bulletin*, **24**, 165–168.

Lejuez C, Hopko D & Hopko S (2001). A brief behavioural activation treatment for depression: treatment manual. *Behaviour Modification*, **25**, 255–286.

McGlashan TH (1988). A selective review of North American long term follow up studies of schizophrenia. *Schizophrenia Bulletin*, **14**, 515–542.

McGrath J, Saha S, Welham J, El Saadi O, MacCauley C & Chant D (2004). A systematic review of the incidence of schizophrenia: the distribution of rates and the influence of sex, urbanicity, migrant status and methodology. *BMC Medicine*, **2,** 13. Available from: www.biomedcentral.com/1741-7015/2/13 [accessed 9 September 2009].

Mairs H & Bradshaw T (2005a). Implementing family intervention following training: what can the matter be? *Journal of Psychiatric and Mental Health Nursing*, **12**, 488–494.

Mairs H & Bradshaw T (2005b). Modernising psychosocial intervention education: the new COPE programme. *Mental Health Practice,* **9**(3), 28–30.

Mairs H, Lovell K & Keeley P (2006). Behavioural activation for psychosis. Unpublished manuscript. Available from the author on request: hilary.j.mairs@manchester.ac.uk.

Malik N, Kingdon D, Pelton J, Mehta R & Turkington D (2009). Effectiveness of brief cognitive-behavioral therapy for schizophrenia delivered by mental health nurses: relapse and recovery at 24 months. *Journal of Clinical Psychiatry*, **70**(2), 201–207.

Marwaha S, Balachandra S & Johnson S (2009). Clinicians' attitudes to the employment of people with psychosis. *Social Psychiatry and Psychiatric Epidemiology*, 44, 349–360.

Morrison A, Renton J, Dunn H, Williams S & Bentall R (2004). *Cognitive Therapy for Psychosis. A Formulation-Based Approach.* Hove: Brunner Routledge.

Nadeem Z, McIntosh A & Lawrie S (2004). EBMH notebook: schizophrenia. *Evidence-Based Mental Health,* **7**, 2–3.

NICE (National Institute for Health & Clinical Excellence) (2009). *Core Interventions in the Treatment and Management of Schizophrenia in Primary and Secondary Care (Update) [National Clinical Practice Guideline Number 82].* London: NICE.

O'Brien M, Singleton N, Sparks J, Melzer H & Troalack B (2002). *Adults with a Psychiatric Disorder Living in Private Households.* London: HMSO.

Pekkala E & Merinder L (2002). Psychoeducation for schizophrenia. *The Cochrane Database of Systematic Reviews*, Issue 2, Article CD002831. Available from: www.cochrane.org [accessed 12 December 2009].

Phelan M, Slade M, Thornicroft G, Dunn G, Holloway F, Wykes T, Strathdee G, Loftus L, McCrone P & Hayward P (1995). The Camberwell assessment of need: the validity and reliability of an instrument to assess the needs of people with severe mental illness. *British Journal of Psychiatry*, **167**, 589–595.

Phelan M, Stradins L, Amin D, Isadore R, Hitrov C, Doyle A & Inglis R (2004). The Physical Health Check: a tool for mental health workers. *Journal of Mental Health*, **13**(3), 277–284.

Pilling S, Bebbington P, Kuipers E, Garety P, Geddes J, Orbach G & Morgain C (2002). Psychological treatments in schizophrenia. I: Meta-analysis of family intervention and cognitive behaviour therapy. *Psychological Medicine*, **32**, 763–782.

Rathod S, Kingdon D & Turkington D (2003). Insight and Schizophrenia. Presentation at Psychological Interventions in Schizophrenia Conference, Oxford.

Richards D, Lovell K, Gilbody S, Gask L, Torgerson D, Barkham M, Bland M, Bower P, Lankshear A, Simpson A, Fletcher J, Escott D, Hennessy S & Richardson R (2008). Collaborative care for depression in UK primary care: a randomised controlled trial. *Psychological Medicine*, **38**, 279–287.

Ritchie JH, Dick D & Lingham R (1994). *The Report of the Inquiry into the Care and Treatment of Christopher Clunis.* London: HMSO.

Robinson D, Woerner MG, Alvir J, Bilder R, Goldman R, Geisler S, Koreen S, Sheitman B, Chakos M, Mayerhoff D & Lieberman JA (1999). Predictors of relapse following response from a first episode of schizophrenia or schizoaffective disorder. *Archives of General Psychiatry,* **56**, 241–247.

Scottish Government (2009). *Towards a Mentally Flourishing Scotland: Policy and Action Plan 2009–2011*. Edinburgh: The Scottish Government. Available from: www. scotland.gov.uk [accessed 12 January 2010].

Scottish Office (1997). *A Framework for Mental Health Services in Scotland*. Available from: www.show.scot.nhs.uk [accessed 9 September 2009].

Selten JP, Sijben NE, van den Bosch RJ, Omloo-Visser J & Warmerdam H (1993). The subjective experience of negative symptoms: a self-rating scale. *Comprehensive Psychiatry*, **34**(3), 192–197.

Sensky T, Turkington D, Kingdon D, Scott JL, Scott J, Siddle R, O'Carroll M & Barnes TE (2000). A randomised controlled trial of cognitive-behavioural therapy for persistent symptoms in schizophrenia resistant to medication. *Archives of General Psychiatry*, **57**, 165–172.

Shorter E (1997). *A History of Psychiatry from the Era of the Asylum to the Age of Prozac*. Chichester: John Wiley & Sons.

Siris, SG (2001). Suicide and schizophrenia. *Journal of Psychopharmacology*, **15**(2), 127–135.

Stahl SM & Buckley PF (2007). Negative symptoms of schizophrenia: a problem that will not go away. *Acta Psychiatrica Scandinavica*, **115**(1), 4–11.

Strassnig M, Miewald J, Keshavan M & Ganguli R (2007). Weight gain in newly diagnosed first-episode psychosis patients and healthy comparisons: one-year analysis. *Schizophrenia Research*, **93**, 90–98.

Tarrier N (1987). An investigation of residual psychotic symptoms in discharged schizophrenic patients. *British Journal of Clinical Psychology*, **26**, 141–143.

Tarrier N (2005). Cognitive behaviour therapy for schizophrenia – a review of development, evidence and implementation. *Psychotherapy and Psychosomatics*, **74**(3), 133–144.

Tarrier N, Beckett R, Harwood S, Baker A & Ugarteburu I (1993). A trial of two cognitive-behavioural methods of treating drug resistant residual psychotic symptoms in schizophrenic patients. I: Outcome. *British Journal of Psychiatry*, **162**, 524–532.

Tarrier N, Yusopoff L, Kinney C, McCarthy E, Gledhill A, Haddock G & Morris J (1998). Randomised controlled trial of intensive cognitive behaviour therapy for patients with chronic schizophrenia. *British Medical Journal*, **317**, 303–307.

Welsh Assembly Government (2002). *Adult Mental Health Services: A National Service Framework for Wales* [pdf]. Available from: www.wales.nhs.uk [accessed 9 September 2009].

Watkins J (1996). *Living with Schizophrenia*. South Yarra: Michelle Anderson Publishing.

Winograd-Gurvich C, Fitzgerald P, Georgiou-Karistianis N, Bradshaw J & White O (2006). Negative symptoms: a review of schizophrenia, melancholic depression and Parkinson's disease. *Brain Research Bulletin*, **70**(4–6), 312–321.

Wykes T, Steel C, Everitt B & Tarrier N (2008). Cognitive behaviour therapy for schizophrenia: effect sizes, clinical models, and methodological rigour. *Schizophrenia Bulletin*, **34**(3), 523–537.

Zubin J & Spring B (1977). A new view of schizophrenia. *Journal of Abnormal Psychology*, **86**, 103–126.

7

Helping People Who Have Acute Mental Health Problems

Sara Munro and John Baker

What will I learn in this chapter?

The aim of this chapter is to explore the 'acute care pathway', i.e. the broad range of services available to those with acute mental health problems. Although the chapter focuses mainly on *inpatient* provision (since inpatient care remains the dominant service for this group of people), there is some discussion of the alternatives to inpatient care that form part of the acute care pathway.

After reading this chapter, you will be able to:

- identify the policy and legislation underpinning acute mental health care provision across the UK;
- appreciate the reasons why individuals might require acute mental health care, the needs they will have and the range of options available to meet those needs;
- identify the different services available within the acute care pathway;
- outline the main interventions used in acute mental health care and understand the evidence base for those interventions.

Introduction

In the preceding three chapters (Chapter 4 on depression, Chapter 5 on anxiety and Chapter 6 on psychosis), we saw that many people with common and/or enduring mental health problems can be successfully treated and managed in a community setting. However, there are times when – for the safety of an individual service user or those around them – it may be necessary to consider treatment in an institutional setting, sometimes against the service user's will. In most cases, this will be because the individual is experiencing an **acute episode** of mental ill health.

Acute episodes of mental ill health can occur in individuals with no previous history of mental health problems or they can be a re-occurring feature of an ongoing mental health problem. They usually cause significant disruption to the individual service user's wellbeing, safety and everyday functioning and they often cause distress and disruption to those closest to the service user, such as family and friends.

Given that a significant proportion of acute episodes of mental ill health continue to be treated in institutional settings in spite of the development of alternatives (Glover et al., 2006; National Audit Office, 2007), the bulk of this chapter will focus on **inpatient care**, acute mental health wards in particular. However, this does not necessarily mean that inpatient care is the only – or, indeed, the best – option for those who are acutely ill. As you will discover, alternatives to inpatient care do exist; moreover, there is a growing consensus that inpatient care should be used only if suitable alternatives are not available.

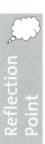

Reflection Point

Home care

According to the Department of Health (DH, 2002), the purpose of an acute inpatient service is 'to provide a high standard of humane treatment and care in a safe and therapeutic setting for service users in the most acute and vulnerable stage of their illness' (p. 5).

Can you think of any reasons why an individual's home cannot be a 'safe and therapeutic setting' even if they are at an 'acute and vulnerable stage of their illness'? Try to think of reasons for allowing people to remain in their homes rather than reasons why they should be admitted.

Policy Context

In the previous chapter we mentioned that there had been a UK-wide, general shift from institutionally based mental healthcare to community-based provision, a shift that began around 60 years ago but has accelerated in recent years. Cynical observers might see this shift merely as a cost-cutting exercise; in recent years, however, there has been a significant *increase* in expenditure on mental health. In England, for example, the advent of the *National Service Framework for Mental Health* (NSF) (DH, 1999a), brought a 47% increase in mental health expenditure between 1999/2000 and 2005/06, a figure representing an average year-on-year rise of 6.7% (Boardman & Parsonage, 2007). Moreover, as far as the care of people with *acute* mental health problems is concerned, it is the change in the proportion spent on hospital inpatient care that is remarkable. Again using England as an example, hospital inpatient services accounted for around 78% of overall spending in 1984/85 compared to just 49% in 2003/04 (Parsonage, 2005). The NSF provides some clues as to where this additional expenditure and the money 'lost' from hospital inpatient services has gone: primarily on increasing the number of *secure* beds (secure provision is discussed in more detail in Chapter 12) and on developing community-based alternatives such as **assertive outreach**, **early intervention** and **crisis resolution/home treatment** (DH, 2001, 2004).

These community-based alternatives are given even greater emphasis in England's recent replacement for the NSF, *New Horizons* (HM Government, 2009). *New Horizons* sees admission to an acute inpatient unit as the exception rather than the rule and it argues that community-based teams – crisis teams in particular – should be the gatekeepers to inpatient care. While the Welsh National Service Framework (Welsh Assembly Government, 2005) isn't as explicit as England's with regard to acute care, it does state that inpatient services need reform, that the estates (buildings) are outdated and that 'inpatient and community developments need to be considered together if the replication of an old model of institutional care within new buildings is to be avoided' (p. 6). Scottish policy parallels much of that in England and Wales in that crisis and home treatment services are seen as first line interventions that can help guard against 'inappropriate' admissions (Scottish Executive, 2006). There is no explicit policy in Northern Ireland in relation to acute mental healthcare but the Bamford Review (DHSSPS, 2005) sets out a need for the reform, renewal and modernisation of mental health services across Northern Ireland with an emphasis on rights, values and partnership.

TABLE 7.1   The acute care pathway

Institutional setting	Community setting
Acute inpatient ward	Crisis resolution and home treatment teams
Psychiatric intensive care ward/unit	Community mental health teams
Low secure unit	Primary care mental health input
Respite unit/time-limited admission	Day services (including independent sector)
	Community-based residential units

The acute care pathway

Much of UK policy on acute mental healthcare encompasses what might be called the **acute care pathway** – 'the journey a service user makes from initial referral to discharge from acute services' (CSIP/NIMHE, 2008, p. 4). Table 7.1 lists some of the services that fall within the acute care pathway. Note that this list is not exhaustive as services will vary according to local needs. As well as being provided by the statutory sector (the NHS and local authorities), these services may be provided by the voluntary and private/ independent sectors.

Although the services in Table 7.1 are categorised according to whether they are institutionally or community based, the division is somewhat artificial since individuals may well receive input from more than one service or team at any one time. As such, effective inter-agency and multidisciplinary team working is essential. Indeed, acute services that are **integrated** – jointly managed and interlinked – are the ones that tend to have the best outcomes for service users (CSIP/NIMHE, 2008).

The bulk of institutionally based acute care is provided by acute inpatient wards and secure units. Since secure units are discussed in more detail in Chapter 12, we will concentrate only on acute inpatient wards here.

Acute inpatient services

While policy may be shifting towards alternatives to inpatient care, inpatient units still have a role to play in the care of people with acute mental health problems – though inpatient admission should be seen as an option of last resort rather than something routine. This policy seems to be reflected in the changes in the availability of acute beds over the past few years. Table 7.2 outlines current and past distribution of acute beds across the four countries of the UK.

In England, the number of short-stay beds has dropped by around 20% between 2000 and 2009, though there has been a parallel rise in the number of medium secure beds available (an 18% rise between 1999 and 2004;

TABLE 7.2 Acute mental health beds for adults of working age

Country (with bed data source)	Acute beds		Change	Population (ONS, 2009)	Ratio 2009
	2000	2009			
England (DH, 2000, 2009)	14,118	11,242	−20%	31.8 million	1:2,827
Wales (StatsWales, 2009)	1,125	881	−22%	1.8 million	1:2,043
Scotland (ISD Scotland, 2009)	3,753	2,458	−35%	3.2 million	1:1,302
NI (DHSSPS, 2009a, 2009b)	1,309	969	−26%	1.1 million	1:1,135
Total UK	20,305	15,550	−23%	37.9 million	

DH, 2004). In Wales, the number of acute beds fell by 22% over the same period and by 26% in Northern Ireland. Scotland has had the biggest reduction, at 35%. Note that there are some marked differences across the four countries in relation to current acute bed provision. Scotland and Northern Ireland have the highest number of beds on a population basis, with roughly one bed to every 1,000 adults of working age; Wales has one bed to around every 2,000 adults and England one bed to almost every 3,000 adults. Indeed, compared to their respective populations, Scotland and Northern Ireland have more than twice the number of beds as England.

The number of acute beds

Can you think of reasons why there should be marked differences across the four countries of the UK in terms of acute bed provision?

Is it because of different philosophies of care within the four countries? Because community services are better developed in England than Scotland or Northern Ireland? Or is it because England hasn't invested as much in acute care as the other three countries have?

Discussion Point

While it has been superseded by *New Horizons*, there is still relevant guidance in the NSF regarding hospital and crisis accommodation. Standard 5 of the NSF states that each service user who requires a period of care away from their home should have: (1) **timely access to an appropriate hospital bed or alternative bed or place**, which is in **the least restrictive environment** consistent with the need to protect them and the public and **as close to home as possible**; and (2) a copy of a written after-care plan, agreed on discharge, which sets out the care and rehabilitation to be provided, identifies the care coordinator, and specifies the action to be taken in a crisis (DH, 1999a). With regard to the standards of *nursing* care, Recommendation 12 of the Chief Nursing Officer's Review of Mental Health Nursing states that 'all individuals receiving inpatient care will receive a service that is safe, supportive and able to respond to individual needs' (DH, 2006, p. 42).

To what extent this guidance has been adhered to is questionable because, while there have been many improvements in the care provided in acute settings in recent years, a range of concerns associated with the quality of inpatient provision remain. A summary of these concerns from a variety of sources (specifically DH, 2004; Rethink et al., 2006; Healthcare Commission, 2008; HM Government, 2009) is contained in Box 7.1.

Box 7.1   Recent concerns relating to acute inpatient care

- Accessing or lack of alternatives to admission
- Overcrowded wards
- High bed occupancy
- Delayed discharges
- The arrangements for safety, privacy and comfort in inpatient areas
- Poor-quality ward environments
- Inequality issues (especially relating to race and gender)
- Insufficient staff contact
- Lack of meaningful activity for service users
- Poor continuity of care between community and inpatient services
- Problems with substance misuse
- The stigma and social exclusion associated with admission
- Overuse of compulsory detention

Alternatives to inpatient care

As we have seen, the principal alternatives to inpatient care are **assertive outreach**, **early intervention** and **crisis resolution/home treatment**. All of these services can be delivered in the service user's own home, which for many is the 'least restrictive environment' in which to provide care and treatment.

Assertive outreach (also known as **assertive community treatment**) is a flexible way of working with people with mental health problems who do not engage effectively with mental health services. The mental health worker sees the service user in his or her chosen environment, whether it be their own home, a café, a park or in the street (SCMH, 2001).

Early intervention, on the other hand, is more of a *strategy for intervening* than a specific intervention. It often refers to the early detection and treatment of real or burgeoning mental health problems in children and young people (see Chapters 9 and 10) but, as we have seen in the previous chapter, the same early detection and treatment principles can also be used in those with ongoing mental health problems in the form of **relapse prevention plans**.

NIMHE (2004) argue that crisis resolution/home treatment (CR/HT) can be defined as a service, choice or opportunity. As a **service**, CR/HT provides a rapid response to, and assessment of, a mental health crisis with the possibility of offering comprehensive acute care at home until the crisis is resolved, usually without hospital admission. As a **choice**, inpatient admission ceases to be the only option. As an **opportunity**, CR/HT can protect individuals from stigma, give greater personal ownership and consequently increase the potential for recovery.

Staffing and skill mix in acute services

In acute inpatient settings it has traditionally been registered mental health nurses and nursing/healthcare assistants who have provided the majority of direct care. In the past, acute mental health services tended to be overseen by consultant psychiatrists, who operated across both inpatient and community services, with the support of specialist registrars (SpRs; in years 4 to 6 of training) and the 'junior doctors', the senior house officers (SHOs; in years 2 to 3 of training). However, there have been a number of significant changes in recent years, including those resulting from the European Working Time Directive (EWTD), the *Modernising Medical Careers* initiative (Four UK Health Departments, 2004), and the *New Ways of Working* programme (DH, 2005, 2007a).

The *Modernising Medical Careers* initiative, implemented between 2005 and 2007, resulted in the creation of **foundation house officers** (or F1/F2 trainees, as they are known; years 1 and 2 of training) and **specialty registrars** (or StRs, as they are known; years 3 to 6 of training) to replace the old SHO and SpR grades. The EWTD set limits on the length of the working week for all employees, including doctors in training, who had traditionally worked very long hours. As we saw in Chapter 3, these changes have led to nurses taking on many of the roles that doctors had previously undertaken, such as physical assessments and prescribing, and they have also created enhanced roles – like advanced practitioner and nurse consultant – for nurses with greater degrees of expertise.

New Ways of Working – also discussed in Chapter 3 – is a flexible, multidisciplinary, workforce programme that encompasses all of the existing professionals (psychiatrists, nurses, psychologists, occupational therapist, pharmacists and social workers) as well as newer workers like graduate primary care mental health workers and assistant practitioners. Its principal goal is to ensure that the right skills are matched to the right aspect of service provision. This means that highly skilled staff (such as psychiatrists and other senior practitioners) can be released from routine work, creating new opportunities for those with intermediate skills whether they be the established or newer types of worker. Because *New Ways of Working* focuses on the needs of service users and carers rather than on the traditional practices of the past, it cuts across both hospital and community settings. Individual workers do not, as such, have to be tied to hospital or community and many workers now work across the entire acute pathway.

Improving acute care

Acute care clearly has its problems but it is also clear that there has been a concerted effort in recent years to try to improve the quality of services that individual service users, their families and carers receive. We will talk more about the role that nurses in particular can play in improving acute care when we talk about assessments and interventions later on. For now, it is worth drawing your attention to the **acute care declaration** (MHN/NMHDU, 2009), which is a consensus statement about the way acute care services should be delivered. A summary of the key points can be found in Box 7.2.

Box 7.2   Key points of the acute care declaration (adapted, with permission, from MHN/NMHDU, 2009)

Published by the Mental Health Network and the National Mental Health Development Unit, and endorsed by, among others, the Royal Colleges of Nursing, Psychiatrists and Occupational Therapists, Star Wards, Rethink and the Sainsbury Centre for Mental Health, the acute care declaration aims:

'to ensure that people with mental health problems who are acutely ill receive the services they need at the time of their greatest vulnerability.'

The declaration itself states that:

'Good quality acute mental health services (inpatient and community) are essential and achievable.'

Furthermore, it outlines that endorsing organisations will work to (emphasis added):

1 Further encourage the commissioning and provision of **high quality** acute care
2 Promote **recovery** and **inclusion** for people using acute mental health services
3 Support the development of a **specialist** acute care workforce
4 Champion **positive perceptions** of acute care services
5 Support **quality improvement**, **service development** and **research** in acute care

Mental health legislation

Since many people are admitted to inpatient acute wards against their will, more often than not it is the acute wards where mental health nurses first come to grips with mental health law. Mental health legislation varies across the four countries of the UK: in England and Wales, the primary legislation is the **Mental Health Act 1983**, as amended by the **Mental Health Act 2007**; in Northern Ireland it is the **Mental Health (Northern Ireland) Order 1986,**[1] which is broadly based on the Mental Health Act 1983 (Heenan, 2009); and in Scotland, the **Mental Health (Care and Treatment) (Scotland) Act 2003**. There are some commonalities across the various pieces of legislation but there are also some differences. The most commonly used parts of the various Mental Health Acts are summarised in Table 7.3.

Additional aspects of the legislation you may encounter in an acute setting include those relating to **leave of absence** from the hospital, e.g. to go to local shops or go home, **compulsory community treatment**, **consent to treatment**, and **police powers**.

Leave of absence

Leave of absence is dealt with by **Section 17** of the English and Welsh Act, and **Article 15** of the Northern Ireland Order. The situation in Scotland is

---

[1] Uniquely in the UK, Northern Ireland is currently in the process of developing combined mental capacity and mental health legislation which will come into force no earlier than 2011 (NI Executive, 2009).

TABLE 7.3 A summary of the most commonly used elements of UK mental health legislation throughout its constituent countries

Section and description	England and Wales		Scotland	Northern Ireland
	Details	**Possible Outcomes**		
Section 5(4) Nurse's holding power	Applies to **inpatients** only Duration 6 hours; not renewable Completed by a nurse with a registration in either mental health or learning disability nursing	Section 5(2). Form 16 completed to cancel 5(4) following assessment by doctor Allowed to lapse	Similar powers, except there is a 2 hour limit; possible extension if the medical practitioner arrives within the second hour (Section 299)	Equivalent 6 hour power under Article 7(3)
Section 5(2) Holding power of doctors and approved clinicians	Applies to **inpatients** only. Duration 72 hours; not renewable Completed by the Responsible Clinician (RC), duty doctor or nominee of the RC	Section 2 Section 3 Allowed to lapse Section rescinded (within the 72 hours)	The equivalent power is emergency detention under section 36 (see below)	Equivalent power under Article 7(2) but of 48 hours duration only
Section 4 Emergency admission to hospital for assessment	Concerned with **admission** only Duration 72 hours; not renewable Applications made by the Approved Mental Health Professional (AMHP; formerly Approved Social Worker)	Assessment for Section 2 (one more medical recommendation required to convert) Discharged by the RC (under Section 23) Allowed to lapse	The equivalent is an Emergency Detention Certificate for 72 hours under Section 36(1) Not renewable Approved Medical Practitioner must examine as soon as practicable	Equivalent power under Article 4 for 7 days if the Responsible Medical Officer produces the detention report; 48 hours for any other doctor

TABLE 7.3 (Continued)

Section and description	England and Wales		Scotland	Northern Ireland
	Details	Possible Outcomes		
Section 2 Short-term detention order for the purpose of assessment	Can be applied to **inpatients** or used to force **admission** Duration 28 days Not renewable	Assessment for Section 3. Discharged by the RC (under Section 23) or the Hospital Managers or the Mental Health Review Tribunal or the nearest relative Allowed to lapse	Short-term detention powers lasting 28 days under Part 6 (Section 44) Extension periods possible to allow late application for a compulsory treatment order (see below) and/or allow time for a Tribunal to hear the case	Initial detention for up to 7 days, which can be renewed for a further 7 days (Article 9)
Section 3 Longer detention order for assessment and treatment (for the first 3 months)	Can be applied to **inpatients** or used to force **admission** Duration 6 months Renewable, initially for 6 months and then for periods of up to one year	Renewal Discharged by the RC (under Section 23) or the Hospital Managers or the Mental Health Review Tribunal or the nearest relative Allowed to lapse Community treatment order	The equivalent is the **compulsory (community or hospital) treatment order** under Part 7 which only a Mental Health Tribunal can approve	Similar powers to England and Wales under Article 12

¹In England and Wales, under the Mental Health Act 2007, the Responsible Clinician can be a mental health professional other than a doctor, though in most cases it will be a doctor. In Scottish and Northern Irish legislation the 'Responsible Medical Officer' must be a doctor.

more complex in that leave of absence is not explicitly referred to; instead **Section 127** of the Scottish Act deals with the temporary suspension of detention orders.

Compulsory community treatment

Linked in with the shift from institutional to community care but also to allay public fears regarding the community care of people with serious mental health problems has been the recent development of compulsory community treatment orders. Northern Ireland currently has no compulsory community treatment powers. In Scotland, however, **compulsory treatment orders** (under Part 7 of the Scottish Act) are generic in that they can be applied to both hospital and community settings. In England and Wales, the Mental Health Act 2007 introduced **community treatment orders** via the insertion of a new section (17A) into the 1983 Act. Community treatment orders contain specific conditions, mostly relating to seeing mental health professionals regularly and, as such, they allow for **supervised community treatment** which is governed by Part 4A of the amended 1983 Act. If the conditions of a community treatment order are broken, the service user can (under **Section 17E**) be recalled back to hospital. Supervised community treatment is controversial: MIND (2007), for example, expressed concerns that it will be used defensively rather than therapeutically, that it will lead to an over-reliance on drug treatments (because drugs are cheaper than community staff). Moreover, they add that there is no evidence that it improves mental state, readmission to hospital, social functioning, likelihood of being arrested, or homelessness.

Consent to treatment

Regarding **consent to treatment**, it is important to bear in mind that 'treatment' can mean not only medication and other physical treatments but also interventions such as nursing care, psychological treatments and training in social or independent living skills. Across the legislation, some treatments have special safeguards regarding consent. In both the English and Welsh Act and the Northern Ireland Order, a detained patient cannot be given psychosurgery without their consent *and* a second opinion (**Section 57**; **Article 63**) and they cannot be given medication beyond three months without their consent *or* a second opinion (**Section 58**; **Article 64**). In England and Wales, electroconvulsive therapy (ECT; see later in this chapter) cannot be given without consent except in an emergency situation (**Section 58A**); in Northern Ireland, ECT requires consent or a second opinion (**Article 64**). In Scotland (under **Part 16** of the Act), those detained cannot be given medication beyond two months, ECT, artificial nutrition or psychosurgery without their consent *or* a second opinion from a 'designated medical practitioner'.

Police powers

In England and Wales, **Sections 135** and **136** of the 1983 Act allow a constable (police officer) to remove a person thought to be suffering from mental disorder to a place of safety from private premises (Section 135) or a public place (Section 136) for up to 72 hours. Section 135 requires permission from a justice of the peace (magistrate). In Northern Ireland, **Articles 129** and **130** of the 1986 Order provide similar powers but the detention period can only be up to 48 hours. In Scotland, similar powers exist under **Part 19** of the 2003 Act, but the detention period can only be up to 24 hours and removal from private premises under **Section 293(1)** requires permission from either a sheriff or justice of the peace. In England, Wales and Northern Ireland a 'place of safety' can be a police station, hospital or special 'Section 136 suite' but in Scotland a police station is not normally seen as a place of safety (Section 300 of the Scottish Act).

Rights to information

All three pieces of legislation (Section 132 of the English and Welsh Act, Article 27 of the Northern Ireland Order and Section 260 of the Scottish Act) impose a duty on hospital authorities to ensure that anybody detained under the legislation is given verbal and written information about the detention, including details of which section or article of the legislation has been implemented, what it means in practical terms and how they can appeal, if such an appeal is allowed by the legislation.

To conclude this section, it's worth noting that while it is important that you are familiar with the key elements of the relevant parts and sections of the legislation applicable to the country you are practising in, a general textbook like this can give only a superficial overview of the legislation and you should look elsewhere for more definitive information and guidance – for instance, to the trained mental health act administrators employed by NHS Trusts, to more specialised texts on mental health law and to government guidance such as the Codes of Practice (see Scottish Executive, 2005; DH, 2008a).

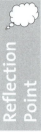

Compulsory detention

Much of our discussion of mental health legislation has focused on compulsory detention. Think about this:

Imagine that you were generally feeling good but for some reason you find yourself compulsorily detained ('sectioned') on an acute inpatient ward. You've never been admitted to hospital for a physical problem before, let alone a mental health problem. You think the staff on the ward haven't explained why you are there, apart from them saying it's 'for your own good', and you're at a loss as to why you can't leave, especially since you are worried about whether you've locked up your flat and whether your two pet cats will be OK.

What sort of thoughts would be running through your head? How would you feel? Would you be passive and accept your admission? Would you try to leave? Fight your way out? If you did that, what judgements do you think the staff would make about you?

More importantly, have your attributions about the behaviour of people admitted to acute wards changed as a result of this exercise?

The Care Programme Approach

All service users admitted to acute mental health wards are subject to the **Care Programme Approach** (CPA) for the duration of their inpatient care. A formal review of their needs must be undertaken prior to discharge to determine whether they will continue to require CPA. CPA is a formal, systematic process used across England, Wales and Scotland (but not Northern Ireland) to coordinate the care of people accessing secondary care mental health services. It was implemented in England in 1991 and updated in 1999 (DH, 1991, 1999b); in Scotland, it was introduced in 1992 with further guidance in 1998 (Scottish Office, 1998); in Wales it was implemented in 2004 following policy guidance in 2003 (Welsh Assembly Government, 2003).

CPA has four elements: (1) a systematic **assessment** of the health and social care needs of service users; (2) a formal, personalised **care plan** to address any assessed needs; (3) a **care coordinator** for each individual service user (i.e. a 'key worker'; more often than not a nurse); and (4) **regular review**.

Originally, CPA had two levels: **standard**, for those with low-level needs who maintained contact with services; and **enhanced**, for those with multiple needs who were likely to disengage from services. However, CPA was 'refocused' on those with more complex needs in England in 2008 (see DH, 2008b) so, in contrast to Scotland and Wales, England currently only has one level of CPA.

CPA becomes particularly relevant in acute care when **discharge** and **aftercare** arrangements are being made, one of its purposes being to ensure that different services and providers within a particular care pathway work together to produce seamless and integrated care for service users. A large proportion of people on acute mental health wards will already have a care coordinator who is based in community mental health services (e.g. a community mental health team, assertive outreach team or early intervention service). Should they not have a care coordinator, the inpatient keyworker normally undertakes this role until either the person is discharged from hospital and from mental health services, or a care coordinator is allocated from a community service.

Typical Problems Requiring Admission to Inpatient Services

Though major mental health problems can be successfully treated and managed in community settings, some people will have mental health problems that are so severe or so intense that it can be difficult to manage those individuals in the community and, as such, a period of hospitalisation may be necessary.

The reasons for admission to acute mental health wards vary. After reviewing the literature, Bowers (2005) identified seven principal reasons for admission to an acute inpatient unit, summarised in Box 7.3.

Box 7.3   Principal reasons for admission to acute inpatient units (after Bowers, 2005)

- **Dangerousness**
- For **assessment**
- For medical **treatment**
- **Severe mental disorder**
- Because of **self-care deficits**
- For **respite for carers**
- For **respite for the service users**

On the whole, acute inpatient mental health services do not have defined inclusion and exclusion criteria. This is fairly unique amongst mental health services and makes it difficult for staff to know what the next admission will bring. This can bring about both challenges and rewards for people who work in acute care.

In terms of specific conditions, there is little analysis of acute ward admission data in the literature. For example, in our recent paper on 'acuity' (Baker & Munro, 2006), we could only find English admission rate data (from SCMH, 1998, Thompson et al., 2004) that was no more recent than the late 1990s. Our findings pointed to mood disorders such as **depression** and **anxiety** being the most common reason for admission in England (more common than psychosis), though London was an exception with **psychosis** accounting for the majority of admissions (but even then, psychosis accounted for only around a third of admissions). We also found that acute ward admissions are not necessarily related to mental health needs since as many as a fifth may be down to **social crises**, including the need for carers to have respite. In a similar vein, Glasby & Lester (2005) observed that up to a third of admissions to inpatient acute wards may be inappropriate (and perhaps even avoidable) because of inadequate assessment by junior or non-specialist staff and a lack of alternatives to inpatient care, especially at night and at weekends.

In terms of **demographics**, admission to acute wards appears to be more common for **men** than women and more common among **younger** age groups (Baker & Munro, 2006). Regarding ethnicity, there is some evidence that **black and minority ethnic** service users stay longer on inpatient wards and that they are more likely to be compulsorily detained than other ethnic groups (DH, 2007b; MHA Commission, 2008).

Assessing Individuals Admitted to Acute Mental Health Wards

Admission to an acute mental health ward is often associated with an intense period of stress and disruption in an individual's life and functioning and it is important to bear this in mind when meeting the person for the first time. Often a range of **immediate** needs has to be taken care of before a more thorough assessment can be carried out. Examples include basic physical needs (food/drink), letting relatives and friends know where the individual is, arranging care for dependants and pets, orienting the individual to the ward, to other service users and to staff and perhaps even just giving the person the opportunity to have ten minutes of peace and quiet. Orienting the service user and allowing

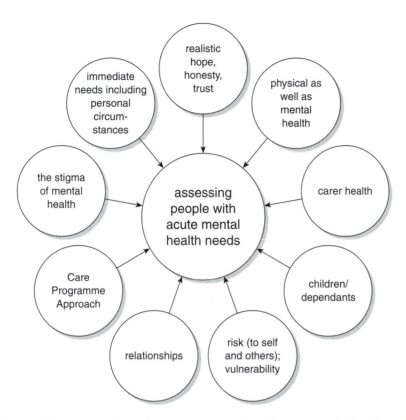

FIGURE 7.1   Things to consider when assessing people with acute mental health needs

him or her to adjust to the change in their environment should be prioritised over the need to attend to paperwork. Remember that he or she may have already been through numerous assessments and interviews prior to arriving on the ward, especially if they have been detained under mental health legislation.

Some of the more important things to consider when you are assessing people in an acute care setting are contained in Figure 7.1.

The assessment process

As with any other area of mental health (perhaps more so), nurses working in acute care need to build a trusting relationship prior to the assessment of a service user's needs. The interpersonal skills and capabilities outlined in Chapter 2 and discussed in the context of assessment in the previous few chapters are essential to the establishment of such a relationship. Once a trusting relationship has been established, the assessment process normally involves both formal and informal assessment, as well as a specific assessment of **risk**. Remember that assessment is an **ongoing** process and, as such, it is good practice to review a service user's progress through regular re-assessment.

Formal assessments

Typically, a global or holistic assessment of the service user is undertaken when they are first admitted to an acute mental health ward, usually involving standardised forms and documents which may also be underpinned by a specific theoretical framework or model, such as the Scottish Capability Framework for Acute Mental Health Care (NES, 2007) or one of the nursing models outlined in Chapter 1.

It is important to note that global or holistic assessments can be difficult for service users. These kinds of assessments are often very broad and may cover numerous areas including, for example, presenting problem, mental and physical health histories, and activities of daily living. Standardised assessments of the service user's mental health may also be carried out using tools such as the Mini-Mental State (an assessment of cognitive functioning; Folstein et al., 1975) or symptom assessment tools such as the Beck Depression Inventory (Beck et al., 1961) or the PSYRATs (Haddock et al., 1999; see Chapter 6). It is especially important that a **baseline** is established and that assessments are repeated during an inpatient stay so that improvements in function and mental state can be identified.

Informal assessments

Because they are present around the clock, nurses are in a unique position to gather valuable information on a service user's general ability and functioning. By using their interpersonal skills to build rapport with the service user, nurses can observe the service user's actions and interactions throughout the day. These informal assessments can help identify a service user's ability to concentrate and process information, their ability to meet their basic physical and self-care needs (food, drink and hygiene) and their ability to communicate and interact with other patients and those who visit them.

Risk assessment and management

Risk assessment is an especially important element of acute mental health care. Risk is one of the main reasons for admission to an acute inpatient unit in that there is often an implicit assumption that the risk the individual poses to themselves or others is too great for them to remain in the community. Risk assessment and management is, therefore, inextricably linked to discharge planning. Risk assessment involves working with a service user to try to esti-mate how likely it is a negative event will occur, how soon it is expected to occur and how severe the outcome will be if it does occur (DH, 2007c). Best practice in managing risk requires knowledge of the **research evidence**, knowledge of the **individual service user** and **their social context**, knowl-edge of the **service user's own experience**, and **clinical judgement** (DH, 2007c). Risk assessment is discussed in much more detail in Chapter 12.

Care planning

Intrinsically linked with assessment is care planning. While care planning is a necessary part of all nursing practice, it is especially important with service users on acute wards because of the enhanced professional and legal demands that often accompany acute admissions (CPA and the issues associated with compulsory detention, for example). Within acute inpatient settings, it is nursing staff who usually take the lead in formulating inpatient care plans. While individual inpatient areas will have devised their own style, format, layout and processes for care planning and while developing effective care planning skills requires support, supervision and lots of practice, there are a number of important principles that can help you produce better care plans. These principles are summarised in Table 7.4.

Remember that care plans are important documents that need to be com-pleted with diligence because they provide evidence of the care and treatment provided. In the unfortunate case of an untoward or serious incident, care plans enable practitioners to account for their practice and the interventions being delivered to service users.

TABLE 7.4 Principles of good care planning

Principle	Details
Service user centredness	Focusing on what the service user's needs are and what *they* want to achieve (their goals)
Clarity	Ensuring that the care plan is understandable and that it is specific in how any such needs or goals can be met
Recovery-focused	Care plans should promote an optimistic future for the service users, informing them there is every chance they will get better, that people with serious mental health problems do, indeed, get better
Collaboration	Care plans should be devised in collaboration with the service user and, wherever possible, with their carers and significant others
Openness	Service users should always be given copies of their care plans and the plans should be reviewed with the service user on a regular basis

Evidence-Based Interventions for Acute Mental Health Problems

The role of the nurse in acute inpatient settings can be varied and complex: he or she will at times be involved in ensuring the **safety of the service user and others**, collecting and communicating **information about service users**, giving and monitoring various **treatments**, tolerating and managing **disturbed behaviour**, providing **personal care**, **supporting relatives and carers**, and **managing the comfort and ambience of the environment** (Bowers, 2005).

Nurses in acute settings can thus be involved in a range of interventions designed to help service users recover from their mental health problems – from those interventions (e.g. pharmaceutical and psychological) that act directly on the service user to those that underpin the creation of an environment conducive to recovery.

Pharmaceutical interventions

Since most service users admitted to acute services will be prescribed psychotropic medication (to reduce arousal or distress, or to stabilise and improve an individual's mental health), medication has a fundamental role to play in acute mental health settings. The most commonly used drugs are the **antipsychotics**, **benzodiazepines**, **hypnotics** (sleeping tablets) and **mood stabilisers** (see Table 7.5).

While medication has been used routinely in inpatient settings for decades, there has been some debate about the effectiveness of its use (Bentall, 2009).

TABLE 7.5 Common medications used in acute care

Medication group	Examples in common use*
Antipsychotics	**'Typical' antipsychotics**, such as chlorpromazine, haloperidol, flupentixol, sulpiride **'Atypical' antipsychotics**, such as olanzapine, risperidone, clozapine
Benzodiazepines	Principally used for agitation and the short-term relief of severe anxiety and alcohol withdrawal: such as diazepam, chlordiazepoxide, lorazepam
Hypnotics	The **benzodiazepines**, such as nitrazepam and temazepam **Non-benzodiazepines**, such as zopiclone and clomethiazole
Mood stabilisers	**Tricyclic antidepressants**, such as amitriptyline and doxepin **Selective-serotonin reuptake inhibitors** (SSRIs), such as fluoxetine, citalopram and paroxetine **Lithium** (used in bipolar disorder)

*Since prescribing varies across the UK, you may not be familiar with some of the specific medications listed; likewise, there may be specific medications you are familiar with which are not listed.

Medication, however, remains a first-line treatment in the NICE guidance on schizophrenia (NICE, 2009a) though with some added conditions such as the avoidance, wherever possible, of polypharmacy, the use of lower doses (certainly not exceeding those recommended in the *British National Formulary*) and the implementation of service user choice, especially given the unpleasant side-effects that are common with many antipsychotic drugs. Medication also features in the NICE guidance on anxiety (NICE, 2004) and depression (NICE, 2009b), though again there are cautions, for example antidepressants are not being recommended for mild-to-moderate depression.

It is important for nurses to know about medication because it is nurses who are most often required to administer (and in some cases prescribe) medications. Nurses also have a co-responsibility (along with the service user) to monitor and manage any side-effects. Harris (2009) identifies a number of principles associated with medicines management that are useful to nurses: first, if medicines are likely to be beneficial, then they should be prescribed at the **lowest dose** to achieve the desired therapeutic effect; secondly, treatment should be seen as a **collaborative** process, one that involves choice and is facilitated through a genuine and trusting relationship with the service user; and thirdly, helping service users develop **self-efficacy** in managing their symptoms should also be a key aspect of medication management.

There are guidelines that can help nurses with the administration and management of medication – regarding rapid tranquilisation, atypical antipsychotics and 'as required' (p.r.n.) medication, for example – many of which are available on the UK Psychiatric Pharmacy Group's website www.ukppg.org.uk (see the list of Web resources at the end of this chapter). Additionally, many employing organisations will have their own policies and procedures in relation to the administration of medicines. Most nurses also find the *British National Formulary* (BNF) a useful resource (see the list of key texts at the end of this chapter).

Electroconvulsive therapy

Electroconvulsive therapy (ECT) is a controversial therapy that you will probably encounter as a treatment option at some point in your career as a mental health nurse. It is used in three main acute conditions: **severe depression**; **catatonia** (a rare condition in which individuals are verbally and physically unresponsive, often maintaining unusual postures for long periods); and **prolonged or severe episodes of mania**.

It is a physical procedure whereby the person is first anaesthetised, after which electrodes are placed against the person's head to induce an artificial seizure. Typically, ECT is given twice a week for three to six weeks. It is controversial for a number of reasons, most notably because of questions over its safety (particularly in terms of long-term brain damage; ECT certainly elicits short-term memory loss) and effectiveness, and because of the ethical questions that surround its use, especially when given without consent (Reisner, 2003). Nevertheless, Cresswell et al. (2007) report survey findings showing that 72% of those having ECT thought that the treatment had helped them (with 14% believing that it had changed or even saved their life) compared to only 5% who stated that they would not want it again.

Specific NICE guidance on ECT can be found in a technology appraisal report (NICE, 2003) and in the NICE guidance on depression (NICE 2009b). The gist of this guidance is summarised in Box 7.4.

Box 7.4   NICE guidance relating to ECT

- ECT should be used for fast-and short-term improvement of **severe** symptoms after all **other treatment options have failed** or where the situation is **life-threatening**.
- Since ECT carries risks (e.g. memory loss), it should be used after a **risk–benefit analysis** has been carried out.
- The issue of **consent** is vital; where discussion and consent are not possible, any **advance directives** should be taken into account.
- Caution should be observed with **older** or **younger** people, and with **pregnant women**.
- The person should be **re-assessed** after every session of ECT.
- The treatment should be stopped as soon as the person has **responded**, if there are **adverse effects** or they withdraw their **consent**.
- ECT should **not** be used routinely for moderate depression.
- It should **not** be used as a long-term treatment to prevent the recurrence of depression, nor should it be used in the general management of schizophrenia.

Adapted from the National Institute for Health and Clinical Excellence Technology Appraisal 59 (ECT; Nice, 2003) and Clinical Guidance 90 (depression; NICE, 2009b)

Psychological and social interventions

As we have seen elsewhere in this book – in Chapters 4 to 6 especially – cognitive behavioural therapy (CBT) and psychosocial interventions (PSI) have a significant evidence base and there is no reason why these interventions cannot be used in inpatient settings, especially once the initial acute phase has begun to subside.

There is some evidence that social interventions such as **befriending** can have similar outcomes to CBT (Sensky et al., 2000) and that, as such, social support merits some attention in psychosis (Milne et al., 2006). Note that befriending is not the same as friendship: friendship is a private, mutual relationship whereas befriending is a *service* that is provided to users (SBDF, 1997).

Observations

This refers to the practice of staff (more often than not, nursing staff) directly observing a service user, his or her whereabouts and his or her behaviour at regular intervals. All provider organisations will have their own local procedures and policies for the use of observations, each containing its own terminology, criteria for employing observations, details of the staff who should carry out observations, and specifications for documentation. Broadly speaking, there are four levels in common use: (1) **no observations**; (2) **general observations** (hourly checks); (3) **intermittent observations** (physical checks on an individual every 10–15 minutes) and (4) **1:1+** (constant nursing presence), which may occur at a distance or within close proximity (arm's length), depending on the risks.

There are four principal reasons for using observations, all of them associated with risk: (1) risk to **self**, because an individual may be suicidal, likely to self-harm, or vulnerable in terms of neglect; (2) risk to **others** (including staff and fellow patients) in relation to physical assault, verbal abuse or displaying inappropriate and over-familiar behaviour that might impact on fellow service users, visitors or staff; (3) risk of **absconding**, which may be coupled with a risk to self or to others; and (4) to **monitor mental state**, which is integral to all of the other reasons.

There have been mixed reports on the therapeutic value of observations over the past decade. The 'refocusing' initiative which was popular in the late 1990s and at the turn of this century was critical of the use of observations because it was seen as a passive intervention that did not promote engagement with service users (Dodds & Bowles, 2001; Bowles & Jones, 2005). As a result of this criticism, attempts were made to remove observations from wards and/or encourage nursing staff to spend productive time with service users. Surprisingly, recent evidence suggests that intermittent observations *are* effective at reducing incidents of self-harm (Bowers et al., 2007; Bowers &

Simpson, 2007). Even if effective, there are still some legitimate criticisms of observations, however. The higher levels of observation are resource-intensive and often it is the least qualified staff who have to spend long periods of time observing service users. Another challenge of observations is conducting them in a manner that causes the least restriction to an individual's privacy and dignity whilst also enabling a therapeutic relationship to flourish.

Case scenario: intermittent observations

Morag, the ward manager of a 26-bedded acute ward, asks Ray, a senior healthcare assistant, to carry out intermittent (15 minute) observations on Michael, a 35-year-old Afro-Caribbean service user who has been detained under a Scottish Mental Health Act 'Emergency Detention Certificate' (roughly equivalent to a Section 4 of the Mental Health Act for England and Wales, or Article 4 of the Northern Ireland Mental Health Order).

The main reason for placing Michael on observations is a concern that he may abscond since he is extremely unhappy about being detained and is openly threatening to leave. Ray approaches Michael, introduces himself and explains to Michael that he will be on intermittent observations and that he will need to check on him every 15 minutes or so. Michael replies to Ray, 'That's what you think; I ain't having no one stalk me; I'll be gone the moment your back's turned.'

Do you think intermittent observation is an appropriate intervention?

Do you think Morag is right to ask a senior healthcare assistant to carry out this activity? Could it have been done by a student nurse? Can you think of any safeguards that need to be in place to protect the staff, Michael, and the other service users on the ward?

Do you think there is anything that can be done to lessen the threats to Michael's privacy and dignity and help build up a therapeutic relationship?

Can you think of any alternative interventions that could be used to reduce the risk that Michael will abscond from the ward?

De-escalation and aggression management

While the management of aggression is considered in more detail in Chapter 12, it is worth briefly examining the evidence base for a couple of commonly used methods of managing aggression in acute settings. **De-escalation** is seen as the first line of action in the NICE guidance on managing aggression and violence (NICE, 2005), even though NICE acknowledges that its evidence base is somewhat limited. De-escalation is a fundamental skill for nurses working in acute settings, its purpose being to prevent the early signs of aggression escalating to more serious aggression or violence. It is not entirely clear what personal qualities and abilities underpin de-escalation and considerably more work is needed to understand how nurses can calm situations rather than act as triggers for violence.

Restraint is another technique for managing aggression, though the NICE guidance again reports that evidence base is limited. Nevertheless, there has been considerable investment in **control and restraint** training as a means of dealing with aggression and violence. Though attempts have been made to standardise this training (by the General Services Association and Broadmoor Hospital, for example), inconsistencies remain across the UK. Like pharmacological interventions, applying 'hands on' restraint should be seen as a last resort in the management of aggression: according to the NICE guidance, staff should only restrain someone if they are **sufficiently trained** and **competent** to do so.

Meaningful activity and structure to the day

A recurring criticism of acute mental health wards is the lack of activity for service users and the associated high levels of boredom. Activity and daily structure are very important for a service user's mental health because meaningful and structured activity can help service users cope with their current difficulties (through distraction or through learning coping strategies), encourage social interaction between service users as well as with staff, and help people regain or learn new skills which can, in turn, improve confidence, motivation and self-esteem. There is some evidence that there is a relationship between structured ward activity, rates of self-harm and the attitudes of nursing staff (Bowers et al., 2007).

Two initiatives that have made an impact in this area are refocusing and *Star Wards*. We mentioned refocusing in the earlier discussion on observations because it is primarily an anti-observation approach. However, because a principal goal of refocusing is giving staff control over their day-to-day elements of their jobs, refocusing can have the knock-on effect of improving meaningful activity on wards that use this approach. There is some limited evidence that refocusing can reduce outcomes such as self-harm and absconding (Dodds & Bowles, 2001) but a recent systematic review of alternatives to traditional acute care (Lloyd-Evans et al., 2009) found little evidence of its effectiveness.

Star Wards – developed by Marion Janner, a service user – aims to increase daily experiences and treatment outcomes for service users in inpatient settings. It collects and shares ideas, no matter how small, from mental health wards that have helped to engage service users or have improved the quality of care: in essence, it is a list of things mental health wards are doing right rather than a list of what is wrong with acute care. The first *Star Wards* publication (Janner, 2006) listed 75 of these ideas and its 'sequel' (Janner, 2008) contains literally hundreds more. Establishing a formal evidence base for *Star Wards* is difficult because each listed idea could in itself be an intervention; nevertheless, the fact that it is **user-led**, that it looks at acute care in a **positive** light, and that it has **spread far and wide** (gaining more than 300 wards as members) means that it is a significant initiative.

Improving communication

Bowers et al. (2009) have produced some guidance for communicating with acutely psychotic people based on interviews with acknowledged expert mental health nurses working in acute settings. Box 7.5 contains a summary of the guidance but since the publication contains a significant amount of detail you may wish to obtain the original document.

Box 7.5 Guidance for communicating with acutely psychotic people (adapted, with permission, from Bowers et al., 2009)

Domain 1: The moral foundations

- **Notice**, do not ignore, the service user; at the same time **do not intrude** and respect their **privacy**.
- Be **warm, empathic** and **concerned**.
- **Respect** the service user and be **honest**, especially in relation to restrictions on their liberty.

Domain 2: Preparing to interact

- **Consult widely**, with records, friends, family and **observe** carefully.
- Consider the **best time of day**, the **best location** and the **right nurse** to make the approach.

Domain 3: Being with the service user

- **Introduce** yourself and **explain** your role.
- **Be with**, or **sit with**, the service user, offering light, causal, normal **conversation** using the here and now as a topic and appropriate humour.

  - For **apathy/withdrawal**, use **comfortable silence** or engage in **one-sided conversations**.
  - For service users actively **hallucinating**, **tolerate** and **make allowances** for such hallucinations in the conversation, **choose simple topics**.
  - For **thought disorder**, **accept** and **listen**, give **reminders** or **prompts**, ask for **clarification**, and keep things **simple**.
  - For **agitation** or **over activity**, **reduce stimulation**, **set interaction limits** and give **positive feedback**.
  - For **upset** or **distress**, normal conversation may be inappropriate.
  - For **irritability** or **aggression**, it may be better to (temporarily) avoid the service user or use a topic that the service user is an expert in to engage them.

Domain 4: Non-verbal communication

- Use a **slow pace**, **slow speech**, **short sentences**, **simple vocabulary** and **repetition**.
- Interactions should be **short** and **frequent**.
- **Tone of voice** should be **caring** and **quiet**.
- **Touch and gesticulation** can be both appropriate and inappropriate.

Domain 5: Emotional responding

- Regulate your own emotional response: be **calm** and **receptive** in the face of psychotic symptoms, service user distress, hostility and aggression.

Domain 6: Getting things done

- When service users need to undertake some task beneficial to their recovery (e.g. eat, get up, take their medication), **suggest**, rather than order, giving **reasons** and breaking tasks down into **smaller steps**.
- Be **flexible**, maximise **choice**, **prompt** and **support** and give **positive feedback**.

Domain 7: Talk about symptoms

- **Hear** what service users' experiences are and seek to **understand** them.

  - For **apathy/withdrawal**, mutually explore causes, develop a **routine** and **purpose** and take **small steps**.

(Continued)

(Continued)

- For service users actively **hallucinating**, consider **stress management, distraction**, and possibly **challenge** the hallucinatory content.
- For **delusions, consider gentle questioning** or **direct challenge.***
- For **agitation** or **overactivity, irritability** or **aggression** consider exercise, distraction, relaxation with explanations and, if necessary, forceful containment.
- For **upset** or **distress**, keeping patients talking to find out the cause, and taking action to relieve the cause.

*Directly challenging delusions is somewhat controversial and requires significant skill on behalf of the nurse. It is an approach that students should use with great caution and always with the guidance and supervision of an experienced mentor.

Alternatives to inpatient care

The evidence base for the three principal alternatives to inpatient care is sketchy. A systematic review (Marshall & Lockwood, 1998) comparing **assertive outreach** with standard care, hospital-based rehabilitation and case management found that assertive outreach is a clinically effective approach to managing the care of people with severe mental health problems and that it could substantially reduce the costs of hospital care.

Regarding **early intervention** services, a systematic review (Marshall & Rathbone, 2006) concluded that there was insufficient evidence to draw any definitive conclusions about their effectiveness. As far as **crisis resolution/ home treatment** services are concerned, there is little contemporary research in this area although an evidence base is beginning to emerge, especially in terms of reduced admission rates and service user preferences (Johnson & Bindman, 2008).

There is also some evidence that community-based *residential* alternatives may be superior to hospital admission. In a systematic review, Lloyd-Evans et al. (2009) compared community-based residential services, time-limited hospital admissions (respite) and residential facilities offering a specific therapeutic model (such as refocusing or the 'Tidal model' discussed briefly in Chapter 1). Of the three types of provision, the best evidence of effectiveness was for community-based residential services such as 'Soteria' houses[2] and

---

[2]Soteria was the Greek goddess of safety and deliverance.

crisis hostels, leading Lloyd-Evans et al. to conclude that community-based residential crisis services are a feasible and acceptable alternative to hospital admission for some people with acute mental illness.

Conclusion

We have seen how acute mental healthcare forms a key component of mental health service provision and that inpatient care is necessary for some individuals in spite of developments in community mental healthcare. In the face of numerous reports criticising acute care provision, we have shown how interventions such as meaningful activity and enhanced communication can bring benefits for both service users and staff.

Acute mental healthcare has the potential to make a significant and positive contribution to the recovery of people who are suffering from mental health problems who also require intensive care and treatment. Moreover, nurses have a key role to play in the ongoing development of acute care services. This is particularly the case when nursing staff display caring and positive attitudes towards service users, spend time interacting and communicating with service users, and when robust, evidence-based interventions are delivered.

Further Reading and Resources

Key texts

Bowers L, Brennan G, Winship G & Theodoridou C (2009). *Talking with Acutely Psychotic People, Communication Skills for Nurses and Others Spending Time with People Who Are Very Mentally Ill. London: City University*. Available from www.acutecareprogramme.org.uk
A comprehensive document that outlines some of the ways in which communication can be enhanced in acute settings.

Harris N, Baker JA & Gray R (eds) (2009). *Medicines Management in Mental Health Care.* Chichester: Wiley–Blackwell.
Recent textbook on medication management edited by three experts in mental health nursing.

Beer MD, Pereira SM & Paton C (eds) (2008). *Psychiatric Intensive Care*, 2nd edition. Cambridge: Cambridge University Press.
Second edition of a key text on psychiatric intensive care, that looks at therapeutic interventions, the interface with other services and the management of psychiatric intensive care services.

Joint Formulary Committee. *The British National Formulary*. London: Royal Pharmaceutical Library of Great Britain/British Medical Association.

Targeted at health professionals, the BNF provides comprehensive details of medicines prescribed in the UK. No publication date is given for this text because it is updated every six months. Section 4 – the Central Nervous System – is of most relevance to those working in mental health. The BNF is also available at www.bnf.org.

Key policy documents

Healthcare Commission (2008). *The Pathway to Recovery: A Review of NHS Acute Inpatient Mental Health Services.* London: Healthcare Commission.

National Institute for Health and Clinical Excellence (2009). *Core Interventions in the Treatment and Management of Schizophrenia in Primary and Secondary Care (Updated).* London: NICE. Available from www.nice.org.uk/CG82

Department of Health (2008). *Code of Practice: Mental Health Act 1983.* London: TSO.

Scottish Executive (2005). *Mental Health (Care and Treatment) (Scotland) Act 2003: Code of Practice. Volumes 1 to 3.* Edinburgh: Scottish Executive.

Web resources

The Star Wards initiative: www.starwards.org.uk
Star Wards is an excellent, user-led initiative that is having a major impact on the quality of care delivered in inpatient settings.

UK Psychiatric Pharmacy Group: www.ukppg.org.uk
Contains lots of useful information relating to mental health medications, including clinical guidelines (at www.ukppg.org.uk/support_clinical.htm). This group also plays a major role in the excellent 'Choice and Medication' website: www.choiceandmedication.org.uk.

The Acute Care Programme: www.virtualward.org.uk
A gateway for news, events, policy and best practice in acute mental health care from the National Mental Health Development Unit.

National Forum for Assertive Outreach: www.nfao.org
Includes FAQs, together with resources on, and information about research into, assertive outreach.

References

Baker JA & Munro S (2006). Factors influencing acuity within inpatient mental health care. *Journal of Psychiatric Intensive Care,* **2**(2), 90–96.

Beck AT, Ward CH, Mendelson M, Mock J & Erbaugh J (1961). An inventory for measuring depression. *Archives of General Psychiatry,* **4**, 561–571.

Bentall RP (2009). *Doctoring the Mind: Is Our Current Treatment of Mental Illness Really Any Good?* London: Penguin.

Boardman J & Parsonage M (2007). *Delivering the Government's Mental Health Policies: Services, Staffing and Costs.* London: Sainsbury Centre for Mental Health.

Bowers L (2005). Reasons for admission and their implications for the nature of acute inpatient psychiatric nursing. *Journal of Psychiatric and Mental Health Nursing*, **12**, 231–236.

Bowers L & Simpson A (2007). Observing and engaging: new ways to reduce self-harm and suicide. *Mental Health Practice*, **10**(10), 12–14.

Bowers L, Brennan G, Winship G & Theodoridou C (2009). *Talking with Acutely Psychotic People: Communication Skills for Nurses and Others Spending Time with People Who Are Very Mentally Ill*. London: City University.

Bowers L, Whittington R, Nolan P, Parkin D, Curtis S, Bhui K, Hackney D, Allan T, Simpson A & Flood C (2007). *The City 128 Study of Observation and Outcomes on Acute Psychiatric Wards*. London: City University (for the NCCSDO).

Bowles N & Jones A (2005). Whole systems working and acute inpatient psychiatry: an exploratory study. *Journal of Psychiatric and Mental Health Nursing*, **12**, 283–289.

Cresswell J, Hood C & Lelliott P (2007). *Electroconvulsive Therapy Accreditation Service (ECTAS) Second National Report: October 2005–October 2007*. London: Royal College of Psychiatrists' Centre for Quality Improvement.

CSIP/NIMHE (Care Services Improvement Partnership/National Institute for Mental Health in England) (2008). *Laying the Foundations for Better Acute Mental Health Care*. London: DH.

DH (Department of Health) (1991). *The Care Programme Approach*. London: DH.

DH (Department of Health) (1999a). *National Service Framework for Mental Health: Modern Standards and Service Models*. London: HMSO.

DH (Department of Health) (1999b*). Effective Care Co-ordination in Mental Health Services: Modernising the Care Programme Approach*. London: DH.

DH (Department of Health) (2000). Hospital Activity Statistics (interactive tables). Available from: www.performance.doh.gov.uk/hospitalactivity/[accessed 12 February 2010].

DH (Department of Health) (2001). *The Mental Health Policy Implementation Guide*. London: HMSO.

DH (Department of Health) (2002). *Mental Health Policy Implementation Guide: Adult Acute Inpatient Care Provision*. London: DH.

DH (Department of Health) (2004). *The National Service Framework for Mental Health – 5 Years On*. London: DH.

DH (Department of Health) (2005). *New Ways of Working for Psychiatrists: Enhancing Effective, Person-Centred Services through New Ways of Working in Multidisciplinary and Multi-Agency Contexts*. London: DH.

DH (Department of Health) (2006). *From Values to Action: The Chief Nursing Officer's Review of Mental Health Nursing*. London: DH.

DH (Department of Health) (2007a). *Mental Health: New Ways of Working for Everyone: Developing and Sustaining a Capable and Flexible Workforce*. London: DH.

DH (Department of Health) (2007b). *Positive Steps: Supporting Race Equality in Mental Healthcare*. London: DH.

DH (Department of Health) (2007c). *Best Practice in Managing Risk: Principles and Evidence for Best Practice in the Assessment and Management of Risk to Self and Others in Mental Health Services*. London: DH.

DH (Department of Health) (2008a). *Code of Practice: Mental Health Act 1983*. London:TSO.

DH (Department of Health) (2008b). *Refocusing the Care Programme Approach: Policy and Positive Practice Guidance*. London: DH.

DH (Department of Health) (2009). Average daily number of available and occupied beds by ward classification, England, 2008–09 [Microsoft Excel file]. London: DH. Available from: www.dh.gov.uk [accessed 10 February 2010].

DHSSPS (Department of Health, Social Services and Public Safety) (2005). *A Strategic Framework for Adult Mental Health Services*. Belfast: DHSSPS. Available from: www.rmhldni.gov.uk [accessed 14 February 2010].

DHSSPS (Department of Health, Social Services and Public Safety) (2009a). *Hospital Statistics by Speciality 1999/2000*. Belfast: DHSSPS. Available from: www.nice.org.uk/CG 90 [accessed 10 February 2010].

DHSSPS (Department of Health, Social Services and Public Safety) (2009b). *Hospital Statistics, 1 April 2008–31 March 2009. Volume 2a: Inpatient Specialty Tables*. Belfast: DHSSPS. Available from: www.dhsspsni.gov.uk [accessed 10 February 2010].

Dodds P & Bowles N (2001). Dismantling formal observation and refocusing nursing activity in acute inpatient psychiatry. *Journal of Psychiatric and Mental Health Nursing*, **8**(2), 183–188.

Folstein MF, Folstein SE & McHugh PR (1975). 'Mini-mental state': a practical method for grading the cognitive state of patients for the clinician. *Journal of Psychiatric Research*, **12**(3), 189–198.

Four UK Health Departments (2004). *Modernising Medical Careers. The Next Steps: The Future Shape of Foundation, Specialist and General Practice Training Programmes*. London: DH.

Glasby J & Lester H (2005). On the inside: a narrative review of mental health inpatient services. *British Journal of Social Work*, **35**, 863–879.

Glover G, Arts G & Suresh K (2006). Crisis resolution/home treatment teams and psychiatric admission rates in England. *British Journal of Psychiatry*, **189**, 441–445.

Haddock G, McCarron J, Tarrier N & Faragher EB (1999). Scales to measure dimensions of hallucinations and delusions: the psychotic symptom rating scales (PSYRATS). *Psychological Medicine*, **29**, 879–889.

Harris N (2009). *Introduction to Medicines Management*. In N Harris, JA Baker & R Gray (eds), *Medicines Management in Mental Health Care*. Chichester: Wiley–Blackwell.

Healthcare Commission (2008). *The Pathway to Recovery: A Review of NHS Acute Inpatient Mental Health Services*. London: Healthcare Commission.

Heenan D (2009). Mental health policy in Northern Ireland: the nature and extent of user involvement. *Social Policy & Society*, **8**(4), 451–462.

HM Government (2009). *New Horizons: A Shared Vision for Mental Health*. London: Department of Health.

ISD (Information Services Directorate) Scotland (2009). Available Beds by Specialty & NHS Board of Treatment [interactive Microsoft Excel document]. Edinburgh: ISD Scotland. Available from: www.isdscotland.org [accessed 12 February 2010].

Janner M (2006). *Star Wards:Practical Ideas for Improving the Daily Experiences and Treatment Outcomes of Acute Mental Health In-Patients*. London: Bright. Available from www.starwards.org.uk [accessed 7 February 2010].

Janner M (2008). *Star Wards 2, The Sequel: Loads More Practical Ideas for Improving the Daily Experiences and Treatment Outcomes of Mental Health Inpatients*. London: Bright. Available from www.starwards.org.uk [accessed 7 February 2010].

Johnson S & Bindman JP (2008). Recent research on crisis resolution teams: findings and limitations. In S Johnson, J Needle, JP Bindman & G Thornicroft (eds), *Crisis Resolution and Home Treatment in Mental Health*. Cambridge: Cambridge University Press.

Lloyd-Evans B, Slade M, Jagielska D & Johnson S (2009). Residential alternatives to acute psychiatric hospital admission: systematic review. *British Journal of Psychiatry*, **195**, 109–117.

Marshall M & Lockwood A (1998). Assertive community treatment for people with severe mental disorders. *Cochrane Database of Systematic Reviews*, Issue 2, Article CD001089.

Marshall M & Rathbone J (2006). Early intervention for psychosis. *Cochrane Database of Systematic Reviews*, Issue 4, Article CD004718.

MHA (Mental Health Act) Commission (2008). *Risk, Rights, Recovery: Twelfth Biennial Report 2005–2007*. London: TSO.

MHN/NMHDU (National Mental Health Development Unit/Mental Health Network) (2009). *Acute Care Declaration*. London: NMHDU/MHN. Available from: www.acute careprogramme.org.uk [accessed 7 February 2010].

Milne D, Wharton S, James I & Turkington D (2006). Befriending versus CBT for schizophrenia: a convergent and divergent fidelity check. *Behavioural and Cognitive Psychotherapy*, **34**, 25–30.

MIND (2007). *Briefing 2: Supervised Community Treatment*. London: MIND. Available from: www.mind.org.uk [accessed 7 February 2010].

National Audit Office (2007). *Helping People through Mental Health Crisis: The Role of Crisis Resolution and Home Treatment Services*. London: National Audit Office.

NES (NHS Education for Scotland) (2007). *A Capability Framework for Working in Acute Mental Health Care: The Values, Skills, and Knowledge Needed to Deliver High Quality Care in a Full Range of Acute Settings*. Edinburgh: NES.

NI (Northern Ireland) Executive (2009). McGimpsey announces single bill approach for mental health [press release 10 September 2009]. Available from: www.northernireland.gov.uk [accessed 7 February 2010].

NICE (National Institute for Clinical Excellence) (2003). *Guidance on the Use of Electroconvulsive Therapy [NICE Technology Appraisal 59]*. London: NICE.

NICE (National Institute for Clinical Excellence) (2004). *Anxiety: Management of Anxiety (Panic Disorder, With or Without Agoraphobia, and Generalised Anxiety Disorder) in Adults in Primary, Secondary and Community Care*. London: NICE.

NICE (National Institute for Clinical Excellence) (2005). *Violence: The Short-term Management of Disturbed/Violent Behaviour in In-patient Psychiatric Settings and Emergency Departments*. London: NICE.

NICE (National Institute for Health and Clinical Excellence) (2009a). *Core Interventions in the Treatment and Management of Schizophrenia in Primary and Secondary Care (Updated)*. London: NICE.

NICE (National Institute for Health and Clinical Excellence) (2009b). *Depression: The Treatment and Management of Depression in Adults (Partial update of NICE clinical guideline 23)*. London: NICE. Available from: www.nice.org.uk/CG90 [accessed 10 February 2010].

NIMHE (National Institute for Mental Health in England) (2004). *Crisis Resolution and Home Treatment*. Birmingham: NIMHE West Midlands/UCE Centre for Community Mental Health. Available from: www.ccmh.uce.ac.uk [accessed 7 February 2010].

ONS (Office for National Statistics) (2009). Key Population and Vital Statistics [2007 data]. Newport: ONS. Available from: www.statistics.gov.uk [accessed 10 February 2010].

Parsonage M (2005). The Mental Health Economy. In A Bell & P Lindley (eds), *Beyond the Water Towers: The Unfinished Revolution in Mental Health Services, 1985–2005*. London: Sainsbury Centre for Mental Health.

Reisner AD (2003). The electroconvulsive therapy controversy: evidence and ethics. *Neuropsychology Review*, **13**(4), 199–219.

Rethink, SANE, the Zito Trust & the National Association of Psychiatric Intensive Care Units (2006). *Behind Closed Doors: The Current State and Future Vision of Acute Mental Health Care in the UK*. London: Rethink. Available from: www.mentalhealthshop.org [accessed 7 February 2010].

SBDF (Scottish Befriending Development Forum) (1997). *Code of Practice: Working Together to Promote Good Practice in Befriending*. Falkirk: SBDF.

SCMH (Sainsbury Centre for Mental Health) (1998). *Acute Problems. A Survey of the Quality of Care in Acute Psychiatric Wards*. London: SCMH.

SCMH (Sainsbury Centre for Mental Health) (2001). *Mental Health Topics: Assertive Outreach*. London: SCMH.

Scottish Executive (2005). *Mental Health (Care and Treatment) (Scotland) Act 2003: Code of Practice. Volumes 1 to 3*. Edinburgh: Scottish Executive.

Scottish Executive (2006). *Delivering for Mental Health*. Edinburgh: Scottish Executive.

Scottish Office (1998). *Implementing the Care Programme Approach: Results of a Joint Survey by the Social Work Services Inspectorate and the Accounts Commission*. Edinburgh: Social Work Services Inspectorate.

Sensky T, Turkington D, Kingdon D, Scott JL, Scott J, Siddle R, O'Carroll M & Barnes TRE (2000). A randomised controlled trial of cognitive-behavioural therapy for persistent symptoms in schizophrenia resistant to medication. *Archives of General Psychiatry*, **57**, 165–172.

StatsWales (2009). NHS beds and their use: summary data, by specialty group [interactive report generator]. Cardiff: Welsh Assembly Government. Available from: www.statswales.gov.uk [accessed 10 February 2010].

Thompson A, Shaw M, Harrison G, Ho D & Verne J (2004). Patterns of hospital admission for adult psychiatric illness in England: analysis of Hospital Episode Statistics data. *British Journal of Psychiatry*, **185**, 334–341.

Welsh Assembly Government (2003). Mental Health Policy Guidance. *The Care Programme Approach for Mental Health Service Users: A Unified and Fair System for Assessing and Managing Care*. Cardiff: Welsh Assembly Government.

Welsh Assembly Government (2005). *Raising the Standard: The Revised Adult Mental Health National Service Framework and an Action Plan for Wales*. Cardiff: Welsh Assembly Government.

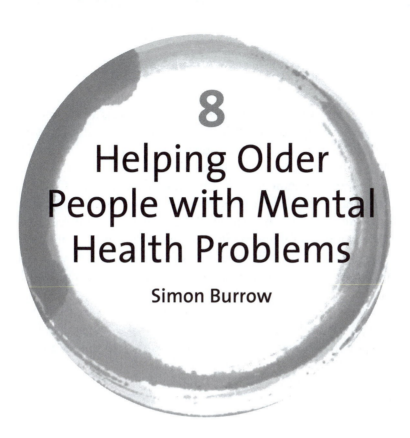

8

Helping Older People with Mental Health Problems

Simon Burrow

What will I learn in this chapter?

This chapter sets out to explore the evidence base by which nurses who are working with older people with mental health problems can pursue best practice. It does so within the wider context of how ageism and other social, psychological and biological factors can impact on the mental wellbeing of older people.

After reading this chapter, you will be able to:

- appreciate the biopsychosocial influences on mental wellbeing in older people;
- reflect on the issue of ageism and the impact this can have on older people and on practice;
- identify the most common mental health problems experienced by older people;
- outline a variety of evidence- and theory-based approaches to assessing and supporting older people with mental health problems.

Introduction

In 1911 there were an estimated 100 centenarians (someone aged at least 100) alive in England and Wales. The number of centenarians is now over 9,000 and is expected to have risen to more than 64,000 by 2033 (ONS, 2009a). In the UK as a whole, the number of people over state retirement age now surpasses the numbers of people under the age of 16 (ONS, 2009b). That we are living longer is a measure of success in our modern age, yet this success brings with it some significant challenges for health and social policy. There are ramifications for employment, income tax revenue (to fund pensions and services) and the availability of a pool of younger workers to provide care for older people with high dependency needs. There is concern that this competition for scarce resources will give rise to tensions across the generations and fuel negative attitudes (see Bengston & Putney, 2006 for a discussion).

The profile of the UK population is one that is ageing and it is the oldest in the population that form the most rapidly expanding segment of all (see Table 8.1). Furthermore, as late old age is the strongest known risk factor in the development of dementia, the numbers of people with dementia are predicted to expand at an exponential rate over the next few decades.

TABLE 8.1   Predicted percentage growth of older people (adapted from Age Concern, 2008a: 2006 figures)

	2018	2028
Over 50s	4.1m (20%)	6.7m (33%)
Over 65s	2.6m (27%)	5.1m (53%)
Over 80s	0.8m (29%)	2.3m (85%)

The ageing population is also becoming more ethnically diverse. Although people from black and minority ethnic (BME) populations in the UK have a younger age profile than the white population (Peace et al., 2007), those people from the waves of economic migration in the 1950s and 1960s are now heading into retirement years and represent 3% of people aged 65 and over (Age Concern, 2008a).

Terminology

The difficulty in using terms such as 'older people' is that we inevitably fall into the trap of classifying a widely differing population by chronological age alone. We run the risk, as such, of making sweeping generalisations on what the needs of 'older people' actually are. As a nurse it is important to be mindful and questioning of the language, labels, values and assumptions we can make around 'older age', and questioning also of the patterns and quality of service we offer older people.

All organisms age, and human beings are no exception. However, ageing is not merely a biological process; in many ways it is also socially constructed, and this social construction of 'old age' can have significant consequences. We see it in the design of health and social care services where separate services frequently exist for the over 65s. We see it also in many dimensions of social policy, perhaps most notably in (enforced) retirement policies, which have a profound impact on individuals and families.

Separate and distinct services

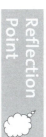

Reflection Point

A person who is 63 years old who has mental health problems is likely to be referred to a different set of services than they would be if they developed the same problems just a few years later. At the age of 66, in the eyes of many services, they would be classified as an 'older person'.

Think of three key advantages and three key disadvantages in maintaining separate and distinct mental health services for 'adults' (18–65 years) and 'older adults' (those over 65).

Emotional wellbeing in later life

There are multiple biological, social and psychological factors that may impact on older people and, in so doing, these factors can influence mental health and wellbeing. In particular, we need to look at **ageism**, material **deprivation**, social **isolation** and **physical ill-health**.

Ageism and stigma

Ageism has been described as: 'The systematic negative stereotyping of older people on the basis of age and the associated prejudice and discrimination ...' (Bond & Cabrero, 2007, p. 117). The effects of ageism are a commonly felt experience and the most widely self-reported form of discrimination in older people (Age Concern/Help the Aged, 2009).

It is possible to consider two separate – if interconnected – manifestations of ageism, the first being the **set beliefs and attitudes people harbour toward older people** and the second could be described as **institutional**

ageism. An example of the former would be perceptions of older people as frail, dependent, inflexible, conservative, cognitively impaired and lacking the physical perfection of youth that dominates Western culture. An example of the latter would be structures and services that discriminate against people on account of their age (though note that discrimination can also be positive, e.g. free or reduced cost transport).

Dobbs et al. (2008) argue that **stigma** – the assignment of negative worth on the basis of individual characteristics or membership of a devalued group – is commonly experienced by older people and has three inter-related components: (1) **dominant cultural beliefs**, where undesirable characteristics are linked to labelled persons; (2) **categorisation**, where labelled persons are placed in distinct categories so as to separate 'them' from 'us'; and (3) **discrimination**, where labelled persons experience status loss and discrimination that result in undesirable outcomes.

As we saw in Chapter 2, it is important to reflect on your own attitudes and values and you should be prepared to challenge (diplomatically) the actions and views of others where appropriate. In a survey, the majority of older people felt that people in very late older age were 'infantilised' (Age Concern/Help the Aged, 2009). This infantilisation is often expressed in the way in which we communicate with older people and there is evidence that such 'baby talk' or 'elderspeak' increases passivity and dependency (Cuddy et al., 2005). In relation to people with dementia, Kitwood (1997) sees infantilisation as an illustration of **malignant social psychology**, a concept we shall return to when discussing dementia.

Material deprivation

Retirement is not a homogenising experience; there is great disparity in material wealth *within* the retired population (Walker & Foster, 2006). Income in later life is tied to income in early life via accumulated pension rights, savings and investments; those who experienced less reward from labour in earlier life tend, in older age, to be the most materially deprived in the population (Vincent, 1999). Thus, social class positioning early in life 'casts a long shadow over future attainment and health outcomes' (Vincent et al., 2006, p. 53) and there is a strong link between occupational and educational status and health (Walker & Foster, 2006).

The 'shadow' described by Vincent et al. has significant impact on the older BME populations who in the 1950s and 1960s arrived in the UK often to take low-paid manual labour with poor security and pension rights. This disadvantage in earlier life may now be translating to a cumulative and complex disadvantage in later life (Nazroo, 2006; Peace et al., 2007).

Social support and social isolation

There is broad recognition of the importance of the strength of family ties and of other social networks on the psychological health of older people (Grundy & Slogett, 2003). A survey of almost a thousand adults over the age of 65 revealed that 7% of participants reported severe loneliness (Victor et al., 2005). A key issue to emerge from qualitative interviews in this study was the importance within the social network of the presence a confidant. Thus, the loss of a confidant, particularly the loss of a long-term partner, can be seen as a major contributor of loneliness (Bond & Corner, 2004).

In a study based on data from almost 2,000 individuals who took part in the British Household Survey, Gray (2009) explored respondents' perceived practical and emotional support. Gray's analysis confirmed a relationship between social class and the quality of social contacts, with higher support scores for retired professionals than for manual workers, and housing tenants had lower perceived support scores than home owners. Kin were seen to generally provide the strongest social support, and childless, single elders had very low support scores.

Thus losses of partners and the absence of kin are key threats to the social and emotional support of older people and factors such as social class, increasing age and ill health may make it increasingly challenging for older people to forge and sustain these important relationships. Supporting and enabling older people who are experiencing mental health problems to develop and/or maintain **social relationships** should be a key consideration for nurses.

Physical ill health and disability

Older people are more likely to experience a range of chronic and acute health complaints, and these are more common still in people in their 80s, 90s and beyond. **Sensory losses**, **arthritis**, **cardiovascular problems** and **cognitive impairment** all become more commonplace. **Chronic pain** is a common experience for older people and is linked to **depression** and **sleep disturbance** (Ersek et al., 2008). Disability and depression commonly co-exist, although the link is not always clear as one may exacerbate the other (Manthorpe & Illiffe, 2005).

The wellbeing paradox

Given the potential to be poorer, more socially isolated, to experience poorer mobility and greater ill health, to suffer bereavements, to be closer to death, to fear the onset of cognitive impairment, and to experience the ill effects of ageism and stigma, you might expect to find study after study revealing older people to be significantly *less* optimistic and showing *greater* evidence of emotional ill health than younger cohorts in the population.

This, however, is simply not the case. Quality of life studies reveal that older people display *higher* levels of life satisfaction than you might expect, or might see in younger people who experience similar deprivations (Marcoen et al., 2007). It appears that as people age it is not uncommon to acquire a degree of **psychological resilience** which may be one factor in explaining what has been coined the **wellbeing paradox** (Windle, 2009), that is the perhaps surprisingly positive relationship between ageing and perceived sense of wellbeing *in spite* of the threats to wellbeing experienced in older age identified above.

It is important, therefore, to hold on to the fact that, for most older people, psychological wellbeing will be the norm. However, mental health problems are, of course, still experienced by many and they are influenced by the complex interplay of biological, psychological and social variables.

Policy Context

The first decade of the new millennium has been witness to a number of significant policy and service improvement initiatives that have had a direct impact on older adult mental healthcare across the UK. In 2001, the *National Service Framework for Older People* (NSF) (DH, 2001) set out to establish national (across England) standards for services for older people through a 10-year programme of action for health and social care services. Standard 7 specifically focused on mental health in older people. *Everybody's Business* (DH/CSIP, 2005) was a detailed service development guide, which aimed to build on the NSF and ensure that mainstream and specialist mental health services were working in a coordinated way to address the needs of older people with mental health problems. This was in recognition of the fact that older people with mental health problems are frequently in receipt of mainstream care – in acute general hospital wards or primary care settings, for example – where systems and skills bases are often not geared towards people with mental health problems.

The Welsh National Service Framework for Older People, issued in 2006, aims to improve the health and social care in Wales through rooting out age discrimination, personalising care, promoting health and wellbeing, challenging dependency and improving specialist services including mental health services for older people (Welsh Assembly Government, 2006). In particular, a key standard of the Welsh NSF is that older people with a high risk of mental health problems have access to primary prevention and integrated services that 'ensure timely and appropriate assessment, diagnosis, treatment and support for them and their carers' (p. 43).

In 2006, the National Institute for Health and Clinical Excellence (NICE) and the Social Care Institute for Excellence (SCIE) produced a set of detailed evidence-based guidelines on supporting people with dementia and their carers in both health and social care environments (NICE/SCIE, 2006). Though the NICE/SCIE guidance has applicability across the whole of the UK, Scotland has some complementary guidance for supporting people with dementia (see *Management of Patients with Dementia*; SIGN, 2006) and a general capability framework for mental health nurses who work with older people (NES, 2008). More recently, and following a public consultation, England has been party to a national dementia strategy, *Living Well with Dementia* (DH, 2009). Rather than detailing clinical guidelines that already exist (in the form of the NICE/SCIE guidance), the strategy aimed to 'ensure that significant improvements are made to dementia services across three key areas: **improved awareness**, **earlier intervention**, and a **higher quality of care**' (p. 9, emphasis added), and set out 17 objectives to achieve these improvements. Scotland's Dementia Strategy was launched in 2010 following a somewhat damning report on the quality of care for people with dementia in Scotland, *Remember I'm Still Me* (Care Commission/MWCS, 2009). The Scottish strategy identifies five key challenges and focuses on two key service delivery areas: improving support after diagnosis and improving hospital care (Scottish Government, 2010). At the time of writing, dementia strategies for Wales and Northern Ireland are in the pipeline.

Mental capacity

Mental capacity refers to the ability of an individual to make their own decisions. It is mentioned here as mental capacity is frequently an issue with people who have dementia. In England and Wales, the law surrounding mental capacity is dealt with through the Mental Capacity Act 2005, which came into force in 2007. In Scotland the Adults with Incapacity (Scotland) Act 2000 applies. In Northern Ireland, no equivalent mental capacity laws exist but mental capacity is being discussed in light of the Bamford Review of Mental Health and Learning Disability (see DHSSPS, 2009).

The mental capacity Acts provide a legal framework for making decisions on behalf of individuals who lack the capacity to make their own informed decisions. In both Acts, 'adults' are defined as people aged 16 and over. The underlying philosophy of both Acts is to ensure that any decision made, or action taken, on behalf of someone who lacks the capacity to make the decision or act for themselves is made in their **best interests**[1] and nurses – especially those working with dementia – should make themselves familiar with the relevant Code of Practice (for England and Wales, see DCA, 2007; for Scotland, see Scottish Government, 2008).

Mental Health Problems in Older People: Anxiety and Depression

Anxiety

Anxiety is a reasonably common disorder in later life, being experienced by about 10–15% of older people (Beekman, 1998). However, since the information presented in Chapter 5 is as applicable to older adults as it is to younger adults when anxiety is the sole or dominant presenting problem, there is little point discussing anxiety in any great detail here. We do know that anxiety often co-exists with **depression** and **dementia** – the two presenting problems we will consider in detail in this chapter – but if these conditions are addressed proactively by healthcare professionals then, more often than not, there will be an associated resolution of, or a reduction in, co-morbid anxiety.

Interventions for anxiety may be categorised as pharmacological or non-pharmacological. With regard to the former, the NICE guidelines (NICE, 2007a) recommend the benzodiazepines (such as chlordiazepoxide and diazepam) for short-term use only while antidepressants (which will discuss in more detail shortly) are recommended for longer courses of treatment. Among the non-pharmacological interventions are relaxation techniques, psychodynamic psychotherapy and cognitive behaviour therapy (CBT). While CBT has been shown to be effective in younger adults (NICE, 2007a), most trials have excluded people over 65 (Wetherell et al., 2003) and consequently, as Ayers et al. (2007) remark, there needs to be much more research on psychological treatments for older adults with anxiety.

Depression

Many people might think that dementia is the most common mental health problem seen in older people. However, the commonest mental health problem in older age is **depression** (one reason why we have considered depression in greater detail than anxiety). According to Age Concern (2007), around a

---

[1]You may recall from Chapter 3 the new role of 'best interests assessor'.

quarter of people over the age of 65 (22% of men and 28% of women) have symptoms of depression which are severe enough to warrant intervention and approximately half of these will meet the criteria for 'clinical depression'. Episodes of depression in older people may have a longer duration with shorter times to relapse than in younger people (Haddad, 2009).

Table 8.2 summarises the main factors associated with depression in older people. A number of these factors (illness and disability; loneliness; care homes; partner relationships and dementia) are of greater relevance to older than younger adults and this goes part of the way to explaining why depression becomes more common in older age groups.

TABLE 8.2   Factors associated with depression in older people

Factor	Remarks
Age	Depression becomes more common in older age groups, with symptoms of depression reaching 40% in the over 85s (Age Concern, 2007)
Illness and disability	There is a strong association between disability and depression in older people (McDougall et al., 2007), particularly impairments of mobility, sight and hearing (Weyerer et al., 2008). The relationship is complex, however, and either condition may precipitate or prolong the experience of the other (Weyerer et al., 2008). Poorer physical functioning is linked with poorer prognosis of people with depression (Licht-Strunk et al., 2009)
Gender	While numerous studies (e.g. McDougall et al., 2007) have found depression to be more common in women than men, after controlling for potential risk-factors, Weyerer et al. (2008) found no gender effect
Loneliness and social isolation	Loneliness in older people is linked to depression (Adams et al., 2004), with rates being particularly high in people who are 'housebound' (Manthorpe & Iliffe, 2005; Sirey, 2008)
Partner relationships	The absence of confiding relationships is linked to higher rates of depression. Lower rates of depression are observed in people who are married (Weyerer et al., 2008) and, in relation to chronic diseases, there is evidence of a 'buffer' effect against depressive symptoms in those with a partner relationship (Bishop et al., 2004)
Material deprivation	McDougall et al. (2007) found an association between deprivation and depression in older people living in the community although they add that the higher rates of depression seen in the more socio-economically deprived groups may be down to the higher rates of illness and disability evident in these groups
Care homes	People in care homes experience high rates of depression, which is often underdiagnosed (Choi et al., 2008)
Educational status	Lower educational status is associated with depression (Weyerer et al., 2008)
BME elders	While elders from minority ethnic groups appear to share prevalence rates similar to the wider population, they appear to receive lower levels of service (Lawrence et al., 2006)
Dementia	Depression commonly coexists with dementia with around 30–50% of people with Alzheimer's being affected (Zubenko et al., 2003)

Assessing older people for depression

Identifying depression in older people can be difficult. It may be that symptoms are not easy to unpick from physical illness or cognitive impairment or that activity levels and mood, for example, are considered to be 'normal' for the person in the eyes of others. As one older person quoted by Age Concern (2008b) remarks: 'I did not know I was depressed, I thought I had a physical health problem and it worried me' (p. 8).

Another difficulty is **stigma**. Some older people may view depression as a sign of weakness and inability to cope. Older people may, as such, have difficulty in admitting there is a problem and in seeking support from health services.

Figure 8.1 outlines some of the things that (mental health) nurses should be aware of when assessing older people for depression. The NICE guidelines (2009) recommend that, in assessing for depression, a person's physical state, living conditions and degree of social isolation should be assessed. These points may be especially relevant to older people. Supporting a person with depression can be particularly challenging: there is evidence that family caregivers (adult children and spouses) who care for depressed older people may suffer poorer mental health themselves as a result of caring (Sewitch et al., 2004).

Assessment, therefore, must be sensitive to the needs of key relationships and carers may require an assessment of their own needs. Indeed, in some circumstances, such an assessment may even be a statutory requirement under the Carers (Recognition and Services) Act 1995 and Carers (Equal Opportunities) Act 2004.

Assessment must also consider the **risk of suicide** in older people. Depression is strongly linked with suicide and 1 in 8 suicides in the UK are by people aged 65 and over, with highest rates of all for men aged 75 and over (Manthorpe & Illiffe, 2005). Box 8.1 outlines some observations regarding suicide in older people.

Box 8.1   Older people and suicide (Age Concern, 2007)

- Older people make fewer suicide attempts than younger people but are more successful at taking their own lives. One in four attempts by older people results in 'completed suicide', compared with one in 15 attempts for the general population.

- Older people, especially men, tend to use more lethal methods such as firearms and hanging. The most common method used by older men is hanging. Older women often die by drug overdose.
- Older people are more likely to be frail and more likely to live alone than younger people. They are less likely to recover from a suicide attempt and less likely to have someone intervene before or during the event.
- Older people who take their own lives are more likely than younger people to have seen their GP in the previous six months. They are more likely to present with symptoms of physical health problems, whereas younger people are more likely to present with symptoms of mental health problems.

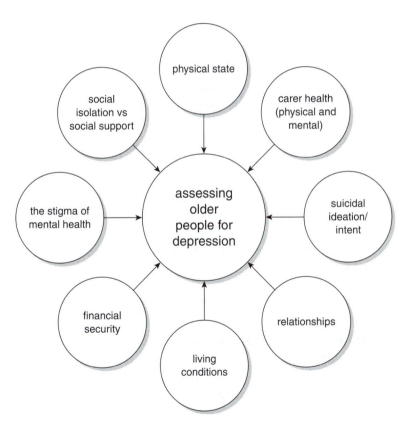

FIGURE 8.1   Things to consider when assessing older people for depression

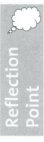

Suicide in older people

Did any of the observations in Box 8.1 surprise you?

How can these observations help you improve your practices when nursing older people? For example, how would you deal with an older person described by others as a 'hypochondriac'? Or with an older person who tells you he or she is lonely?

The NICE guidelines recommend that healthcare professionals should always ask people with depression directly about suicidal ideas and intent, and there is absolutely no reason why this guidance should not apply to older as well as younger adults.

Evidenced-based interventions for depression

Since most of the evidenced-based interventions for depression outlined in Chapter 4 are as relevant to older adults as they are to younger adults, we will not dwell on them too much here other than to make some specific comments in relation to older people. The NICE guidelines on depression (NICE, 2009) are applicable across the whole of the UK (in partnership with NHS Quality Improvement Scotland in Scotland and the DHSSPS in Northern Ireland) and you should familiarise yourself with the range of evidence-based interventions detailed in this guidance and how they might fit in with the 'stepped care model' of service provision.

Interventions for older people with depression can broadly be divided into three categories: **physical treatments**, **psychological treatments** and **social interventions**.

Physical treatments

There are two principal physical treatments: **medication** and **electroconvulsive therapy** (ECT). Treatment with **antidepressants** is considered to be as effective as with younger adults but longer treatment times are often necessary to achieve therapeutic effects (Haddad, 2009). Antidepressant medication should be individually tailored with a 'start low and go slow' approach in the more frail. Nurses need to be aware that some older people may fear drug dependence, recall prior negative experiences of medication, not view their symptoms as a medical illness, and be concerned that antidepressants will prevent natural feelings (Givens et al., 2006). As such, nurses should ensure that older people are given clear information and guidance if medication is recommended.

The NICE guidance (2009) notes that there is an increased risk of gastro-intestinal bleeding in older people prescribed selective serotonin reuptake inhibitors (SSRIs) and that a gastroprotective drug should be given to older people who are also taking non-steroidal anti-inflammatory drugs (NSAIDs) or aspirin. The guidance also recommends that older people prescribed anti-depressants should be specifically monitored for side-effects.

In ECT, a seizure is induced under general anaesthetic through the application of a brief electric current to the brain. As we mentioned in Chapter 7, ECT is a controversial treatment that has supporters and opponents within each of the professional groups, among individual service users and within the general public. Regarding the evidence for ECT in *older people*, Frazer et al. (2005) found, in a systematic review, that ECT was an effective treatment for older people with *severe* depression, although the side-effects of ECT – memory deficit, confusion, cardiovascular problems and an increased risk of falls – are by no means trivial. There are also the attendant risks associated with having a general anaesthetic. The 2009 NICE guidance makes a general recommendation that ECT be considered for 'severe depression that is life-threatening and when a rapid response is required, or when other treatments have failed' (NICE, 2009, section 1.10.4.1), although it does add that caution should be employed when using ECT with older people.

Social interventions

Social interventions to combat loneliness and isolation and strengthen relationships with kin (where these relationships exist) are very important and should be considered alongside other interventions, although the Social Exclusion Unit (2006) acknowledges that society as a whole has a role to play here since factors as varied as access to transportation, material deprivation and fear of crime can have an impact on isolation. Strategies to increase social contacts have been shown to improve mental wellbeing (Stevens & Tilburg, 2000). Establishing trust and developing a relationship with the older person may make it easier over time for them to **access community and religious groups**, **befriending schemes** or more traditional **day centres** and **lunch clubs**.

Psychological interventions

There is evidence suggesting psychotherapeutic treatments designed for younger adults can be effective in treating mild depression in older people but there has been limited research in this area to date (Haddad, 2009). Wilson et al. (2009) undertook a systematic review of psychotherapeutic treatments for depression in older people finding only a very small number of trials. These trials, moreover, involved only two types of intervention: CBT and psychodynamic therapy. Of the seven trials included in the review, only five had any degree of 'independent' control and all of these involved CBT compared to a waiting-list control. The remaining two trials compared CBT with psychodynamic psychotherapy. Wilson et al. found some evidence that CBT was more effective than a waiting-list control in helping older people with depression but there was no difference in outcomes in the two trials comparing CBT and psychodynamic therapy. As Wilson et al. remark, further research is needed into the potential of psychotherapeutic approaches though it does seem that the evidence for CBT in the treatment of depression in older people, while limited, is more robust than that for psychodynamic therapy. If CBT (or, indeed, other psychotherapeutic approaches) are to be used with older people then some factors may need to be adapted. Manthorpe & Illiffe (2005), for example, comment that there would need to be some flexibility around pacing and structure and that adjustments for comfort and sensory impairment would need to made.

In 2007, the NICE guidance for depression remarked that 'the full range of psychological interventions should be made available to older adults with depression, because they may have the same response to psychological interventions as younger people' (NICE, 2007b, section 1.2.4.3). We can see no reason to counter this statement and see it as an appropriate summary to this section although we should point out that it has disappeared from the recently introduced 2009 guidance (NICE, 2009).

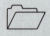 Case scenario: depression

Greg is 78; he is a widower of three years and lives alone. Greg's dog, Pip, died two months ago: 'We reared him from a pup and he was part of the family – the three of us against the world. He kept me going after Flo passed on; he was my link to her if you like.'

Soon after the death of Pip, Greg began having problems sleeping; he was not eating well, had low energy and was no longer taking regular walks. He was seen by his GP who prescribed a low dose SSRI for 'depressive symptoms'. Greg has been taking these for four days. The GP made a referral to the Community Mental Health Team as Greg had made mention of not seeing 'much point' in going on following the death of his dog.

What will be your main concerns? How would you as a Community Mental Health Nurse approach your first visit to Greg? What will be the important elements of your assessment?

Mental Health Problems in Older People: Dementia

Dementia is one of the health and social care challenges of the modern age. The number of people with dementia in the UK is expected to double (to 1.2 million) by 2031 and triple (to 1.8 million) by 2051 (see Figure 8.2).

It is estimated that dementia costs the UK economy £17 billion a year with costs expected to treble to £50 billion over the next 30 years in real terms as the UK population of people with dementia rises to 1.4 million (DH, 2009). The bulk of these figures are related to supported accommodation costs and to informal care (Alzheimer's Society, 2007). It has been estimated that there are 4 million carers in England, a million of whom are

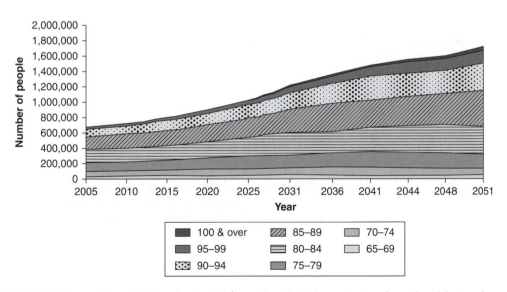

FIGURE 8.2 Dementia projections for the UK (reproduced, with permission, from the Alzheimer's Society, 2007)

TABLE 8.3 Prevalence of dementia in the UK (adapted, with permission, Alzheimer's Society, 2010)

Age group	Prevalence
40–64 years	1 in 1400 (< 0.1%)
65–69 years	1 in 100 (1%)
70–79 years	1 in 25 (4%)
80+ years	1 in 6 (17%)

providing in excess of 50 hours a week of care; of these carers, around 70% care for older people (Audit Commission, 2004).

Age is the key (known) risk factor for dementia: it is comparatively rare in younger age groups and increases significantly with advancing years (see Table 8.3).

Dementia has been described as:

> A collection of symptoms, including a decline in memory, reasoning and communication skills, and a gradual loss of the skills needed to carry out daily activities. These symptoms are caused by structural and chemical changes in the brain as a result of physical diseases such as Alzheimer's disease. (Alzheimer's Society, 2007)

The causes of dementia are wide and varied, as many as 200 different causes having been identified (Stephan & Brayne, 2007). There are, however, several common subtypes (see Table 8.4), though it should be noted that the distinction between these subtypes – in terms of both pathology and presentation – is often blurred.

TABLE 8.4 Types of dementia

Type of dementia	Proportion of overall dementias[a]	Brief description
Alzheimer's disease	62%	Brain cells are destroyed and there are changes to brain chemistry. A pattern of neuritic plaques and neurofibrillary tangles is evident at post-mortem. The hippocampus is commonly affected early in the condition affecting short-term memory with recall. People go on to experience a progressive loss of a wide array of functional abilities, which may include: increasing expressive and receptive difficulties with speech (aphasia), visuo-spatial impairment, problems with recognition (agnosia) and purposeful movements and sequenced actions (apraxia)

TABLE 8.4 (Continued)

Type of dementia	Proportion of overall dementias[a]	Brief description
Vascular dementia (VaD)	17%	Takes a more unpredictable path with cognitive damage resulting from the areas where strokes have occluded blood supply to areas of the brain. A steplike decline, where people experience plateaus and periods of sudden deterioration, is typical
Mixed (Alzheimer's and VaD)	10%	Features of both Alzheimer's and vascular dementia are present
Dementia with Lewy Bodies (DLB)	4%	Caused by tiny spherical proteins occurring within brain cells. People typically experience hallucinations, fluctuations in cognition, spatial disorientation and physical effects akin to Parkinson's disease. People with DLB are particularly vulnerable to the Parkinsonian side-effects of neuroleptic (antipsychotic) medications
Fronto-temporal lobe dementia (FTD)	2%	The brain primarily experiences damage in the frontal and temporal lobe areas before progressing to other areas of the cortex. Includes Pick's disease and commonly affects people under 65. Memory may not be affected in the earlier stages but people commonly experience personality and behavioural changes including compulsive behaviours and reduced empathy and/or difficulties with speech
Other dementias	5%	

[a]*Source*: Alzheimer's Society (2007).

Viewing dementia holistically

Dementia has been the subject of wide interest and debate, particularly since the early 1990s. While much progress has been made in understanding the neuropathology of dementia, there have also been explorations of the psychosocial basis of dementia and of the implications for care. Arguably, one of the most significant developments in recent years has been the growing 'voice' of people with dementia via a variety of platforms including: first-person accounts of living with dementia, such as *Dancing with Dementia* (Bryden, 2005); people with dementia actively engaging in – and 'co-constructing' – research (Keady et al., 2007); organisations run by – and for – people with dementia, such as the Scottish Dementia Working Group and the Dementia Advocacy Support Network (DASNI); and website forums such as *Talking Point* (see the further reading and resources at the end of this chapter).

It is of course harder for people in later dementia to tell us what we need to hear, but as Goldsmith (1996) and Killick & Allan (2001) point out, people with dementia *are* communicating with us; the question is, are we always listening?

A biopsychosocial approach to understanding dementia is key to the provision of holistic support. Sabat (2008) describes how it does not make sense to see all the behaviours of a person with dementia as 'symptoms' – in other words, as a consequence of the neuropathology (brain damage) resulting from the disease process. Instead, the behaviour of people with dementia is likely to be affected by at least four things: (1) brain damage; (2) the person's reaction to the effects of the brain damage; (3) the ways in which the person is treated by healthy others; and (4) the reactions of the diagnosed person to the ways in which he or she is treated by others. As such, important as it is to understand the complex impairments people are experiencing as a result of neuropathology, it is equally vital to recognise that the person will have a *psychological* reaction to the impairments and will, in addition, be profoundly affected by how they are supported – or not supported – by 'healthy' others.

Tom Kitwood, a leading force in the development of 'person-centred care' in dementia care, emphasises the importance of human relationships in maintaining the 'personhood' of someone with dementia and the potential harm that could be caused by what he terms **malignant social psychology** (Kitwood, 1997). Person-centred care involves care that is centred on the whole person (not just the dementia), their remaining abilities and the person in the context of their family, culture and society (Cheston & Bender, 1999). The 'malignant' interactions Kitwood refers to (such as out-pacing, labelling, infantilising or ignoring people with dementia) are not necessarily deliberate but may arise out of a lack of insight or lack of knowledge of the negative effects of the interactions. Brooker (2007) explores Kitwood's ideas in more detail, presenting a model to support implementation of these ideas in order to improve services for people with dementia.

Assessing older people with dementia

Nurses may work with people with dementia and their carers in a variety of settings including: **pre- and post-diagnosis support**, specialised **memory clinics**, **early intervention** services, **ongoing support in the community**, specialist support into **care homes** and **general hospitals** or hospital-based care and **day hospitals**. The type of assessments nurses will be involved in will, of course, vary, however, a number of fundamental issues and values

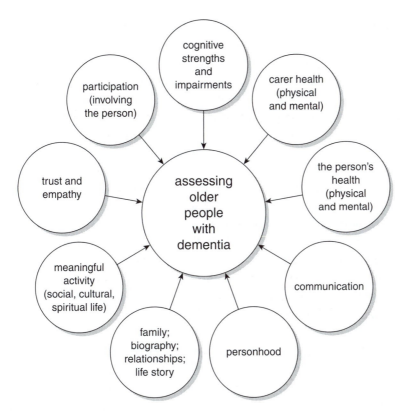

FIGURE 8.3   Things to consider when assessing older people with dementia

underpin any assessment and a few of these are summarised in Figure 8.3 and discussed here.

An understanding of the person's **key relationships** is central to understanding needs and informing positive interventions for people with dementia and their carers (Nolan et al., 2004). Caring for a person with dementia can place huge emotional, physical, social and financial demands on families and friends. Carers will have complex needs in their own right and may well be entitled to their own local authority assessment of need under the Carers (Recognition and Services) Act 1995 and Carers (Equal Opportunities) Act 2004.

You will recall from Chapter 2 the importance of communication and interpersonal skills in mental health nursing. Communication is at the heart of dementia care. People with dementia will frequently struggle with different aspects of verbal communication. You may need to **adapt your style of speech**, **reduce the length of sentences** accordingly, **avoid abstract concepts**,

avoid distractions and **avoid situations involving too many people**. Above all, you will need to **communicate at a pace that works for the person**. This may also mean repeated visits. For thorough and thought-provoking accounts of communication with people with dementia, see Killick & Allan (2001) and Goldsmith (1996).

Building **trusting**, **empathic** relationships should underpin engagement and assessment. Given that assessment will have an emotional impact on the individual, commonly used tools to assess cognition such as the Mini Mental State Examination (Folstein et al., 1975) may feel disempowering, threatening and, by turns, humiliating to those on the receiving end. Good dementia care avoids exposing people to failure. If these are likely consequences of specific assessment tools then you will need to work hard to allay such feelings (see Cheston & Bender, 1999, pp. 196–214). Every opportunity should be given to enable the person to **use their own words** to define their problems and goals. You should always endeavour to **see the person's perspective**; where a person is unable to express clearly in words their thoughts and feelings you should use all your capabilities to 'look behind the words' and to 'read' non-verbal meaning.

Understanding a person's **biography/life story** is essential to person-centred care and to understanding people in the here and now (Bruce & Schweitzer, 2008). As memory and verbal communication become increasingly impaired such information can be lost and it is vital to find meaningful ways to understand and engage with the person as the dementia progresses. **Cultural and spiritual needs** are also central to our identities and our sense of belonging and these should be captured in the assessment.

As with depression, **physical health** needs to be considered. It is important therefore that any assessments undertaken are truly **holistic**, that is, they consider the person's physical needs as well as their social, psychological and spiritual needs. Some of the nursing models outlined in Chapter 1, such as the *Activities of Daily Living* (see Roper et al., 2000), are particularly well suited to the assessment of physical care (one reason that they are often criticised by mental health nurses) and you might find assessment schedules based on such models useful as an adjunct to any mental health assessments you carry out. In addition, polypharmacy is often a reality for many older people and it is important that any medications used, and their reasons for prescription, are detailed.

People with dementia may begin to lose confidence in getting out and about, and keeping up **occupational** or **leisure interests** or friendships. Sometimes families (or service providers) may curtail a person's independence and freedoms through concerns for their safety. This can have an impact on self-esteem and wellbeing and as such assessment should address a person's activity and involvement at home and in the wider **community**.

People with dementia are sometimes viewed – or 'positioned' – by others in relation to their *deficits*, for example a wife introducing her husband to you as 'This is my husband; he's the patient' (Sabat, 2008, p. 80). Assessments will flag up risks and deficits but you also need to focus on **strengths** and **abilities** and on the 'person' (Sabat, 2008). Without this focus, it will be difficult to obtain the information necessary to support and provide care that enhances the whole person.

 Case scenario: dementia

Working in a hospital liaison team you are called to a medical ward to assess and advise on the care of an 86-year-old woman with dementia, Mabel, who has been described as 'agitated' and 'aggressive'. Mabel was admitted with a broken collar bone and bruising following a fall at home, she also has a urine infection, which may have been a factor in her fall. Psychotropic medication has been prescribed p.r.n. following the most recent incident but has yet to be given.

You sit and talk with Mabel. She clearly has some receptive and expressive verbal communication difficulties and has difficulty retaining information. She comes across as being anxious and uncertain as to her surroundings, but when talking about familiar matters such as her grandchildren, she appears much more relaxed. You notice as you observe staff interact with her that their speech is rushed and you feel she is clearly 'out-paced' in both communication and the conduct of some of the procedures.

You speak to her son for further information and he reveals how she is a very private person; he suspects that since her husband died 20 years previously no one will have seen her naked. Together you hypothesise that Mabel may feel either intimidated, violated or acutely embarrassed when helped with personal care and may be struggling to make sense of what is happening to her.

What further information will you seek to build up an informed picture and to either confirm or eliminate your hypotheses?

What thoughts will you already be having at this stage on advice/care planning for ward staff?

Evidence-based interventions for dementia

Because of the variety of roles and settings nurses may occupy in caring for people with dementia and their carers, and the constantly evolving nature of these roles, the following section on evidence-based interventions presents only a snapshot of early and later stage interventions for people with dementia. For an exploration of the breadth and complexity of nursing roles in *community* mental health teams and evidence-based interventions in meeting the needs of people with dementia and carers, see Keady, Clarke & Adams (2003) and Keady, Clarke & Page (2007).

Early interventions for dementia

Within the NICE/SCIE guidelines and the English dementia strategy mentioned earlier, there is a growing emphasis on early diagnosis for those with dementia, and post-diagnostic support for families and carers. The focus has very much been on health promotion, education and the provision of emotional and social support. In this section, we will consider a few early interventions for dementia that mental health nurses are frequently involved in; in particular, we will look at **medication monitoring and support**, **psychological interventions** and **social support**.

Medication monitoring and support

The cholinesterase inhibitors (such as donepezil, galantamine and rivastigmine) appear to have some benefits for people with Alzheimer's (Birks, 2006). A key role for most nurses is to support people on medication and the support of people on anti-dementia medication should be no exception. This may involve monitoring the effectiveness of the drugs and monitoring also for side-effects. The nurse will need adequate knowledge of the risks and benefits of these medications (and their interactions with other medications, since polypharmacy is common amongst older people) so that she or he can help people with dementia and their carers make informed choices about whether to continue with the medication or not. For an exploration of the nurse's role in cholinesterase inhibitor treatment from the perspective of a community mental health nurse working in a memory clinic, see Page (2003).

Psychological interventions

Although rigorous evaluations of psychological interventions for dementia are still needed, an evidence base is beginning to emerge (Moniz-Cook & Manthorpe, 2009). A systematic review of psychological approaches to treat neuropsychiatric symptoms[2] of dementia (Livingston et al., 2005) found evidence that **behaviour management techniques** (including cognitive behavioural approaches) that centred on the individual's behaviour had positive effects that often lasted for months. There was also evidence of the effectiveness of **psychoeducation** in changing caregiver's behaviour (these were more effective in individual rather than group settings) and of other structured education programmes designed for residential staff and informal carers.

The review found that **reminiscence therapy** (where a variety of approaches are used to share experiences and memories, sometimes involving props such as old photographs, newspapers and household items) had some limited evidence; however, two other dementia interventions that were popular in the 1980s and 1990s – **validation therapy** and **reality orientation** – were found to be ineffective. A good critique of validation therapy can be found in Morton (1999). While the review found a lack of evidence for reality orientation, there was some evidence for **cognitive stimulation**, a technique that has grown out of reality orientation but which also contains some elements of reminiscence. Cognitive stimulation is recommended in the NICE/SCIE guidelines (2006) and appears not only to improve cognitive function, but also quality of life (Spector et al., 2003). Cognitive stimulation aims to slow the overall rate of cognitive decline by concentrating on cognitive 'reserve' capacity (Cantegril-Kallen et al., 2008). The method takes the form of facilitated group sessions with different themes each week and comprises mixed activities that include songs, reminiscence and a range of failure-free mental activities in a supported social setting. The goals of cognitive stimulation are to preserve cognitive function for as long as possible, to enhance performance of everyday living activities and to increase or re-establish self-worth by improving self-confidence and providing motivation to perform activities that require cognitive effort.

A cognitive therapy not mentioned in Livingston et al.'s review is **cognitive rehabilitation**. In contrast to the group approach of cognitive stimulation, cognitive rehabilitation tends to be a more individualised therapy. Cognitive rehabilitation is about 'optimising remaining cognitive functioning, finding ways around difficulties, reducing their impact or helping someone to live more comfortably with their limitations' (Oyebode & Clare, 2008, p. 160). It has parallels with, and uses similar techniques to, the rehabilitation processes

---

[2]We mentioned earlier that it is problematic to view dementia in terms of symptoms because terminology like 'neuropsychiatric symptoms' can be construed to imply that behaviours are the direct consequence of disease; to be 'managed' without necessarily giving any emphasis to the influence of external factors. Unfortunately, this is the terminology that the review used.

employed in other forms of brain damage in that a whole range of techniques and approaches are used to strengthen remaining abilities and compensate for those lost. The techniques and approaches may include, for example, the use of external memory aids, which may be message boards, calendars or a range of 'assistive technologies' (for further information on assistive technologies in dementia, see ATDementia, 2007). Cognitive rehabilitation has potential but there is currently insufficient evidence to support its use in dementia (NICE/ SCIE, 2006), mainly owing to a complete absence of randomised controlled trials (Clare & Woods, 2003).

Social support and peer support groups

Since social isolation can have a profound emotional impact on older people, it makes sense to see social and peer support as an integral part of the English dementia strategy. Peer support in dementia was pioneered by Robyn Yale, an American social worker. Peer support groups can have very different aims and may have a clear time-structured psychotherapeutic focus or they may be more socially focused, enabling members to 'steer' the group and its aims and objectives. Peer support seems to be valued by participants: participants often speak of the importance of being able to share feelings and no longer feeling alone (Yale, 1998). Other forms of social support include voluntary sector support, such as the support provided by 'Alzheimer's cafés', an idea that originally developed in the Netherlands (Morrissey, 2006).

Empirical data around the outcomes of social and peer support for people with early stage dementia is scarce. Mason et al. (2005) undertook a study involving 11 members of two support groups. The overall experience was described as 'positive', with the groups providing a forum for personal disclosure and story-telling, but importantly also, they were seen as an opportunity for social contact, making new social ties and friendships. Some people, however, will not feel comfortable with these forms of group support so it is important to remember that working with people with **sensitivity** and arriving at **shared goals** are what really counts.

Later interventions for people with dementia

Dementia is a progressive condition and as cognitive impairment worsens, care and support focused on maintaining **personhood** and **promoting wellbeing** becomes paramount. May et al. (2009) have produced a valuable practice guide on 'enriched care planning' which aims to support the delivery of person-centred dementia care. It builds on the work of Kitwood (1993), who argued how the experience of a person with dementia was influenced by a complex interplay between neurological impairment, physical health, personality, biography (the person's life history) and social psychology (the impact of relationships, social interactions, care and other environmental factors on the person). According to May et al., care should be based around an informed understanding of 'life story, lifestyle and future wishes, personality, health, capacity for doing, cognitive ability and life at the moment' (p. 22). Interventions then may be many and varied and might, for example, include **life-story work** (see Moos and Bjorn, 2006, for a review of the literature on life story work), facilitating **meaningful occupation**, **supporting relationships**, **sensory stimulation**, **physical care**, and **creative art therapies or music**, to name but a few.

Another useful framework for informing care, particularly in formal care settings, is the **Senses Framework**. Davies & Nolan (2008) describe how this can be helpful in facilitating **relationship-centred care**. 'Relationship-centred care' builds on 'person-centred care' and focuses on the importance of personal relationships in maintaining personhood and wellbeing. In care services this is very much about the quality of relationships between the person with dementia, family and care staff. The Senses Framework suggests that effective care should involve the creation of a set of senses/experiences for the person, family carers *and* care staff (see Box 8.2).

Box 8.2   The Senses Framework (reproduced, with permission, from Davies & Nolan, 2008)

- A sense of **security** – of feeling safe and receiving or delivering competent and sensitive care
- A sense of **continuity** – the recognition of biography, using the past to contextualise the present
- A sense of **belonging** – opportunities to form meaningful relationships or feel part of a team
- A sense of **purpose** – opportunities to engage in purposeful activities or to have a clear set of goals to aspire to
- A sense of **achievement** – achieving meaningful or valued goals and feeling satisfied with one's efforts
- A sense of **significance** – to feel that you matter, and that you are valued as a person

Nurses may find themselves advising on interventions for people whose behaviour is said to be 'challenging' to families or care staff. Actions by people with dementia such as **shouting**, **apathy**, **wandering**, **agitation** or **aggression** are often described as 'challenging behaviours' and nursing responses subsequently described as the *management* of challenging behaviours. You might have thoughts on whether or not these descriptions are helpful, especially in light of our earlier discussion about being mindful of seeing such behaviours as the inevitable 'symptoms' of dementia rather than as a means of **communicating underlying need**.

Kitwood's view of dementia as a complex interplay of factors can help us understand the potential for multiple meanings of 'challenging' behaviour. If, for example, a person is observed pacing up and down a hospital corridor and shouting an unintelligible word, this behaviour could actually be rooted in a multitude of internal or external factors. It could, for example, be closely related to specific cognitive damage (as in **perseveration**, which is when a person gets 'stuck' in a repetitive action of some sort, e.g. repeating a word or gesture); alternately the person may have a physical need and be in pain, they may be thirsty or hungry, or needing the toilet. It is equally possible they may be feeling bored, lonely, anxious, frightened, lost, or perhaps, as past and present begin to lose definition, they are seeking the comfort or attention of a person from much earlier in their life (their mother or father?).

Identifying the underlying *meaning* behind such behaviour will then inform our responses. Without seeking the meaning, any intervention may be wholly inappropriate and may even make matters worse for the person (an anti-psychotic medication for example would be of no help if the person was experiencing pain). Simply viewing the behaviour as 'a symptom of dementia' tells us very little and does not help us connect with – and respond appropriately to – the needs of the *person*. Stokes (2008) provides a fascinating collection of case studies/stories about people with dementia and the quest to discern the underlying meaning in what on the surface may seem strange or puzzling behaviour. Another useful read in helping both carers and professionals understand and, indeed, rethink one frequently highlighted 'behaviour' – wandering – is *Dementia: Walking Not Wandering* (Marshall & Allan, 2006). Marshall and Allan illustrate how the actions of people with dementia (in this case, walking) can be pathologised and labelled (as 'wandering') and how, without looking at the meaning and motivations behind actions, we can unintentionally respond in ways that may only further disable.

Mental Health Problems in Older People: Delirium

Delirium, or acute confusion, is a disturbance of **consciousness** and **cognition**, with rapid onset, fluctuating course and an underlying cause (Siddiqi et al., 2007). It is common in older people (hence its discussion here), particularly in hospitals, and occurs secondary to a medical condition (the underlying cause). Box 8.3 lists the common causes of delirium.

Box 8.3   Common causes of delirium (adapted, with permission, from Royal College of Psychiatrists, 2009)

- A urine or chest infection
- Having a high body temperature
- Side-effects of drugs like pain killers and steroids
- Chemical problems in the body, such as dehydration or low salt levels
- Liver or kidney problems
- Suddenly stopping drugs or alcohol
- Major surgery
- Epilepsy
- Brain injury or infection
- Terminal illness
- Constipation
- Being in an unfamiliar place

Delirium is associated with outcomes such as falls, fractures and pressure ulcers and it can interfere with hydration and nutrition (Schofield, 2007). Since these are outcomes that nurses frequently encounter in older people, all nurses working with older people – mental health nurses included – need to be able to spot delirium and know what action to take. Delirium often co-exists with dementia, but it is easily missed as any 'confused', changeable or unusual behaviour may be associated with the dementia rather than a delirium caused by, for example, an underlying infection or other primary cause. A person with delirium may be **hyper**-active and **hyper**-alert; on the other hand they may be **hypo**-active, quiet and listless (Schofield, 2007) and therefore easy to miss.

According to the British Geriatrics Society and Royal College of Physicians (2006), the features listed in Box 8.4 must be present for a diagnosis of delirium. While the first three criteria are necessary, a diagnosis can be made without the fourth, though having direct evidence of physiological changes as a result of a general medical condition lessens the risk of misdiagnosis.

Box 8.4   Criteria for a diagnosis of delirium

- There is a disturbance of consciousness, with reduced ability to focus, sustain or shift attention.
- There is a change in cognitive ability (e.g. memory deficit, disorientation, language disturbance) or the development of a perceptual disturbance not accounted for by a pre-existing or evolving dementia.
- The disturbance develops over a short period of time (usually hours to days) and tends to fluctuate during the course of the day.
- There is evidence from the person's history, physical examination, or laboratory findings that the disturbance is caused by the direct physiological consequences of a general medical condition, substance intoxication or substance withdrawal.

Reproduced from: British Geriatrics Society and Royal College of Physicians. *Guidelines for the prevention, diagnosis and management of delirium in older people. Concise guidance to good practice series*, No 6. London: RCP, 2006. Copyright © 2006 Royal College of Physicians. Reproduced with permission.

Treatment for delirium is simply treatment of the underlying cause, hence prompt diagnosis is essential. Thus, when assessing older people, mental health nurses should give **due consideration to the general physical health of older people**, as well as their mental health, and be cognisant of the way in which delirium can present. Moreover, since delirium is often (but not always) an early sign of dementia and/or a serious underlying physical illness (British Geriatrics Society and Royal College of Physicians, 2006), it is important that older people with delirium are – once stabilised – suitably followed up and supported. Such follow up and support will depend on whether there is any previous history of delirium and/or dementia and could include, for example, referral to a physician or psychiatrist dealing with old age, a community mental health nurse, occupational therapist or social worker.

People who recover from an episode of delirium may retain memory of some of the delusions, hallucinations and behaviour experienced and many who recall the experience describe it as a highly distressing experience (Breitbart et al., 2002). This has implications for the need for emotional support both during and following the experience. For a fascinating first-person insight into the experience of delirium, see Crammer (2002).

 ## Case scenario: delirium

Mary lives with her husband Sahid. Sahid is 74 and has Alzheimer's. Sahid no longer has the ability to communicate verbally. Both manage with little input from outside services. Over the course of a few days Sahid became unusually tense, agitated and restless. Mary was unable to deduce what was wrong.

Sahid is seen by his GP who feels he is progressing to another 'phase' of his dementia and that Mary should consider further support. The GP makes a referral to the Community Mental Health Team (CMHT). Eighteen hours after seeing the GP (and before the case has been allocated with the CMHT), Mary, in desperation at Sahid's level of confusion, rushes him into the A&E department of the local hospital. Sahid receives a battery of tests, including an endoscopy, which reveals a perforating duodenal ulcer.

Why do you think the underlying illness was not spotted earlier?

What lessons are there from this scenario for professionals engaged in the care of older people?

A consideration of delirium serves to remind nurses of the importance of **physical assessment** and **physical care** in older people since, as you have seen, it is clear that physical ill health and/or physiological deficiencies can both cause and exacerbate mental health problems. Regarding physical care, the Nursing and Midwifery Council's Essential Skills Clusters (NMC, 2007), referred to in note 3 in Chapter 2 (admittedly in the context of the potential for confusion with the ten Essential Shared Capabilities) are helpful in identifying core physical nursing skills. The textbook by Nash (2010) also provides some excellent guidance on physical nursing in mental health care.

Conclusion

We are experiencing a profound shift in the age structure of our population. Although ageing does not necessarily equate with problems in mental ill health, we can expect to see a proportional increase in the numbers of older people with mental health needs that will challenge our health and social care services. One of the key challenges for health and social policy is not just the extension of life, but the extension of a healthy, active life and the shortening of the period of life before death spent in frailty and dependency (DH, 2001).

We have tried to emphasise that alongside biological factors, there is a complexity of social and psychological factors that can influence mental wellbeing. Material deprivation, which is linked to social class and deprivation in earlier life, social isolation and loneliness, bereavement and the ageist attitudes of others, can all impact on wellbeing and may be subtly implicated in either causing or prolonging mental ill health.

The focus of this chapter has been on the commonest causes of mental ill health in older people: depression, anxiety, dementia and delirium. Naturally older people will experience the whole range of mental health problems that have been addressed elsewhere in this book. Younger people with ongoing mental health problems and substance misuse problems will, of course, age and may receive support from 'older adult' mental health services, which returns us to the question posed at the beginning of the chapter over whether we need specialist services for older adults at all.

Dependency on alcohol – which may be as high as 12% in men over 60 (Dyson, 2006) – is another potentially significant issue for older people. Alcohol dependence may be partly responsible for some of the falls, confusion and depression seen in older people although health professionals are more likely to attribute these to the conditions highlighted in this chapter (Minardi et al., 2007). The discussion on alcohol misuse in Chapter 11 is, as such, as relevant to older people as it is to younger people.

One thing we should all be aware of is that the older population will continue to evolve and change. We are going to see an increasingly ethnically diverse population and, as the 'baby-boomer' generation reaches retirement age, it is quite likely we will increasingly see a population who are more vocal and politically aware (Minardi et al., 2007). Changes to health and social care systems will surely continue apace, perhaps most notably with the personalisation of social care services, with older people in greater control of budgets and how to spend and organise their care, and legislation to outlaw age discrimination. Working with older people with mental health problems will continue to be a dynamic and challenging area of practice for nurses.

Further Reading and Resources

Key texts

Downs M & Bowers B (eds) (2008). *Excellence in Dementia Care: Research into Practice.* Maidenhead: Open University Press.
An excellent collection of chapters from a range of experts on a broad range of evidence-based issues in dementia care.

Keady J, Clarke C & Page S (2007). *Partnerships in Community Mental Health Nursing and Dementia Care.* Maidenhead: Open University Press.
An extensive collection of contributions from a wide range of practitioners and researchers exploring the contribution of nursing in community-based dementia care.

Neno R, Aveyard B & Heath H (eds) (2007). *Older People and Mental Health Nursing: A Handbook of Care.* London: Oxford–Blackwell.
Comprehensive evidence-based guide to nursing older people with mental health needs.

NHS Education for Scotland (2009). *An Educational Resource to Support Early Interventions for People Receiving a Diagnosis of Dementia.* Edinburgh: NHS Education for Scotland.
Excellent workbook focusing on early interventions in dementia care, prepared by the Dementia Services Development Centre, University of Stirling. Freely available from www.nes.scot.nhs.uk.

Stokes G (2008). *And Still the Music Plays: Stories of People with Dementia.* London: Hawker Publications.
Fascinating collection of story-based accounts of people with dementia in which the meanings behind often complex and puzzling behaviours are explored.

Key policy documents

Audit Commission (2004). *Support for Carers of Older People: Independence and Well-Being.* London: Audit Commission.

Department of Health (2001) *National Service Framework for Older People.* London: Department of Health.

Welsh Assembly Government (2006). *National Service Framework for Older People in Wales.* Cardiff: Welsh Assembly Government.

National Institute for Health and Clinical Excellence/Social Care Institute for Excellence (2006). *Dementia: Supporting People with Dementia and their Carers in Health and Social Care. NICE Clinical Guideline 42.* London: NICE. Available from www.nice.org.uk/CG42

Department of Health (2009). *Living Well with Dementia: A National Dementia Strategy.* London: Department of Health.

Scottish Government (2010). *Scotland's National Dementia Strategy.* Edinburgh: Scottish Government.

Web resources

AgeUK: www.ageuk.org.uk
> *The UK's largest charity working with, and for, older people formed as a result of a merger between Age Concern and Help the Aged.*

Alzheimer's Society (England Wales and Northern Ireland) and Alzheimer Scotland: www.alzheimers.org.uk and www.alzscot.org
> *Information, advice, support and campaigning on all forms of dementia. The Alzheimer's Society hosts* Talking Point, *an online community for people with dementia and their carers, family and friends* (see http://forum.alzheimers.org.uk).

ATDementia: www.atdementia.org.uk
> *Searchable database of assistive technologies for people with dementia.*

Dementia Advocacy and Support Network International (DASNI): www.dasninternational.org
> *An Internet-based support network 'by and for those diagnosed with dementia'.*

The Social Care Institute for Excellence (SCIE) Dementia Gateway: www.scie.org.uk/publications/dementia/index.asp
> *A set of resources including information on a range of dementia topics, on-line e-learning resources, videos and other resources.*

Office of the Public Guardian: www.publicguardian.gov.uk/index.htm
> *Supporting decision making for those who lack capacity or would like to plan for their future within the framework of the Mental Capacity Act 2005.*

Scottish Anti-Ageism Initiative: www.seetheperson.info
> *Website aiming to tackle ageism in Scotland but also useful to the other nations of the UK.*

References

Adams K, Sanders S & Auth E (2004). Loneliness and depression in independent living retirement communities: risk and resilience factors. *Aging and Mental Health,* **8**(6), 475–485.

Age Concern (2007). *Improving Services and Support for Older People with Mental Health Problems.* London: Age Concern.

Age Concern (2008a). *Older People in the United Kingdom: Key Facts and Statistics.* London: Age Concern.

Age Concern (2008b). *Undiagnosed, Untreated and At Risk: The Experiences of Older People with Depression.* London: Age Concern.

Age Concern/Help the Aged (2009). *One Voice: Shaping our Ageing Society.* London: Age Concern/Help the Aged.

Alzheimer's Society (2007). *Dementia UK: A Report into the Prevalence and Cost of Dementia Prepared by the Personal Social Services Research Unit (PSSRU) at the London School of Economics and the Institute of Psychiatry at King's College London, for the Alzheimer's Society.* London: Alzheimer's Society.

Alzheimer's Society (2010). *Demography*. London: Alzheimer's Society. Available from: www.alzheimers.org.uk [accessed 30 September 2010].

ATDementia (2007). What do we mean by assistive technology? [pdf]. Available from: www.atdementia.org.uk [accessed 2 November 2009].

Audit Commission (2004). *Support for Carers of Older People: Independence and Well-Being*. London: Audit Commission.

Ayers C, Sorrell J, Thorp S & Wetherell J (2007). Evidence-based psychological treatments for late-life anxiety. *Psychology and Aging*, **22**, 8–17.

Beekman A, Bremmer M, Deeg D, van Balkom A, Smit J & de Beurs E (1998). Anxiety disorders in later life: a report from the Longitudinal Aging Study Amsterdam. *International Journal of Geriatric Psychiatry*, **13**, 717–726.

Bengston VL & Putney NM (2006). Future 'conflicts' across generations and cohorts? In JA Vincent, CR Phillipson & M Downs (eds), *The Futures of Old Age*. London: Sage.

Birks J (2006). Cholinesterase inhibitors for Alzheimer's disease. *Cochrane Database of Systematic Reviews*, Issue 1, Article CD005593.

Bishop I, Kriegsman D, Beekman A & Deeg D (2004). Chronic diseases and depression: the modifying role of psychosocial resources. *Social Science and Medicine*, **59**, 721–733.

Bond J & Cabrero G (2007). Health and dependency in later life. In J Bond, SM Peace, F Dittmann-Kohli & G Westerhof (eds), *Ageing in Society*. London: Sage.

Bond J & Corner L (2004). *Quality of Life and Older People*. Maidenhead: Open University Press.

Breitbart W, Gibson C & Tremblay A (2002). The delirium experience: delirium recall and delirium-related distress in hospitalized patients with cancer. *Psychosomatics*, **43**, 183–194.

British Geriatrics Society and Royal College of Physicians (2006). *Concise Guidance to Good Practice No. 6: The Prevention, Diagnosis and Management of Delirium in Older People*. London: Royal College of Physicians.

Brooker D (2007). *Person-Centred Dementia Care: Making Services Better*. London: Jessica Kingsley.

Bruce E & Schweitzer P (2008). Working with life history. In M Downs & B Bowers (eds), *Excellence in Dementia Care: Research into Practice*. Maidenhead: Open University Press.

Bryden C (2005). *Dancing with Dementia*. London: Jessica Kingsley.

Cantegreil-Kallen I, de Rotrou J & Rigaud A-S (2008). Cognitive stimulation for people with mild cognitive impairment and early dementia. In E Moniz-Cooke & J Manthorpe (eds), *Early Interventions in Dementia Care: Evidence-Based Practice*. London: Jessica Kingsley.

Care Commission/MWCS (Mental Welfare Commission for Scotland) (2009). *Remember I'm Still Me: Care Commission and Mental Welfare Commission Joint Report on the Quality of Care for People with Dementia Living in Care Homes in Scotland*. Dundee: Care Commission/Edinburgh: MWCS.

Cheston R & Bender M (1999). *Understanding Dementia: The Man with the Worried Eyes*. London: Jessica Kingsley.

Choi G, Ransom S & Wyllie J (2008). Depression in older nursing home residents: the influence of nursing home environmental stressors, coping, and acceptance of group and individual therapy. *Aging and Mental Health*, **12**(5), 536–547.

Clare L & Woods B (2003). Cognitive rehabilitation and cognitive training for early-stage Alzheimer's disease and vascular dementia. *Cochrane Database of Systematic Reviews*, Issue 4, Article CD003260.

Crammer JL (2002). Subjective experience of a confusional state. *British Journal of Psychiatry*, **180**, 71–75.

Cuddy A, Norton M & Fiske S (2005). This old stereotype: the pervasiveness and persistence of the elderly stereotype. *Journal of Social Issues*, **61**(2), 267–285.

Davies S & Nolan M (2008). Attending to relationships in dementia care. In M Downs & B Bowers (eds), *Excellence in Dementia Care: Research into Practice*. Maidenhead: Open University.

DCA (Department for Constitutional Affairs) (2007). *Mental Capacity Act 2005: Code of Practice*. London: TSO.

DH (Department of Health) (2001). *National Service Framework for Older People*. London: DH.

DH (Department of Health) (2009). *Living Well with Dementia: A National Dementia Strategy*. London: DH.

DH/CSIP (Department of Health/Care Services Improvement Partnership) (2005). *Everybody's Business. Integrated Mental Health Services for Older Adults: A Service Development Guide*. London: DH.

DHSSPS (Department of Health, Social Security and Public Safety) (2009). *Delivering the Bamford Vision: The Response of the Northern Ireland Executive to the Bamford Review of Mental Health and Learning Disability. Action Plan 2009–2011*. Belfast: DHSSPS. Available from: www.dhsspsni.gov.uk [accessed 2 November 2009].

Dobbs D, Eckert J, Rubinstein B, Keimig L, Clark L, Frankowski A & Zimmerman S (2008). An ethnographic study of stigma and ageism in residential care or assisted living. *The Gerontologist*, **48**(4), 517–526.

Dyson J (2006). Alcohol misuse and older people. *Nursing Older People*, **18**(7), 32–35.

Ersek M, Turner JA, Cain KC & Kemp CA (2008). Results of a randomized controlled trial to examine the efficacy of a chronic pain self-management group for older adults. *Pain*, **138**(1), 29–40.

Folstein M, Folstein S & McHugh P (1975). 'Mini-mental state': a practical method for grading the cognitive state of patients for the clinician. *Journal of Psychiatric Research*, **12**, 189–198.

Frazer CJ, Christensen H & Griffiths KM (2005). Systematic review: effectiveness of treatments for depression in older people. *Medical Journal of Australia*, **182**(12), 627–632.

Givens J, Datto C, Ruckdeschel K, Knott K, Zubritsky C, Oslin D, Nyshadham S, Vanguri P & Barg F (2006). Older patients' aversion to antidepressants: a qualitative study. *Journal of General Internal Medicine*, **21**, 146–151.

Goldsmith M (1996). *Hearing the Voice of People with Dementia – Opportunities and Obstacles*. London: Jessica Kingsley.

Gray A (2009). The social capital of older people. *Ageing and Society*, **29**, 5–31.

Grundy E & Sloggett A (2003). Health inequalities in the older population: the role of personal capital, social resources and social economic circumstances. *Social Science and Medicine*, **56**(5), 935–947.

Haddad M (2009). Mental health and older people. In R Newell & K Gournay (eds), *Mental Health Nursing: An Evidence-Based Approach*, 2nd edition. London: Churchill Livingstone.

Keady J, Clarke C & Adams T (2003). *Community Mental Health Nursing and Dementia Care*. Maidenhead: Open University Press.

Keady J, Clarke C & Page S (2007). *Partnerships in Community Mental Health Nursing and Dementia Care*. Maidenhead: Open University Press.

Keady J, Williams S & Hughes J (2007). Making mistakes: using co-constructed inquiry to illuminate meaning and relationships in the early adjustment to Alzheimer's disease – a single case study approach. *Dementia*, **6**(3), 343–364.

Killick J & Allan K (2001). *Communication and the Care of People with Dementia*. *Maidenhead:* Open University Press.

Kitwood T (1993). Person and process in dementia. *International Journal of Geriatric Psychiatry*, **8**(7), 541–545.

Kitwood T (1997). *Dementia Reconsidered: The Person Comes First*. Maidenhead: Open University Press.

Lawrence V, Banerjee S, Bhugra D, Sangha K, Turner S & Murray J (2006). Coping with depression in later life: a qualitative study of help-seeking in three ethnic groups. *Psychological Medicine*, **36**(10), 1375–1383.

Licht-Strunk E, Van Marwijk H, Hoekstra T, Twisk J, De Haan M & Beekman A (2009). Outcome of depression in later life in primary care: longitudinal cohort study with three years' follow-up. *British Medical Journal*, **338**, a3079 [BMJ Online First].

Livingston G, Johnston K, Katona C, Paton J & Lyketsos CG (2005). Systematic review of psychological approaches to the management of neuropsychiatric symptoms of dementia. *American Journal of Psychiatry*, **162**, 1996–2021.

Manthorpe J & Iliffe S (2005). *Depression in Later Life*. London: Jessica Kingsley.

Marcoen A, Coleman P & O'Hanlon A (2007). Psychological ageing. In J Bond, SM Peace, F Dittmann-Kohli & G Westerhof (eds), *Ageing in Society*. London: Sage.

Marshall M & Allan K (2006). *Dementia: Walking not Wandering. Fresh Approaches to Understanding and Practice*. London: Hawker Publications.

Mason E, Clare, L & Pistrang N (2005). Processes and experiences of mutual support in professionally-led support groups for people with early-stage dementia. *Dementia*, **4**(1), 87–112.

May H, Edwards P & Brooker D (2009). *Enriched Care Planning for People with Dementia*. London: Jessica Kingsley.

McDougall F, Kvaal K, Matthews F, Paykel E, Jones P, Dewey M & Brayne C (2007). Prevalence of depression in older people in England and Wales: The MRC CFA study. *Psychological Medicin*, **37**(12), 1787–1795.

Minardi H, Heath H & Neno R (2007). Mental health and well-being for older people in the future: the nursing contribution. In R Neno, B Aveyard & H Heath (eds), *Older People and Mental Health Nursing: A Handbook of Care*. Chichester: Wiley.

Moniz-Cook E & Manthorpe J (eds) (2009). *Early Psychosocial Interventions in Dementia: Evidence-Based Practice*. London: Jessica Kingsley.

Moos I & Bjorn A (2006). Use of the life story in the institutional care of people with dementia: a review of intervention studies. *Ageing and Society*, **26**(3), 431–454.

Morrissey MV (2006). Alzheimer's cafe for people with and affected by dementia. *Nursing Times*, **102**(15), 29–31 [Apr 11–17].

Morton I (1999). *Person-Centred Approaches to Dementia Care*. Bicester: Speechmark.

Nash M (2010). *Physical Health and Well-Being in Mental Health Nursing: Clinical Skills for Practice*. Maidenhead: Open University Press.

Nazroo J (2006). Ethnicity and old age. In JA Vincent, CR Phillipson & M Downs (eds), *The Futures of Old Age*. London: Sage.

NES (NHS Education for Scotland) (2008). *Working with Older People in Scotland: A Framework for Mental Health Nurses*. Edinburgh: NES.

NICE (National Institute for Health and Clinical Excellence) (2007a). *Anxiety: Management of Anxiety (Panic Disorder, with or without Agoraphobia, and Generalised Anxiety Disorder) in Adults in Primary, Secondary and Community Care (Amended). Nice Clinical Guideline 22 (Amended)*. London: NICE.

NICE (National Institute for Health and Clinical Excellence) (2007b). *Depression: Management of Depression in Primary and Secondary Care (Amended). NICE Clinical Guideline 23*. London: NICE.

NICE (National Institute for Health and Clinical Excellence) (2009). *Depression: The Treatment and Management of Depression in Adults (Update). NICE Clinical Guideline 90*. London: NICE.

NICE/SCIE (National Institute for Health and Clinical Excellence/Social Care Institute for Excellence) (2006). *Dementia: Supporting People with Dementia and their Carers in Health and Social Care. NICE Clinical Guideline 42*. London: NICE.

NMC (Nursing and Midwifery Council) (2007). Introduction of Essential Skills Clusters for Pre-registration Nursing programmes. NMC Circular 07/2007. London: NMC. Available from www.nmc-uk.org [accessed 21 April 2010].

Nolan M, Davies S, Brown S, Keady J & Nolan J (2004). Beyond 'person centred' care: a new vision for gerontological nursing. *Journal of Clinical Nursing*, **13**(9), 45–53.

Oyebode J & Clare L (2008). Supporting cognitive abilities. In M Downs & B Bowers (eds), *Excellence in Dementia Care: Research into Practice*. Maidenhead: Open University Press.

ONS (Office for National Statistics) (2009a). *Centenarians: The Fastest Growing Age Group* [Web document]. Available from: www.statistics.gov.uk [accessed 28 October 2009].

ONS (Office for National Statistics) (2009b). *Statistical Bulletin: Population Estimates, August 2009* [pdf]. Available from: www.statistics.gov.uk/pdfdir/pop0809.pdf [accessed 16 October 2009].

Page S (2003). From screening to intervention: the community mental health nurse in the memory clinic setting. In J Keady, C Clarke & T Adams (2003). *Community Mental Health Nursing and Dementia Care*. Maidenhead: Open University Press.

Peace S, Dittmann-Kohli F, Westerhof G & Bond, J (2007). The ageing world. In J Bond, S Peace, F Dittmann-Kohli & G Westerhof (eds), *Ageing in Society*. London: Sage.

Roper N, Logan WW & Tierney AJ (2000). *The Roper–Logan–Tierney Model of Nursing: Based on Activities of Living*. Edinburgh: Churchill Livingstone.

Royal College of Psychiatrists (2009). *Factsheet: Delirium*. London: Royal College of Psychiatrists Public Education Editorial Board. Available from: www.rcpsych.ac.uk [accessed 2 November 2009].

Sabat S (2008). A bio-psycho-social approach to dementia. In M Downs & B Bowers (eds), *Excellence in Dementia Care: Research into Practice*. Maidenhead: Open University Press.

Schofield I (2007). Delirium. In R Neno, B Aveyard & H Heath (eds), *Older People and Mental Health Nursing: A Handbook of Care*. Chichester: Wiley.

Scottish Government (2008). *Adults with Incapacity (Scotland) Act 2000: Revised Code of Practice for Persons Authorised under Intervention Orders and Guardians*. Edinburgh: The Scottish Government.

Scottish Government (2010). *Scotland's National Dementia Strategy*. Edinburgh: The Scottish Government. Available from www.scotland.gov.uk [accessed 26 June 2010].

Sewitch M, McCusker J, Dendukuri N & Yaffe M (2004). Depression in frail elders: impact on family care-givers. *International Journal of Geriatric Psychiatry*, **19**, 655–665.

Siddiqi N, Holtz R, Britton M & Holmes J (2007). Interventions for preventing delirium in hospitalised patients. *Cochrane Database of Systematic Reviews*, Issue 2, Article CD005563.

SIGN (Scottish Intercollegiate Guidelines Network) (2006). *Management of Patients with Dementia: A National Clinical Guideline*. Edinburgh: SIGN.

Sirey J, Bruce M, Carpenter M, Booker D, Reid D, Newell M, Carrington K-A & Alexopoulos G (2008). Depressive symptoms and suicidal ideation among older adults receiving home delivered meals. *International Journal of Geriatric Psychiatry*, **23**(12), 1306–1311.

Social Exclusion Unit (2006). *A Sure Start to Later Life: Ending Inequalities for Older People*. London: Office of the Deputy Prime Minister.

Spector A, Thorgrimsen L, Woods B, Royan L, Davies S, Butterworth M & Orrell M (2003). Efficacy of an evidence-based cognitive stimulation therapy programme for people with dementia. *British Journal of Psychiatry*, **183**, 248–254.

Stephan B & Brayne C (2007). Prevalence and projections of dementia. In M Downs & B Bowers (eds), *Excellence in Dementia Care: Research into Practice*. Maidenhead: Open University Press.

Stevens N & Tilburg T (2000). Stimulating friendship in later life: a strategy for reducing loneliness among older women. *Educational Gerontology*, **26**, 15–35.

Stokes, G (2008). *And Still the Music Plays: Stories of People with Dementia*. London: Hawker Publications.

Victor C, Scambler S, Bowling A & Bond J (2005). The prevalence of, and risk factors for, loneliness in later life: a survey of older people in Great Britain. *Ageing and Society*, **25**(3), 357–375.

Vincent J (1999). *Politics, Power and Old Age*. Oxford: Open University Press.

Vincent JA, Phillipson CR & Downs M (eds) (2006). *The Futures of Old Age*. London: Sage.

Walker A & Foster L (2006). Ageing and social class: an enduring relationship. In JA Vincent, CR Phillipson & M Downs (eds), *The Futures of Old Age*. London: Sage.

Welsh Assembly Government (2006). *National Service Framework for Older People in Wales*. Cardiff: Welsh Assembly Government.

Wetherell J, Gatz M & Craske M (2003). Treatment of generalized anxiety disorder in older adults. *Journal of Consulting and Clinical Psychology*, **71**, 31–40.

Weyerer S, Eifflaender-Gorfer S, Köhler L, Jessen F, Maier W, Fuchs A, Pentzek M, Kaduszkiewicz H, Bachmann C, Angermeyer MC, Luppa M, Wiese B, Mösch E & Bickel H (2008). Prevalence and risk factors for depression in non-demented primary care attenders aged 75 years and older. *Journal of Affective Disorders*, **111**(2–3), 153–163.

Wilson K, Mottram P & Vassilas C (2009). Psychotherapeutic treatments for older depressed people. *Cochrane Database of Systematic Reviews*, Issue 2.

Windle G (2009). What is mental health and well-being? In Cattan M (ed.), *Mental Health and Well-Being in Later Life*. Open University Press.

Yale R (1998). *Developing Support Groups for Individuals with Early-stage Alzheimer's Disease: Planning Implementation and Evaluation*. Baltimore, MD: Health Professions Press.

Zubenko GS, Zubenko WN, McPherson S, Spoor E, Marin DB, Farlow MR, Smith GE, Geda YE, Cummings JL, Petersen RC & Sunderland T (2003). A collaborative study of the emergence and clinical features of the major depressive syndrome of Alzheimer's disease. *American Journal of Psychiatry*, **160**, 857–866.

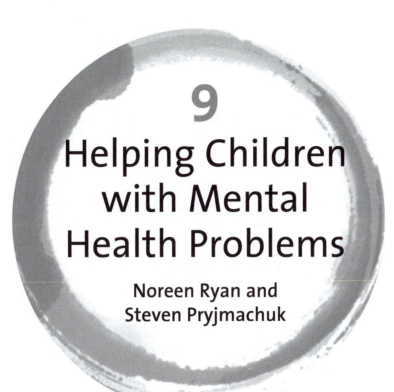

9
Helping Children with Mental Health Problems

Noreen Ryan and Steven Pryjmachuk

What will I learn in this chapter?

This chapter aims to provide an overview of mental health difficulties in younger children (the under-12s) by focusing upon the developmental stages of childhood, the interplay between nature and nurture, psychosocial considerations of the family, and the wider context in which children live and grow.

After reading this chapter, you will be able to:

- appreciate the factors influencing emotional and psychological wellbeing in younger children and the common mental health difficulties that present in this age group;
- understand how child and adolescent mental health services are organised and delivered across the UK;
- identify a range of evidence-based interventions available to younger children with mental health problems and their families;
- reflect upon the role that nurses have in promoting emotional wellbeing in children.

Introduction

This chapter and the next are concerned with the **mental health of children and young people** and the services provided by **child and adolescent mental health services** (or 'CAMHS' as they are known). The UK, like most signatories to the Convention on the Rights of the Child (United Nations General Assembly, 1989), defines a child as a person below the age of 18 years. You might, as such, wonder why we have chosen to split the topic of child mental health into two chapters: this chapter on younger children and the next on older children. The answer is that there are qualitative and quantitative differences in the way younger and older children experience the world around them and in the way services are provided for them. An arbitrary cut-off point that reflects a very crude division between younger children and older children is the **age of 11 years**, an age at which puberty often begins (or when a child becomes an **adolescent** or, to use a term more acceptable to this group, a **young person**), where education often changes (from primary to secondary school) and where healthcare services – including child mental health services – are often separated.

Mental health and mental health problems in children

Children's mental health matters. Untreated mental health problems in children lead to **family/relationship problems and breakdown**, **educational failure**, **crime** and **antisocial behaviour**, the costs of which are not only borne by health services but by the wider social, education and youth justice services (CAMHS Review, 2008).

It is difficult to conceptualise mental health problems in children without some idea of what we mean by mental health. The CAMHS Review (2008) found the World Health Organisation definition of mental health helpful: 'a state of well-being in which the individual realises his or her abilities, can cope with the normal stresses of life, can work productively and fruitfully, and is able to make a contribution to his or her community' (WHO, 2004). The influential NHS Health Advisory Service report *Together We Stand* (NHS HAS, 1995) is less explicit in its definition instead identifying some characteristics that are indicative of a mentally healthy child (see Box 9.1).

> ## Box 9.1 Characteristics of child mental health (NHS HAS, 1995)
>
> - A capacity to enter into and sustain mutually satisfying personal relationships
> - The continuing progression of psychological development
> - An ability to play and to learn so that attainments are appropriate for age and intellectual level
> - A developing moral sense of right and wrong
> - The degree of any psychological distress suffered, and any maladaptive behaviour that manifests, being within normal limits for the child's age and context

In child mental health, 'deviations' from mental health tend to be referred to as **mental health problems** or **mental disorders**. The NHS HAS (1995) defines mental health problems as 'a broad range of emotional or behavioural difficulties which cause concern or distress'. All children will, as such, experience a mental health problem at some point since emotional and/or psychological upheavals like starting school, the death of a loved grandparent or pet, frustration in learning new things, forming relationships and so on are a normal part of childhood. Most children get through these upheavals relatively easily but some will have an intensity or persistence that requires intervention from a child care (not necessarily mental health) specialist. If these upheavals cause **substantial** interference with the child's personal functioning or that of his or her carers, then it may be indicative of a diagnosable mental disorder or, at the very least, a severe mental health problem[1].

Your childhood

Think about your own childhood and consider whether there were times when your emotional or psychological wellbeing was compromised (e.g. the death of

(Continued)

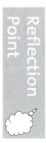

Reflection Point

---

[1]The distinction between what might be a 'diagnosable mental disorder' and what might be a 'severe mental health problem' is discussed in more detail when we talk about diagnostic frameworks shortly.

(Continued)

a loved one or pet, trouble at school, friendships or relationships that went sour, issues with shyness or being overly embarrassed about yourself).

How did you deal with any issues? Who did you turn to (family, friends, other significant adults like teachers or neighbours)? Were you supported (or not, as the case may be) by anyone in particular? Who listened to your concerns? Did you keep things to yourself?

It has been estimated that around one in five children and young people will have (mild to moderate) mental health problems (Mental Health Foundation, 1999). More concerning is that one in ten children and young people aged between 5 and 15 years in England, Scotland and Wales will have a diagnosable mental disorder (Meltzer et al., 2000; Green et al., 2005; CAMHS Review, 2008). A 2004 survey of young people in Great Britain (Green et al., 2005) provides us with some valuable information about mental disorder (that is, the most serious mental health problems) in children, a summary of which can be found in Box 9.2.

Box 9.2   Some characteristics of mental disorder in children (Green et al., 2005)

- Children rarely present with one disorder: as many as **1 in 5 have more than one disorder**, the most common combinations being conduct and emotional disorder and conduct and hyperkinetic disorder.
- Overall, problems are more common in **boys**.
- Problems are more common in older (aged 11–15) than younger (aged 5–10) children.
- The most common problems fall into three categories: **emotional** disorders, **conduct** disorders and **hyperkinetic** disorders.
- Children who have more than three stressful life events are at three times greater risk of developing emotional and behavioural problems.
- 50% of **children in care** ('looked after' children) have a diagnosable mental disorder compared with 10% of children in the rest of the population.
- Children who attend **special schools** for emotional and behavioural difficulties are at a greater risk of mental disorder.

- Over one-third of children with a **learning disability** have a diagnosable mental disorder.
- Children who have **physical disabilities** are twice as likely to develop psychological problems as those who do not.
- Children who experience **serious and chronic illnesses** are also more susceptible to psychological disorder.

It is also useful to consider what factors might influence the presence of mental health problems in children. A child's mental health is directly determined – both positively and negatively – by his or her own individual makeup, the relationships he or she has with his or her parents, family and carers, and by aspects of the wider communities to which he or she belongs. Some of these factors increase the **risk** of mental health problems; others **protect** against mental health problems and, as such, may well play a role in **resilience**. Table 9.1 outlines some of the risk and protective factors identified in child mental health.

Diagnostic frameworks

The use of diagnostic frameworks in CAMHS can be controversial amid concern about the 'medicalisation' of childhood and the stigma that is often

TABLE 9.1   Risk and protective factors in child mental health (CAMHS Review, 2008)

Focus	Risk factors	Protective factors
Child	Learning difficulty, low IQ, academic failure, low self-esteem, difficult temperament, physical illness, communication difficulties, genetic influences	Gender (female), good communication skills, being in control, humour, religious faith, capacity to reflect, higher intelligence
Family	Parental conflict, family breakdown, inconsistent discipline, hostile and rejecting relationships, physical, sexual and emotional abuse, severe parental mental health difficulties, parental offending, death, loss	At least one good parent/carer–child relationship, affection, supervision, authoritative discipline, support for education, absence of discord in parental relationship
Community	Socio-economic disadvantage, homelessness, disaster, discrimination and unemployment	Good housing, good school with academic and non-academic opportunities, high standard of living, leisure activities, wide supportive networks

associated with mental illness. This is why some people prefer to think in terms of children having mild, moderate or severe mental health problems rather than a diagnosable mental disorder. As you may recall from Chapter 1, the two main diagnostic frameworks employed in mental health are ICD-10 (WHO, 2007) – the preferred system in the UK and Europe – and DSM-IV (American Psychiatric Association, 2000), used mainly in North America. While these frameworks are used in British CAMHS (largely, but not exclusively, by psychiatrists), less medical – and some would say more woolly – classifications also exist. For example, both Green et al. (2005) and the NHS HAS (1995) advocate the use of a **problem–centred approach** in classifying mental health problems in children and young people. Here, consideration of the presenting problem is seen as more useful than a formal diagnosis. An example of such as classification is given in Table 9.2.

TABLE 9.2   Classifying mental health problems in children by presenting problem (after NHS HSA, 1995)

Nature of presenting problem	Includes
Emotional	Anxiety, phobias, depression and separation disorders (including school refusal)
Conduct	Behaviour problems, non-compliance, defiance (oppositional defiant disorder), fire setting, temper tantrums
Hyperkinetic	Attention deficit disorder
Developmental	Delays in developing skills in, for example, speech, social ability, bladder and bowel control
Eating related	Anorexia, bulimia, overeating, obesity
Self-harm	Cutting, self-poisoning, substance misuse
Psychotic	Schizophrenia

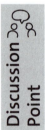

Discussion Point

To diagnose or not?

While on placement in a community CAMHS service, you find yourself working with a team of nurses who say that they prefer not to label children with psychiatric diagnoses but instead prefer to think of children having 'a range of emotional, psychological and behavioural problems'. You get talking to Rena, one of the child psychiatrists on the team. Rena says that she understands why the nursing staff choose to avoid a formal diagnosis, but she thinks it is always better to offer such a diagnosis because you can then easily identify appropriate treatments for the child and family.

What do you think are the advantages and disadvantages of Rena's view? Compare these with the advantages and disadvantages of the nursing staff's view? When thinking about this, try to see things from the child and family's perspective as well as that of the professionals.

Policy Context

The development of modern CAMHS

During the latter half of the 1990s, two major reviews of CAMHS provision in the UK stimulated a period of change that is still ongoing. In 1995, the NHS Health Advisory Service (a body offering advice and support on all aspects of mental health service provision, now called the independent Health and Social Care Advisory Service), published *Together We Stand*, a complete review of British CAMHS provision. This report called for major changes in the commissioning, management and organisation of CAMHS provision and is perhaps best known as the report that established the 'four-tier' organisational model that underpins most CAMHS provision in the UK.

A few years later, in 1999, the Audit Commission published *Children in Mind*, a review of CAMHS provision focusing mainly on the value for money of such provision (the Audit Commission is, after all, the statutory body charged with ensuring that public money is spent wisely). Despite the guidance offered by *Together We Stand* some years earlier, the Audit Commission reported variable levels of CAMHS provision with generally poor investment, little inter-agency working, long waiting lists and services restricting access to those in need.

Every Child Matters

In 2000, Victoria Climbié, an eight-year-old child living in London, died of cruelty and neglect despite being assessed by various children's services on numerous occasions. The death caused a public outcry and, in response, a public inquiry was held under the chairmanship of Lord Laming. The subsequent Laming Report (DH/Home Office, 2003) led to the development of an overarching children's strategy for England called *Every Child Matters* (DES, 2003). *Every Child Matters* focuses on five outcomes central to children's general health and wellbeing and marks out four broad areas of work to support these outcomes (see Box 9.3).

Box 9.3   Every Child Matters

Every Child Matters outcomes

- Be healthy
- Stay safe
- Enjoy and achieve
- Make a positive contribution
- Achieve economic wellbeing

Every Child Matters work streams

- Supporting parents and carers in their parenting role
- Early intervention and effective protection of children, especially in terms of improving interagency communication
- Accountability and integration in children's services (such as establishing Children's Trusts and Children's Commissioners)
- Workforce reform

The following year, the Children Act 2004 was passed. This Act provided the specific legal framework for *Every Child Matters* in England as well as some UK-wide obligations such as the requirement that Children's Commissioners be established in each of the UK's four constituent countries. While *Every Child Matters* is an **overarching children's strategy** encompassing all aspects of childcare, specific **health-related** aspects of *Every Child Matters* are further developed in the *National Service Framework for Children, Young People and Maternity Services* (DES/DH, 2004). Standard 9 of this Framework – the psychological and emotional wellbeing of children – is of particular relevance to child mental health. Box 9.4 outlines the standard in full, together with some markers of good practice.

Box 9.4   Standard 9 and markers of good practice (adapted from DES/DH, 2004)

Standard 9: 'All children and young people, from birth to their eighteenth birthday, who have mental health problems and disorders have access to timely, integrated, high quality, multi-disciplinary mental health services to ensure effective assessment, treatment and support, for them and their families.'

Markers of good practice:

- All staff working directly with children and young people have sufficient knowledge, training and support to promote the psychological wellbeing of children.
- Protocols for referral, support and early intervention are agreed between all agencies.
- In order to improve access, CAMHS professionals should provide a balance of direct and indirect services and be flexible about where children and young people are seen.
- Children and young people are able to receive urgent mental healthcare when required.
- CAMHS are able to meet the needs of **all** children, including young people aged 16–17.
- The needs of children and young people with complex, severe and persistent behavioural and mental health needs are met through a multi-agency approach.
- Arrangements are in place to ensure that specialist multidisciplinary teams are of sufficient size and have an appropriate skill-mix, training and support.
- Children and young people who require admission to hospital for mental healthcare are cared for in an environment suited to their age.
- When children and young people are discharged from inpatient services into the community or transferred from child to adult services, their continuity of care is ensured by use of the care programme approach.

In late 2007, the government published *The Children's Plan* (DCSF, 2007), a ten-year plan for developing children's service in England that built upon *Every Child Matters*. Notable within this plan was the announcement that an independent CAMHS review would be undertaken. The review was to: (1) take stock of CAMHS developments to date; (2) identify how universal services (such as schools) could play a more effective role in child mental health; (3) help develop priority actions for the government's vision of emotional health and wellbeing in children; and (4) examine the development of robust local and national outcome measures. The CAMHS Review was published in 2008.

The CAMHS Review

The CAMHS Review found that there had been some progress over the last few years in the development of services contributing to the mental health and psychological wellbeing of children and young people. However, the Review concluded that these services were not as comprehensive, as consistent or as good as they could have been. The Review found that children and young people didn't see many services as responsive, accessible or as child-centred as they could be. It also found unhelpful legal and administrative processes in accessing services, unacceptable variations in service provision between regions and within local areas, and busy professionals who had little time to understand the research and evidence underpinning effective interventions. Many of these findings echoed those of the Audit Commission report issued almost a decade before.

Other nations of the UK

CAMHS policy in Scotland has been driven largely by the Scottish *Needs Assessment Report on Child and Adolescent Mental Health* (PHIS, 2003), which in turn led to Scotland's own CAMHS Framework (Scottish Executive, 2005), a framework designed to assist agencies with planning and delivering integrated approaches to children and young people's mental health. Scotland has its equivalent to *Every Child Matters*, entitled *Getting It Right for Every Child* (Scottish Government, 2008). *Getting It Right* has slightly different outcomes from those of England, having eight rather than five: **being healthy**, **achieving**, **nurtured**, **active**, **respected**, **responsible**, **included** and **safe**. Having mentally healthy infants, children and young people has also been identified as a priority of Scotland's over-arching mental health policy, *Towards a Mentally Flourishing Scotland* (Scottish Government, 2009).

Following identified limitations in CAMHS provision in Wales (such as historical patterns of service provision rather than ones based on need, poor cooperation between education, health and social care, little specialist training and services under enormous pressure), the Welsh Assembly published an all-Wales CAMHS strategy in 2001 (National Assembly for Wales, 2001). However, a recent report from the Wales Audit Office and Health Inspectorate Wales (2009) concluded that despite some improvements, CAMHS were still failing many children and young people. As such, it is likely that CAMHS policy will be reviewed again in Wales in the near future.

In Northern Ireland, CAMHS provision is being reviewed through the generic Bamford Review of Mental Health and Learning Disability (see DHSSPS, 2009), though the four-tier model common to the whole of the UK (see below) is very likely to stay.

The organisation of CAMHS in the UK

Despite differences in policy across the four countries of the UK, mental health services for children and young people across the UK tend to be organised according to a four-tier model developed by the NHS Health Advisory Service in 1995. The four tiers are not designed to demarcate between services, but instead allow services to describe what they do and at what specific level of need. When a child's needs cannot be met by a specific tier, advice and intervention is sought from the next tier up. As Figure 9.1 shows, this organisational model is intended to make the best use of different practitioners, and to improve the availability and accessibility of services. Mental health specialists are clustered in Tiers 3 and 4, at the more severe end of the spectrum of mental health problems. **Tier 4** services are normally inpatient services, whether generic or more specialized, such as eating disorders units or units for young people with mental health problems who have committed crimes. **Tier 3** services are for children and young people with severe, persistent and complex disorders and are usually provided by a

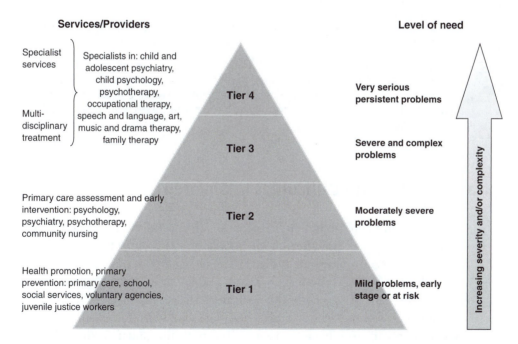

FIGURE 9.1   The four-tier framework for the delivery of CAMHS in the UK (adapted, with permission, from Kendal, 2009)

multidisciplinary team who may well make use of more specialized services such as day-patient, or even inpatient, facilities.

Tier 2 practitioners are usually CAMHS specialists working individually in primary care (for example, in a outpatient or community CAMHS clinic) and may offer early intervention and outreach services. **Tier 1** CAMHS services are provided by **anyone who has contact with children**. Some Tier 1 CAMHS practitioners may not have mental health training. They provide general advice, health promotion, early assessment and referral and include GPs, school nurses, teachers and voluntary agencies. Tier 1 professionals may well be involved in promoting **emotional health and wellbeing**, one of the four key targets of the national 'Healthy Schools Programme' (DH/DCSF, 2007). As such, nurses might find themselves working across a spectrum of child mental health services that encompasses mental health promotion and illness prevention as well as the provision of intensive, specialized mental health treatments (Kendal, 2009).

Discussion Point

The role of nurses in CAMHS

Thinking about the four-tier model illustrated in Figure 9.1, where do you think *nurses* might fit in?

You might find it helpful to think about nurse in its broadest sense – one that encompasses specialist nurses other than mental health nurses, such as children's nurses, health visitors, school nurses, nurses working in A&E, and so on. What different qualifications and skills do you think nurses working in each tier might require?

Typical Mental Health Difficulties in Children

Emotional and behavioural problems are relatively common in children, being seen in at least 10% of the school population in England (Cooper, 2005). Many mild or even moderate problems can be dealt with by Tier 1 professionals and typically only those with severe and/or persistent problems tend to require the help of mental health specialists. Because sources of support may be different for pre-school and school-age children (for example, **health visitors** are far more likely to be involved with the under-5s than CAMHS staff), it is helpful to separate pre-school (0–4 years) children from school-age (5–11 years) children when looking at childhood mental health problems.

Pre-school mental health difficulties in children

Postnatal depression and attachment disorders

The presence of severe postnatal depression in mothers can have a catastrophic impact on the development of the child if untreated. It is relatively common for new mothers to have mild depression – the 'baby blues' – as a consequence of childbirth; in some women, however, there is also a risk of **severe depression** or a specific form of psychosis – **puerperal or post-partum psychosis** – which may require hospitalisation. (Information about depression and psychosis in adults can be found Chapters 5, 6 and 7.) Mothers who are depressed tend to be less responsive, less attentive and more critical towards their babies, putting the healthy development of the mother–child relationship into jeopardy (Murray & Cooper, 1997). There is, as such, a risk of **attachment disorders** developing whereby the mother–child relationship lacks warmth and sensitivity, becoming intrusive, distant, resistant or ambivalent. Attachment disorders can have a serious impact on the ability to develop long-term secure relationships in both childhood and adulthood. Healthy, **secure attachment** is demonstrated by children seeking proximity (closeness) and care from caregivers; in **insecure-avoidant attachment** the child actively avoids the parent, while in **insecure-ambivalent attachment** (or insecure-resistant attachment) the child shows active or passive hostility towards the parent, often through difficult behaviour and negative interactions.

Separation anxiety

Children become anxious when they have to separate from an attachment figure like a parent, sibling or member of their extended family. This normal response is known as **separation anxiety**. It starts at about the age of 9 months and lasts until about the age of 4 years. When children have separation anxiety, they are typically clingy, fear people they don't know and become distressed when separated from an attachment figure. They may worry because they do not feel safe being away from the attachment figure, and they may not want to go to school or they may be afraid of sleeping or being at home alone. The child may feel sick, anxious or have nightmares about the possibility of separation. Like many mental health problems, separation anxiety only becomes problematic when a normal response gets out of control, is inappropriate or when it impairs the child or carer's everyday functioning. **School refusal** (or school phobia) is a specific form of separation anxiety that affects some school-age children. We will look at school refusal later in this chapter.

Sleep difficulties

Sleep difficulties in small children are common. Many children wake during the night and find that they are unable to settle themselves back to sleep without comfort from a parent or carer. In some cases, sleep may be disturbed by **sleep-walking**, **night terrors** or **nightmares**; if these difficulties are severe and persistent they may generally need deeper investigation by and specialist help from paediatricians to rule out an organic/physical cause such as epilepsy. In assessing sleep problems, it is important to identify any emotional reason for a child's sleeplessness. Any assessment, as such, needs to be thorough and should include assessment of sleep pattern, the bedtime routine, knowing what happens before bed and while settling in bed, what time the child sleeps from, whether they wake, what happens when they do wake and what time they wake in the morning. Assessing how the parents manage the night time routine is also important.

Most sleep difficulties can be overcome by establishing a regular sleep routine, including a wind down period from normal, boisterous play to more quiet play, an actual countdown to bedtime, a bath, supper, bedtime story and planned leaving of the child after hugs and kisses.

Feeding problems

Feeding problems are also common in young children and can range from an inability to tolerate the texture of certain foods, a lack of interest in food, only being willing to accept a limited choice of food stuffs (faddiness), poor table manners (usually down to poor social skills), an inability or unwillingness to feed themselves and pica eating (eating inappropriate stuff such as foam, material, dirt, etc.).

Feeding difficulties can arise for many reasons and, often, these can be determined from a comprehensive assessment of the child and family's experience of early feeding. Typical questions that might be asked are: What was breast feeding or bottle feeding like for mother and child? Was this pleasurable or fraught with anxiety and distress? Was the child keen to learn to feed him or herself? Was he or she weaned to solid foods at the right time and given a varied diet? Did the parents/carers allow the child to make a mess when learning the skill of feeding? How do the parents/carers engage with meal times? Is it a social situation where the family meets together? Does the family have table and chairs to sit together? Does the child refuse to eat or is the family too busy to sit down? If the parents are feeding the child, is this a rewarding experience, so much so that the child does not want to give it up?

Like sleep difficulties, feeding difficulties respond well to routine: establishing a good mealtime routine where the family comes together in a positive way will often resolve the problem.

School-age difficulties in children

Enuresis and encopresis

Enuresis and **encopresis** often referred to as, respectively, **wetting** and **soiling**, are common disorders of childhood resulting in distress for the child and their family (Butler, 2008).

Enuresis is defined as the involuntary passing of urine after the age at which a child is normally expected to have gained bladder control. Enuresis can be **primary**, where bladder control has never been established, or **secondary**, where bladder control was achieved for at least six months and then lost. Enuresis happens most commonly at night (**nocturnal enuresis**) and occasionally during the day (**diurnal enuresis**). Bedwetting is more common in boys and daytime wetting more common in girls. Before considering enuresis to be an emotional problem, physical causes for the problem need to be excluded by a GP or paediatrician.

Encopresis is the involuntary or voluntary passing of faeces in inappropriate places after the age that normal bowel function is expected. Paradoxically, **constipation** can cause soiling due to an 'overflow' of faecal matter from the colon; consequently (and unsurprisingly), some parents treat the child for diarrhoea with over-the-counter medications making the constipation – and the soiling – worse. As with enuresis (and perhaps more so), encopresis frequently causes distress to children and their families.

In assessing children who soil, it is always necessary to exclude any physical cause, particularly constipation. It is also important to consider that any child who soils may be suffering **abuse** or **maltreatment**. When assessing children who soil, the following questions are typically asked: What is the child's experience of toilet training? Has there been any experience of pain when defecating or is the child fearful of going to the toilet? What is the parent/carer's response to the soiling? Is it managed in a sensitive and non-punitive way? Is the child helped to clean him or herself up or is he or she ridiculed and humiliated by his family and peers? What toilet facilities does the child have access to at home and school? What has already been tried to stop the soiling?

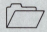 Case scenario: soiling

Emily is an 8-year-old girl living at home with her mother. Her parents separated in acrimonious circumstances when she was 3 years old; before this their relationship was volatile and violent. Emily has two older brothers, Paul 14 and Philip 11, whom she does not get on with. She attends a local mainstream school where she is an unpopular child as she often smells. She is often picked on and teased by the other children and she can be nasty to her peers.

Emily was referred to CAMHS by a paediatrician for assistance with soiling. The paediatrician had treated Emily for chronic constipation for many years; she had never managed to pass a stool into the toilet, preferring to use pull-up nappies to defecate in. She had periods of constipation with overflow diarrhoea, which led to low self-esteem and anxiety about going out of the house without a pull-up nappy in case she soiled herself. The paediatrician has ruled out any physical reasons for soiling. This has caused some parent–child conflict as her parents find it hard to understand why she will not go on the toilet. They see no alternative other than to buy pull-up nappies for Emily.

What things might you need to be aware of or ask Emily and her parents during assessment? What about relationships, environment (both home and at school), history, current behaviour and Emily's feelings and those of her parents?

Reflect upon your own views about working with children who wet and/or soil themselves. Consider your thoughts, feelings and responses to working with this client group.

Attention deficit hyperactivity disorder

Attention deficit hyperactivity disorder (ADHD) is a common disorder of childhood. It is a neuro-developmental disorder characterised by a persistent pattern of **hyperactivity**, **impulsivity** and **inattention** that is more frequent and severe than in individuals at a comparable level of development, which cannot be explained by any other disorder and which impairs the child in their psychological, social and educational development and functioning (Ryan & McDougall, 2008; NCCMH, 2009). While ADHD is the most widely used term for this disorder, you might also see **attention deficit**

disorder (ADD) and **hyperkinetic disorder** (HKD) in use. ADHD in not only a disorder of childhood: it can persist into adolescence, adulthood and older age. ADHD is often associated with other problems, such as behaviour problems, family/relationship issues, tics and Tourette's syndrome, learning difficulties, anxiety and depression. It affects far more boys than girls.

ADHD is a complex disorder that has been associated with a variety of issues, including the 'nature/nurture' debate, diet, poor childrearing practices and family breakdown (Banerjee et al., 2007; Ryan & McDougall, 2008; NCCMH, 2009).

Behaviour problems

A very common complaint in childrearing is that children do not do what parents or those in authority ask. Sometimes there is no real problem, only a mismatch between the child's actual behaviour and high parental expectations or the child's actual behaviour and parental misunderstandings of what is 'normal' for the child's age. A good example is **temper tantrums**: these are developmentally acceptable in toddlers but more worrying in older children and of particular concern in teenagers. Where there is a real problem, the child may be said to have an **oppositional defiant disorder** (ODD) or a **conduct disorder**, the latter being more serious. These behavioural disorders entail more than a child's being occasionally naughty, difficult, stubborn or aggressive, the child has to present with a **persistent, repetitive pattern** of not sticking to the rules or disobeying socially accepted norms.

ODD is characterised by unusually frequent temper outbursts, arguing with adults, actively refusing to do what is asked, disobedience, deliberately annoying others, blaming others for their mistakes, being easily annoyed, angry, resentful, spiteful and vindictive. The behaviour is more likely to present in the under-11s and is likely to have caused upset at home and complaints from the child's teachers. Conduct disorder is much more severe than ODD and children with conduct disorder present with an array of poor behaviours, including telling lies, frequent fighting, destruction of other people's property, bullying, staying out late, running away from home, playing truant, being cruel to people or animals and criminal behaviour such as stealing, breaking into other people's property, fire setting, rape and using weapons to threaten or intimidate others. This type of behaviour often results in the child being in trouble with the police and the youth justice system. Conduct disorders can be **socialised** or **unsocialised**. In **socialised conduct disorder**, the child or young person has friends who also act in an antisocial way: the child and his (it is nearly always boys) friends often act together as a group, engaging in behaviours such as shoplifting or stealing cars. A child with an **unsocialised conduct disorder** lacks any real friends and typically engages in solitary antisocial activities. Unsocialised conduct disorder is seen more frequently in teenagers than younger children.

Emotional disorders: depression and anxiety-related disorders

Emotional disorders such as **depression**, **anxiety**, **phobias** and **obsessive–compulsive disorder** are relatively common in children and our understanding of these difficulties is growing.

Depression is characterised by feelings of sadness, irritability and loss of interest which last for most of the day and persist over a period of time. Depression is associated more with adolescents, but can be seen in younger children. Other features may be tiredness, altered appetite, weight loss or gain, insomnia, agitation, frustration, feelings of worthlessness or guilt, poor concentration, thoughts of death and recent talk or experience of self-harm. It is important to bear in mind that children and young people present to healthcare services in a variety of ways and there is no clear-cut consistency in the presentation of depression (NCCMH, 2005a).

Generalised anxiety presents as worries about a wide range of past, present or future events and situations. The child may worry about school work and exams, disasters and accidents, his/her own health, weight or appearance, bad things happening to his or her parents, family or others, the future, making and keeping friends, death and dying, being bullied and teased.

Phobias are an anxiety disorder where the focus of the anxiety (fear) is some specific object or situation. Most children with a specific phobia will have a fear of animals, insects, noise, the dark and school (but see also the discussion on school refusal below). This fear is characterised by persistent and excessive anxiety: the child becomes very upset each time the fear object or situation is encountered (sometimes merely by thinking about the object or situation) and tries to avoid the object or situation. **Social phobia** is a specific phobia where the anxiety is about social activities: meeting new or large groups of people; eating in front of others; reading or writing in front of others; speaking in class and so on. The child is often able to socialise with familiar people in small numbers but is frightened of interacting with other adults or children in unfamiliar situations. The child becomes distressed, cries, blushes or feels sick and will try to avoid such social situations. Where a child refuses to go to school because of such anxieties, the child may develop **school refusal/school phobia**. School refusal may also be underpinned by other anxieties such as a fear of real or potential bullying, or a fear of being separated from a parent or carer (separation anxiety). Note that school refusal is very different from **truancy**, which is a wilful, unauthorised absence from school, normally because some other activity is seen to be more interesting or exciting.

Obsessive–compulsive disorder (OCD) is another anxiety disorder that frequently begins in childhood or adolescence, the prevalence in this group being around 1% (NCCMH, 2006). It consists of two elements: an **obsession**, which is an involuntary, intrusive thought often accompanied by an implicit demand for action; and a **compulsion**, which is a desire to act on the demands of the intrusive thought. OCD behaviours include rituals and repetitive behaviour; common examples of such behaviour include **hand washing** (the obsession is a sense of being dirty or contaminated; the compulsion, the need to wash your hands) or over-zealous **checking** (the obsession is 'did I do such-and-such?'; the compulsion, a need to check whether such-and-such has actually been done). As with many mental health problems, OCD tends to become a problem when it seriously interferes with the child or carer's everyday functioning.

Post-traumatic stress disorder (PTSD) is a disorder that some people experience following a traumatic experience such as violent crime, war, torture, major accidents and disasters. A particular trauma that can affect children and young people is **childhood sexual abuse**. Symptoms in older children tend to be the same as is in adults – **flashbacks** (the re-experiencing of the trauma), **emotional numbing** and **increased physiological arousal** – but in younger children, PTSD may also manifest in overt aggression and destructiveness.

Anxiety and depression are particularly associated with the so-called **somatoform disorders** – disorders that are characterised by physical symptoms (such as persistent headaches, stomach aches or vomiting) but without any identifiable physical cause. (These disorders may also be referred to as **medically unexplained symptoms**.) Girls generally report more somatoform symptoms than boys and their reports generally increase as they move towards adolescence; the opposite is true for boys (Eminson, 2001). Eminson also identifies associations between somatoform symptoms and traits in children such as perfectionism, conscientiousness and low self-esteem.

Tics and Tourette's syndrome

Tics are involuntary muscle contractions that result in either a movement (a **motor tic**) or a sound (a **vocal tic**). Tics are common in childhood, boys being more affected than girls, and most are mild, transient or episodic. Unless they bother the child, tics do not usually require specialist attention although sometimes tics develop during adolescence into **Tourette's syndrome**, a condition whereby tics are coupled with other features, particularly those of ADHD and OCD.

Autistic spectrum disorders

Autistic spectrum disorders (ASDs) – which include both **autism** and **Asperger syndrome** – are a controversial set of disorders that span the fields of education, psychiatry, genetics and learning disability. According to the Autism Working Group (DES/DH, 2002), those with ASDs are impaired in three ways: (1) in their ability to understand and use non-verbal and verbal communication; (2) in their ability to understand social behaviour (which affects their ability to interact with other children and adults); and (3) in the way in which they think and behave, which may be demonstrated by restricted, obsessional, or repetitive activities.

You may well come into contact with children with ASD in CAMHS. Sometimes this is because of concerns regarding co-occurring conditions such as ADHD, social skills deficits or behaviour disorder. More often, it is because a school-age child requires an assessment of 'social difficulties', 'communication difficulties' or 'developmental difficulties', perhaps because an ASD has not been picked up during a routine early childhood assessment in a child development clinic.

No one really knows what causes ASDs. Since both the medical and educational/psychological communities have laid claim to ASDs, both biomedical (genetic; neurological) and educational-psychological (socialisation; learning; behavioural) theories of ASDs exist and the plethora of treatments around tend to be split along medical/educational-psychological lines.

Referral and assessment in CAMHS

Referral

Children are referred to CAMHS by many agencies. Currently the child's GP is the most frequent referrer, but professionals such as paediatricians,

TABLE 9.3   The Common Assessment Framework

Section of the CAF	Includes information on
1. Development of the infant, child or young person *Scottish IAF: 'How I grow and develop'*	Health Emotional and social development Behavioural development Identity, including self-esteem, self-image and social presentation Family and social relationships Self-care skills and independence Learning
2. Parents and carers *Scottish IAF: 'What I need from people who look after me'*	Basic care, ensuring safety and protection Emotional warmth and stability Guidance, boundaries and stimulation
3. Family and environment *Scottish IAF: 'My wider world'*	Family history, functioning and wellbeing Wider family Housing, employment and financial considerations Social and community elements and resources, including education

school nurses, social workers, educational psychologists and youth justice workers are often in a good position to refer. The referral process is normally through letter or, increasingly, through completion of the **Common Assessment Framework** (CAF), a universal tool developed to ensure that services for children are both integrated and focus on the needs of the child (DES, 2003). Although the CAF applies specifically to England, Wales is piloting and developing its own version of the CAF, and in Scotland, the similar **Integrated Assessment Framework** (IAF) exists. In Northern Ireland there is, at the time of writing, no equivalent framework despite calls for such from the NSPCC as far back as 2004 (Bunting, 2004). The common assessment frameworks (CAF and IAF) provide a standard process for the holistic assessment of the child's needs as well as of his or her strengths. They also consider the role of parents/carers and environmental influences (see Table 9.3).

Assessment

The purpose of assessment in CAMHS is to place the child's current and past functioning in the context of family dynamics and relationships so as to determine whether intervention or support is required. It is rare for children to seek referral and assessment directly; more often than not, it is worried parents or carers who seek out specialist help. As we mentioned earlier, children rarely present with a single discrete disorder but with a combination of problems, and to understand the complexity of these problems, a **comprehensive** assessment is necessary.

No single professional is likely to be able to provide the breadth and depth of knowledge and expertise required to accurately assess child mental health difficulties, hence a range of professionals is usually involved in the assessment process. For example, **paediatricians** and **child psychiatrists** might carry out medical tests, **psychologists** (educational and clinical) might perform formal psychometric tests while **social workers** may provide a background social-economic assessment. Learning difficulties, particularly specific learning difficulties such as dyspraxia or speech and language problems, can also contribute to mental health problems in children. Assessment in CAMHS is, as such, usually undertaken by a multidisciplinary team and **nurses** – especially those with a background in **mental health** or **children's (paediatric) nursing** – form an important part of this multidisciplinary team, accounting for approximately 25% of the CAMHS workforce (Audit Commission, 1999). Indeed, the NHS HAS (1995) sees nurses specialising in child mental health as one of the three key child mental health professionals along with child psychiatrists and child psychologists.

In order to carry out a comprehensive nursing assessment, nurses working in CAMHS need to have knowledge about normal child development (i.e. physical and psychological **milestones**) so that they can differentiate between 'normal' experiences and behaviours and those that we might call 'abnormal'. Nurses also need to have the necessary communication and interpersonal skills required to work with children, young people and their families. Figure 9.2 outlines some of things that nurses need to consider when assessing children with mental health problems.

The assessment process

A clinical consultation and interview is the primary assessment tool in CAMHS. As we have seen in previous chapters, the main tasks at the beginning of the interview are those of **engagement**, putting the child and family at ease and establishing a **therapeutic relationship**. Since many child mental problems are complex, a comprehensive assessment is best obtained via a **structured** rather than non-directive interview (where the child and his or her family are invited to talk freely about their concerns).

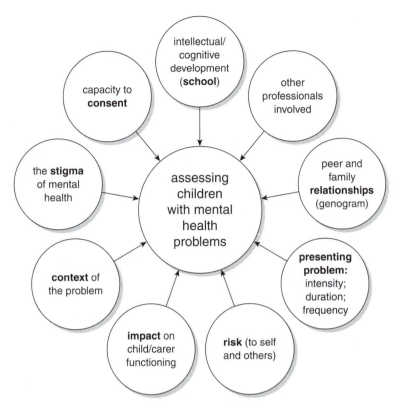

FIGURE 9.2   Things to consider when assessing children with mental health problems

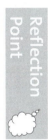

Reflection
Point

Assessment

Assessment isn't always an easy process. Here are a number of common issues that occur with assessment. Have a think about what you would do if:

- A child refuses to speak to you
- A child is unable to separate from their parent/carer
- A parent/carer became hostile and critical about the child when the child was present
- A parent/carer says that the child's view of the problem isn't important 'because they're only a child'.

TABLE 9.4   A suggested outline for interviewing in CAMHS (after Rutter & Taylor, 2002)

Interview stage	Guidance
1. Presenting problems	Establish, for example: Who initiated the referral? Why was the referral made and why now? Whose problem is it? What do the child and family understand by coming to see a child mental health professional
2. Background to the problems	Ask about the **duration** and **severity** of problems and who is the **most concerned** about them (child? parent? school?)
3. Family and social history	Draw a **genogram**. Ask about family and social history; the mental and physical health of family members
4. Developmental history	Ask about: Conception and maternal health during pregnancy Parental use of medication, illicit drugs, alcohol and tobacco Labour and delivery (including any complications), birth weight and any need for special care Post natal history (including attachment and any neonatal complications) Developmental milestones Medical history Educational achievement and progress
5. Observations of child and family	Including how the family members interact with one another; where possible, carry out separate parental and child interviews
6. Use of formal assessment tools	For example, the Conners scales (see Kollins et al., 2004) and the Strengths and Difficulties Questionnaire (SDQ; Goodman, 1997)
7. Information from other sources	So long as child and parental consent has been obtained, information from **school-based staff** such as teachers and school nurses, as well as other professionals like **social workers**, **speech and language therapists**, **educational psychologists** and **paediatricians**, will be helpful
8. Summary, formulation and intervention	Summarising helps capture the problem and ensures that CAMHS is the right service for the family (i.e., there is clear evidence of clinically significant impairment in behavioural, emotional, social, academic or occupational functioning). Diagnosis and formulation needs to be discussed with the child and family/carers in a sensitive way as do intervention options

A suggested outline for structured interviewing can be found in Table 9.4. Before engaging with a child the nurse should ensure that the environment is age-appropriate, use language that is sensitive to the child's needs and provide a statement to the child and family about confidentiality and safe-guarding their health. Any room used for interview should be **quiet**, **private** and **free from distractions**, with chairs that are **comfortable** and that avoid creating barriers in the interview. It should be well equipped with **age-appropriate toys** and **paper and pens** so that **rapport** develops. Observations made during the interview about the child's ability or inability to use the toys appropriately or occupy themselves for periods of time is useful. The interview aims to collect other important information about the child and family, not just the facts. Therefore it is important that the nurse has **good interview techniques** and **interpersonal and communication skills**. The nurse also needs to show **genuine interest** in the problems presented by the child and family as well as gathering relevant clinical information and their own observations during the interview.

The interview should commence with non-threatening or non-contentious questions. **Open communication** should be used to **engage** the child and family and to encourage reciprocal rapport, for example, everyone should tell each other their names, the child should be asked the name of the school they attend, how old they are and what they like to do. Having toys and paper and pens can help with this open communication as well as giving some understanding of the child's developmental stage through drawing, play and writing. Particular note should be taken of **inattention**, **hyperactivity** and **impulsivity** presented by the child on interview. Interviewing the child separately (interview stage 5) can help assess the child's **ability to separate**, **physical appearance**, **motor behaviour**, **speech** and **use of language**, **social interactions**, **mood**, **cognitive functioning** and **developmental level**.

When using formal assessment tools (interview stage 6), remember that all assessment tools have their limitations and those using particular assessment tools should be aware of their relative strengths and weaknesses. Some tools may only be available to suitably qualified or trained individuals. Because many child mental health problems are complex, it may not be possible to arrive at a full formulation (the last interview stage) in a single, initial interview and further interviews may need to be arranged and/or information sought from elsewhere, from grandparents, health visitors, school staff and other childcare professionals, for example (interview stage 7).

Case scenario: ADHD

Kyle is a 7-year-old boy who lives at home with his mother, Lizzie, aged 27, and her partner, Steven, aged 31. They have been together for five years. Kyle does not have any contact with his natural father. Kyle and Lizzie lived with his maternal grandparents for the first 18 months of his life before they set up home with Steven. Kyle was cared for by his maternal grandmother after Lizzie returned to work soon after Kyle's birth. His grandmother is very important to Kyle. There are no other siblings and Kyle's care continues to be shared between his mother and her partner and his grandparents.

Kyle's GP referred Kyle to CAMHS because his teachers have been expressing concern about his behaviour in the classroom, stating that he could not sit still and was disrupting the other pupils' learning. He was falling behind with his academic progress. He did not have many friends and his attempts to be friendly with his peers were rejected, leaving Kyle feeling left out and sad. During the GP consultation, Kyle was described as being 'hyperactive, but warm and friendly on a 1:1'.

During assessment by a CAMHS nurse consultant, Kyle found it difficult to occupy himself with age-appropriate toys, asking the adults in the room to play with him. He was not disruptive or oppositional but was active, restless, boisterous and noisy. His parents related in a warm, calm and consistent manner on interview. There were some differences in opinions between his parents and maternal grandmother, but the family handled these in a sensitive way.

What things would you need to be aware of or ask Kyle and his family about during assessment? What about relationships, environment (both home and at school), history, current behaviour and Kyle's feelings and those of his parents?

(We shall return to this case scenario later.)

Consent and confidentiality: safeguarding vulnerable children

When helping children and their families – through assessment and through intervention – **consent** is as much an issue as it is for adults. However, consent is a bit more complicated in children than in adults so some brief discussion of the topic is warranted here. The gist of the law is that children aged 16 and over are presumed to be 'competent' in law, that is, have the capacity to consent for themselves without parental knowledge or approval. Children under the age of 16 are not presumed to have such competency but they may be competent if they have 'sufficient understanding and maturity to enable them to understand fully what is proposed' (this is often referred to as **Gillick competence**, after a judgment made by the House of Lords). Such competence is unlikely in younger children but may be something nurses have to deal with in the over-12s and we will pick this up again in the next chapter.

In any nurse–patient relationship, confidentiality is usually a given. There are, however, two situations when a child's confidentiality may need to be breached without necessarily obtaining the child's consent. The main indication is where there is information disclosed that suggests that the child may be **at significant risk of harm or abuse**. In these circumstances, it is good practice for the nurse to support the child or young person to make the disclosure themselves. However, if the child is unable or unwilling to do this, the nurse has a professional obligation to report the disclosure on the child's behalf. In addition, where a competent young person or child is refusing treatment for a life-threatening condition, the duty of care requires that confidentiality be breached and those with parental responsibility be told so that they can provide the necessary consent for treatment. In both scenarios, nurses must have a clear understanding of their duties and have ready access to local policies on confidentiality and information sharing. NHS trusts usually have access to legal advice where there are complex legal or ethical dilemmas. For routine advice about confidentiality, consent and information sharing, nurses should also be able to access professional advice from their employing organisation or from a professional body such as the Royal College of Nursing. For safeguarding children or child protection matters, nurses should have access to **named and designated professionals** who can assist them to make safe and competent decisions that may affect the welfare of a child. Guidance for nurses and other professionals related to safeguarding and protecting vulnerable children is available for England (HM Government, 2006; NICE, 2009a), Wales (AWCPPRG, 2008), Scotland (Scottish Executive, 2004) and Northern Ireland (DHSSPS, 2003).

Evidence-Based Interventions for Child Mental Health Problems

Resources for healthcare are limited; there is, as such, a need to ensure that the interventions on offer in CAMHS are those shown to have demonstrable benefits for the child and his or her family. Though many interventions used in CAMHS have little or no evidence base (CAMHS Review, 2008), research into CAMHS interventions has increased in recent years and a picture of effective CAMHS interventions is beginning to emerge (see, for example, Fonagy et al., 2002; Wolpert et al., 2006). NICE – the National Institute for Health and Clinical Excellence – has also begun to focus on interventions in child mental health in a much more discrete way. Whereas in the past NICE may have included some information for children and young people in its general guidance for specific mental health problems (as was the case with its guidance for OCD; NICE, 2006a), it has in recent years issued separate, specific guidance for mental health problems in children and young people.

Most of the interventions we will discuss can be – indeed, are – undertaken by *nurses* working in CAMHS, though some may require a specific level of expertise and/or additional specialist training. For example, the prescribing of medications would require, as you may recall from Chapter 3, completion of a nurse-prescribing course in order to become an independent prescriber, and cognitive behavioural therapy and eye movement desensitisation and reprocessing both normally require that the therapist has had additional training. Though children's nurses are eligible to work in CAMHS as well as mental health nurses, the principles of many of the interventions listed will be familiar to most mental health nurses who have completed training but not to most children's nurses. It should come as no surprise, therefore, to find that by far the majority of nurses working in CAMHS are mental health nurses.

It is important for the child and family to be committed to treatment as improved outcomes are unlikely without motivation (Basu & Padmore, 2009); since families are more likely to be motivated when there is mutual engagement with professionals, this observation reinforces the importance of establishing a therapeutic relationship when working in CAMHS.

Problems in preschool children

The best evidence is for **information and advice**, especially when coupled with a **parenting programme**. 'Parenting programme' is an overarching term that encapsulates parent support, parent education and parent training

(Utting et al., 2006). These programmes are designed to help parents develop positive strategies for managing behaviour, but also give praise and reward to children, encourage parents to play and spend time with their child and set limits and rules. A Cochrane Review of parenting programmes (Barlow et al., 2010) found some support for the use of group-based parenting programmes to improve the emotional and behavioural adjustment of the under-4s but, like many Cochrane Reviews, it also called for further research. Two specific parent training programmes that have good evidence are **Triple-P: Positive Parenting Programme** (Sanders, 2003) and **The Incredible Years** (Webster-Stratton, 2005). The Incredible Years is especially notable since it is a programme developed by a nurse, Carolyn Webster-Stratton. Less formally, working with parents and children to establish routines and using behavioural contingency approaches (e.g. reward or star charts) may also be helpful. Since every family with a child under the age of 5 will have a named health visitor, interventions for pre-school children are often instigated by **health visitors**.

Enuresis and encopresis

Physical causes should always be excluded first and, with encopresis in particular, the possibility of abuse or maltreatment should also be ruled out. Psychological treatments for enuresis include parent and child reassurance, diary keeping of the times and frequency of wetting, reward charts, bladder training and enuresis alarms. Pharmacological treatment with **desmopressin** – a synthetic version of vasopressin, a hormone that regulates the body's retention of water – can be helpful (Butler, 2008). NICE guidance on nocturnal enuresis is scheduled for publication in late 2010.

For encopresis, treatments in use include a well-balanced diet, psychoeducation, behavioural programmes to develop good toilet routine, praise/reward for sitting on the toilet, and a positive and sensitive approach from parents. Medications for constipation are often managed in collaboration with a medical practitioner such as a GP or paediatrician. The best evidence is for **behavioural techniques**; laxatives alone are ineffective (Matson & LoVullo, 2009).

ADHD

At one time, food additives were thought to play a causal role in ADHD and their removal from the diet was seen to be the answer. For example, in the mid- 1970s, the 'Feingold diet' (Feingold, 1975) advocated restricting some

3,000 additives in the diets of hyperactive children, including artificial colourings and flavourings as well as the natural salicylates (chemicals similar to aspirin). While there is little evidence to support this theory in its extreme, there is some evidence that some children respond negatively to caffeine found in tea, coffee and carbonated drinks and some evidence that certain food additives – like the food colouring tartrazine (E102), and the food preservative sodium benzoate – can trigger behaviour problems in children (Rowe, 1988; Rowe & Rowe, 1994). In a recent, well-designed, randomised controlled trial, McCann et al. (2007) found that additives commonly found in children's food **did** increase the average levels of hyperactivity in a general population sample of children. In other words, it seems that there are some additives that can cause hyperactivity in normal children and logic would imply that these additives could also make children with ADHD worse.

Apart from removing additives from the diet, there has also been some interest in supplementing the diets of children with ADHD, particularly with **omega 3 fatty acids** (Voigt et al., 2001; Richardson & Puri, 2002; Richardson & Montgomery, 2005; Johnson et al., 2009). This follows some hints in the literature that fatty acid deficiencies may contribute to a range of adult psychiatric and neurological disorders, and to common neurodevelopmental disorders including ADHD, dyslexia, dyspraxia and autistic spectrum disorders (Richardson, 2004). The position on diet and ADHD, however, is best summed up by the full version of the NICE guidelines which state that 'the quality of the evidence for dietary interventions is generally poor', adding further that 'the evidence that elimination or supplementation diets ... may reduce ADHD symptoms is inconclusive' (NCCMH, 2009, p. 229). It is worth noting, however, that this statement does not specifically say that diet shouldn't necessarily be considered in treating ADHD, just that the evidence is weak and/or inconclusive. As such, it is understandable that parents might want to restrict a certain food group if they think that it makes the behaviour of their child worse (Spender et al., 2001) and nurses should be sensitive to these concerns.

The evidence for a **multimodal approach** – one that includes psychosocial interventions, parent management training, social skills group training and classroom management – is, on the other hand, much more robust (MTA Cooperative Group, 1999; NCCMH, 2009). **Pharmacological treatments** for ADHD also have an evidence base in that stimulant medication (methylphenidate) and non stimulant medication (atomoxetine) can increase concentration span and reduce hyperactivity and impulsivity in children with

ADHD (NCCMH, 2009). These benefits, however, have to be balanced against the downsides of giving young children regular doses of psychotropic medication.

 Case scenario: ADHD revisited

Remember Kyle from earlier? The nurse consultant's formulation is that Kyle is a boy who presents with pervasive evidence of poor concentration, hyperactivity, impulsivity and distractibility on interview and in his general life, which is causing impairment to his day-to-day functioning. He does not present with any evidence of social communication difficulties, although he finds peer relationships difficult. The nurse consultant adds that these symptoms can be understood in terms of attention deficit hyperactivity disorder (ADHD).

The nurse consultant suggests the following line of treatment:

- Psychoeducation (through verbal discussion and written information) for the parents and teachers about the symptoms and treatment of ADHD.
- Referral to an educational psychologist and behaviour support service so that Kyle's school can help Kyle access his education fully.
- Behaviour management advice to parents.
- Trialling ADHD medication.

Do you think the nurse consultant's recommendations are appropriate? Are they evidence-based? Can you think of any alternatives or additional advice, guidance and support that might be offered?

Behaviour problems/conduct disorder

Group-based, parent-training/education programmes which are structured, informed by social learning theory, include relationship-enhancing strategies, enable parents to identify their own parenting objectives, incorporate role play and homework and are delivered by appropriately trained and skilled facilitations are the most effective interventions for these disorders (NICE, 2006b; Wolpert et al., 2006).

Emotional disorders

Depression

Depression in children is treated in similar ways to how depression is treated in adults (see Chapter 4), although additional caution needs to be observed. Specific NICE guidelines exist for the treatment and management of depression in children and young people as follows: 'watchful waiting' in Tier 1 for a few weeks; if no change and the depression is mild, then offer a course of **non-directive supportive therapy**, **group CBT** or **guided self-help**; if no change or the depression is moderate-severe, refer to Tier 2 or 3 for assessment and a specific psychological therapy such as **CBT of at least 3 months' duration**; if no change, and following multidisciplinary review, then consider the SSRI **fluoxetine** (Prozac) but use **with caution** in the under-12s (NICE, 2005a).

Anxiety disorders

There are no specific treatment guidelines for anxiety in children (that is, no current NICE guidelines), though many of the psychological and behavioural strategies used with adults (see Chapter 5) can be equally useful with children so long as they are made age-appropriate. There is evidence that **behavioural approaches** and **individual or group CBT** work well for generalised anxiety and social anxiety (Wolpert et al., 2006; Silverman et al., 2008), and individual CBT may work for school refusal (Silverman et al., 2008).

Phobias

Careful and sensitive handling by parents or carers is often all that is required for many phobias but, as with most child mental health problems, some children will experience difficulties that seriously interfere with their or their carers' lives and so may require help from a mental health specialist. In these more serious cases, there is some evidence for **exposure therapy** and **CBT approaches** (Wolpert et al., 2006; Silverman et al., 2008).

Obsessive – compulsive disorder

Guidance on treating OCD in children is contained in the general NICE guidelines for OCD (NICE, 2006a) and OCD is discussed in more detail (albeit in adults) in Chapter 5. The NICE guidelines recommend: **guided self-help** in the first instance; if no change, then a course of **age-appropriate group or individual CBT** should be offered; if no change, the addition of a SSRI may be useful but, as with depression, SSRIs should be used with caution.

Post-traumatic stress disorder

The evidence base for interventions for PTSD in children and young people is contained in some general NICE guidelines on PTSD (NICE, 2005b). The full NICE guidelines (NCCMH, 2005b) suggest that psychological interventions – **especially trauma-focused CBT** – are effective for PTSD stemming from sexual abuse but *not* necessarily for PTSD stemming from other causes. The NICE guidelines also suggest that **eye movement desensitisation and reprocessing** (EMDR) – a therapy that uses eye movements to 'reprocess' traumatic memories so that they lose their sensory and emotional intensity – may also have some potential in the treatment of PTSD in children and young people.

Autistic spectrum disorders

Common educational-psychological treatments include parenting programmes, communication training, behavioural analysis and training, and music therapy. Common biomedical treatments include diet and nutritional supplements, as well as medications such as the stimulant methylphenidate, the antipsychotic risperidone and the antidepressant fluoxetine. NICE are writing clinical guidance for England that is scheduled for publication in late 2011. Scottish guidance (SIGN, 2007), however, has identified some evidence for **parenting programmes**, **communication training**, the **Lovass Programme** (an intensive behavioural intervention) and **risperidone** (to control aggression and self-injury). There is also evidence for **early intervention** that incorporates **applied behaviour analysis** with developmental and relationship-based approaches (Dawson et al., 2010).

Mental health promotion

An evidence based intervention that sometimes gets lost when the focus is on child mental health *problems* rather than child mental *health* is that of **health promotion**. Schools, in particular, can have an essential role to play in mental health promotion (HM Government, 2009) and NICE have produced guidance on the role that primary and secondary schools can play in enhancing children's social and emotional well-being through 'whole-school' and universal approaches that also incorporate targeted interventions for children and young people with mild-to-moderate mental health problems, the education and training of both pupils and the workforce, collaborative working between schools, parents, children and other professionals, and the provision of pastoral support (NICE, 2008, 2009b). Nurses can play a role here either directly with the children and young people (as a school nurse or outreach CAMHS nurse, for example) or indirectly (by training other education and childcare workers in child mental health issues, for example).

Conclusion

In this chapter we have looked at the provision of child mental health services, the sorts of children who need access to these services and the kinds of interventions on offer. In doing so, we have explored contemporary policy and research that suggested that there is often a mismatch between CAMHS provision and the needs of the children, young people and families they serve. We have outlined how a comprehensive, multidisciplinary, child-and-family-focused assessment is essential if nurses and other health professionals are to help those families most at need.

We have also seen how the evidence base in CAMHS is relatively weak but moving in the right direction and we have briefly touched on the role that health promotion and early intervention might be able to play in lessening the emotional distress and pain experienced by many children and their families. Above all, we hope that we have demonstrated the significant and varied role that nurses can play in guiding, supporting and helping children and young people with mental health difficulties and their families.

Further Reading and Resources

Key texts

McDougall T (2006). *Child and Adolescent Mental Health Nursing*. London: Blackwell.
A comprehensive British textbook edited by, and with contributions from, a number of nurse consultants working in CAMHS.

Rutter M, Bishop D, Pine D, Scott S, Stevenson J, Taylor E & Thapar A (2008).
Rutter's Child and Adolescent Psychiatry, 5th edition. London: Blackwell.
*The standard text on child **psychiatry** (so obviously has a medical slant), but still very useful to nurses and other CAMHS professionals.*

Ryan N & McDougall T (2008). *Nursing Children and Young People with ADHD.* London: Routledge.
The only British textbook specifically about nursing in ADHD.

Claveirole A & Gaughan M (2011) (eds) *Understanding Children and Young People's Mental Health*. Chichester: John Wiley and Sons.
A comprehensive British text that refreshingly avoids an English-centric bias since it is written by Scottish CAMHS Specialists.

Wolpert M, Fuggle P, Cottrell D, Fonagy P, Phillips J, Pilling S, Stein S & Target M (2006). *Drawing on the Evidence: Advice for Mental Health Professionals Working with Children and Adolescents*, 2nd edition. London: CAMHS Evidence-Based Practice Unit. Available from: www.annafreudcentre.org.
A guide for CAMHS professionals on current evidence-based interventions for a range of mental health problems affecting children and young people.

Key policy documents

CAMHS Review (2008). *Children and Young People in Mind: The Final Report of the National CAMHS Review*. London: Department for Children, Schools and Families/ Department of Health.

Department for Children, Schools and Families (2007). *The Children's Plan: Building Brighter Futures*. London: HMSO.

National Collaborating Centre for Mental Health (2005). *Depression in Children and Young People: Identification and Management in Primary, Community and Secondary Care*. London: British Psychological Society/Royal College of Psychiatrists. Available from: www. nice.org.uk/CG28

National Collaborating Centre for Mental Health (2009). *Attention Deficit Hyperactivity Disorder: The NICE Guideline on Diagnosis and Management of ADHD in Children, Young People and Adults*. London: British Psychological Society/Royal College of Psychiatrists. Available from www.nice.org.uk/CG72

National Institute for Health and Clinical Excellence (2006). *Parent-Training/Education Programmes in the Management of Children with Conduct Disorders. NICE Technology Appraisal Guidance 102*. London: NICE. Available from: www.nice.org.uk/TA102

Web resources

Young Minds: www.youngminds.org.uk
'The UK's leading charity committed to improving the emotional wellbeing and mental health of children and young people and empowering their parents and carers.'

Royal College of Psychiatrists Young People's resources: www.rcpsych.ac.uk/ mentalhealthinfo/youngpeople.aspx
This website provides a series of leaflets suitable for professionals, parents and children in relation to children's mental health and wellbeing.

Parenting programme websites: www.incredibleyears.com and www.triplep.net
The websites of two effective, evidence-based, parenting programmes.

ADDISS: www.addiss.co.uk
> *Website of the National Attention Deficit Disorder Information and Support Service, the UK's leading ADHD charity.*

National Autistic Society: www.nas.org.uk
> *The UK's foremost charity for people with autistic spectrum disorders.*

References

AWCPPRG (All Wales Child Protection Procedures Review Group) (2008). *All Wales Child Protection Procedures.* Available from: www.awcpp.org.uk [accessed 18 January 2010].

APA (American Psychiatric Association) (2000). *Diagnostic and Statistical Manual of Mental Disorders, 4th Edition* (Text Revised) (DSM-IVR). Washington: APA.

Audit Commission (1999). *Children in Mind: Child and Adolescent Mental Health Services.* London: Audit Commission.

Banerjee T, Middleton F & Faraone S (2007). Environmental risk factors for attention deficit hyperactivity disorder. *Acta Paediatrica*, **96**, 1269–1274.

Barlow J, Smailagic N, Ferriter M, Bennett C & Jones H (2010). Group-based parent-training programmes for improving emotional and behavioural adjustment in children from birth to three years old. *Cochrane Database of Systematic Review,* Issue 3, Article Number CD003680.

Basu R & Padmore J (2009). Mental health problems in childhood and adolescence. In I Norman & I Ryrie (eds), *The Art and Science of Mental Health Nursing*, 2nd edition. Maidenhead: Open University Press.

Bunting L (2004). *Assessment of Children in Need in Northern Ireland.* Belfast: National Society for the Prevention of Cruelty to Children.

Butler RJ (2008). Wetting and soiling. In M Rutter, D Bishop, D Scott, J Stevenson, E Taylor & A Thapar (eds), *Rutter's Child and Adolescent Psychiatry*, 5th edition. London: Blackwell.

CAMHS Review (2008). *Children and Young People in Mind: The Final Report of the National CAMHS Review.* London: Department for Children, Schools and Families/Department of Health.

Cooper P (2005). Biology and behaviour: the educational relevance of a biopsychosocial perspective. In P Clough, P Garner, JT Pardeck & F Yuen (eds), *Handbook of Emotional and Behavioural Difficulties.* London: Sage.

Dawson G, Rogers S, Munson J, Smith M, Winter J, Greenson J, Donaldson A & Varley J (2010). Randomized, controlled trial of an intervention for toddlers with autism: the Early Start Denver Model. *Pediatrics*, **25**(1), e17–e23.

DCSF (Department for Children, Schools and Families) (2007). *The Children's Plan: Building Brighter Futures.* London: HMSO.

DES (Department for Education and Skills) (2003). *Every Child Matters.* London: HMSO.

DES/DH (Department for Education and Skills/Department of Health) (2002). *Autistic Spectrum Disorders: Good Practice Guidance. 01 Guidance on Autistic Spectrum Disorders.* Annesley: DES Publications.

DES/DH (Department for Education and Skills/Department of Health) (2004). *The National Service Framework for Children, Young People and Maternity Services*. London: HMSO.

DH (Department of Health)/Home Office (2003). *The Victoria Climbié Inquiry: Report of an Inquiry by Lord Laming* [The Laming Report]. London: HMSO.

DH/DCSF (Department of Health/Department for Children, Schools and Families) (2007). *Introduction to the National Healthy Schools Programme*. London: HMSO.

DHSSPS (Department of Health, Social Security and Public Safety) (2003). *Co-operating to Safeguard Children*. Belfast: DHSSPS.

DHSSPS (Department of Health, Social Security and Public Safety) (2009). *Delivering the Bamford Vision: The Response of the Northern Ireland Executive to the Bamford Review of Mental Health and Learning Disability. Action Plan 2009–2011*. Belfast: DHSSPS. Available from: www.dhsspsni.gov.uk [accessed 2 November 2009].

Eminson M (2001). Somatising in children and adolescents. 1. Clinical presentations and aetiological factors. *Advances in Psychiatric Treatment*, **7**, 266–274.

Feingold BF (1975). *Why Your Child Is Hyperactive*. New York: Random House.

Fonagy P, Target M, Cottrell D, Phillips J & Kurtz Z (2002). *What Works for Whom? A Critical Review of Treatments for Children and Adolescents*. London: Guilford Press.

Goodman R (1997). The Strengths and Difficulties Questionnaire: a research note. *Journal of Child Psychology and Psychiatry*, **38**, 581–586.

Green H, McGinnity A, Meltzer H, Ford T & Goodman R (2005). *Mental Health of Children and Young People in Great Britain, 2004*. Basingstoke: Palgrave Macmillan.

HM Government (2006). *Working Together to Safeguard Children: A Guide to Inter-agency Working to Safeguard and Promote the Welfare of Children*. London: TSO.

HM Government (2009). *New Horizons: A Shared Vision for Mental Health*. London: DH. Available from: www.dh.gov.uk [accessed 14 February 2010].

Johnson M, Östlund S, Fransson G, Kadesjö B & Gillberg C (2009). Omega-3/omega-6 fatty acids for attention deficit hyperactivity disorder: a randomized placebo-controlled trial in children and adolescents. *Journal of Attention Disorders*, **12**(5), 394–401.

Kendal SE (2009). *The Use of Guided Self Help to Promote Emotional Wellbeing in High School Students*. Unpublished PhD thesis. Manchester: University of Manchester.

Kollins SH, Epstein JN & Conners CK (2004). Conners' rating scales – revised. In ME Maruish (ed.), *The Use of Psychological Testing for Treatment Planning and Outcome Assessment: Volume 2, Instruments for Children and Adolescents*. Hillsdale, NJ: Erlbaum.

Matson JL & LoVullo, SV (2009). Encopresis, soiling and constipation in children and adults with developmental disability. *Research in Developmental Disabilities*, **30**(4), 799–807.

McCann D, Barrett A, Cooper A, Crumpler D, Dalen L, Grimshaw K, Kitchin E, Lok K, Porteous L, Prince E, Sonuga-Barke E, Warner JO & Stevenson J (2007). Food additives and hyperactive behaviour in 3-year-old and 8/9-year-old children in the community: a randomised, double-blinded, placebo-controlled trial. *The Lancet*, **370**, 1560–1567.

Meltzer H, Gatward G, Goodman R and Ford T (2000). *Mental Health of Children and Adolescents in Great Britain*. London: TSO.

Mental Health Foundation (1999). *Bright Futures*. London: Mental Health Foundation.

MTA Cooperative Group (1999). A 14-month randomised clinical trial of treatment strategies for attention–deficit hyperactivity disorder. *Archives of General Psychiatry*, **56**, 1073–1086.

Murray L & Cooper PJ (1997). Effects of postnatal depression on infant development. *Archives of Disease in Childhood*, **77**, 97–101.

National Assembly for Wales (2001). *Child and Adolescent Mental Health Services: Everybody's Business* [strategy Document]. Cardiff: National Assembly for Wales.

NCCMH (National Collaborating Centre for Mental Health) (2005a). *Depression in Children and Young People: Identification and Management in Primary, Community and Secondary Care*. London: British Psychological Society/Royal College of Psychiatrists.

NCCMH (National Collaborating Centre for Mental Health) (2005b). *Post-Traumatic Stress Disorder (PTSD): The Management of PTSD in Adults and Children in Primary and Secondary Care*. London: Gaskell/British Psychological Society.

NCCMH (National Collaborating Centre for Mental Health) (2006). *Obsessive Compulsive Disorder: Core Interventions in the Treatment of Obsessive Compulsive Disorder and Body Dysmorphic Disorder*. London: British Psychological Society/Royal College of Psychiatrists.

NCCMH (National Collaborating Centre for Mental Health) (2009). *Attention Deficit Hyperactivity Disorder: The NICE Guideline on Diagnosis and Management of ADHD in Children, Young People and Adults*. London: British Psychological Society/Royal College of Psychiatrists.

NHS HAS (NHS Health Advisory Service) (1995). *Together We Stand: The Commissioning, Role and Management of Child and Adolescent Mental Health Services*. London: HMSO.

NICE (National Institute for Health and Clinical Excellence) (2005a). *Depression in Children and Young People: Identification and Management in Primary, Community and Secondary Care*. London: NICE.

NICE (National Institute for Health and Clinical Excellence) (2005b). *Post-Traumatic Stress Disorder (PTSD): The Management of PTSD in Adults and Children in Primary and Secondary Care*. London: NICE.

NICE (National Institute for Health and Clinical Excellence) (2006a). *Obsessive Compulsive Disorder: Core Interventions in the Treatment of Obsessive Compulsive Disorder and Body Dysmorphic Disorder*. London: NICE.

NICE (National Institute for Health and Clinical Excellence) (2006b). *Parent-Training/ Education Programmes in the Management of Children with Conduct Disorders. NICE Technology Appraisal Guidance 102*. London: NICE.

NICE (National Institute for Health and Clinical Excellence) (2008). *Promoting Children's Social and Emotional Wellbeing in Primary Education. NICE Public Health Guidance 12*. London: NICE.

NICE (National Institute for Health and Clinical Excellence) (2009a). *When to Suspect Child Maltreatment. NICE Clinical Guideline 89*. London: NICE.

NICE (National Institute for Health and Clinical Excellence) (2009b). *Promoting Young People's Social and Emotional Wellbeing in Secondary Education. NICE Public Health Guidance 20*. London: NICE.

PHIS (Public Health Institute of Scotland) (2003). *Needs Assessment Report on Child and Adolescent Mental Health*. Glasgow: PHIS.

Plumb J, Anderson Y & Street C (2007). *Maintaining the Momentum: Towards Excellent Services for Children and Young People's Mental Health.* London: The NHS Confederation.

Richardson A (2004). Clinical trials of fatty acid treatment in ADHD, dyslexia, dyspraxia and the autistic spectrum. *Prostaglandins, Leukotrienes and Essential Fatty Acids*, **70**(4), 383–390.

Richardson A & Montgomery P (2005). The Oxford–Durham study: a randomized controlled trial of dietary supplementation with fatty acids in children with developmental coordination disorder. *Pediatrics*, **115**(5), 1360–1366.

Richardson AJ & Puri BK (2002). A randomized double-blind, placebo-controlled study of the effects of supplementation with highly unsaturated fatty acids on ADHD-related symptoms in children with specific learning difficulties. *Progress in Neuropsychopharmacology and Biological Psychiatry*, **26**(2), 233–239.

Rowe K (1988). Synthetic food colourings and hyperactivity. *Australian Paediatric Journal*, **24**(2), 143–147.

Rowe K & Rowe K (1994). Synthetic food coloring and behaviour: a dose response effect in a double-blind, placebo-controlled, repeated-measures study. *Journal of Pediatrics*, **125**, 691–698.

Rutter M & Taylor E (2002). Clinical assessment and diagnostic formulation. In M Rutter & E Taylor (eds), *Child and Adolescent Psychiatry*, 4th edition. London: Blackwell.

Ryan N & McDougall T (2008). *Nursing Children and Young People with ADHD.* London: Routledge.

Sanders MR (2003). Triple P - Positive Parenting Program: A population approach to promoting competent parenting. *Australian e-Journal for the Advancement of Mental Health*, **2**(3), 9–25. Available from: amh.e-contentmanagement.com [accessed 18 January 2010].

Scottish Executive (2004). *Protection of Children (Scotland) Act 2003: Guidance for Organisations.* Edinburgh: The Scottish Executive.

Scottish Executive (2005). *The Mental Health of Children and Young People: A Framework for Promotion, Prevention and Care.* Edinburgh: The Scottish Executive.

Scottish Government (2008). *A Guide to Getting It Right for Every Child.* Edinburgh: The Scottish Government. Available from: www.scotland.gov.uk [accessed 18 January 2010].

Scottish Government (2009). *Towards a Mentally Flourishing Scotland: Policy and Action Plan 2009–2011.* Edinburgh: The Scottish Government. Available from: www.scotland.gov. uk [accessed 18 January 2010].

SIGN (Scottish Intercollegiate Guidelines Network) (2007). *Assessment, Diagnosis and Clinical Intervention for Children and Young People with Autism Spectrum Disorders: A National Clinical Guideline.* Edinburgh: SIGN.

Silverman WK, Pina AA & Viswesvaran C (2008). Evidence-based psychosocial treatments for phobic and anxiety disorders in children and adolescents: a review and meta-analyses. *Journal of Clinical Child & Adolescent Psychology*, **37**, 105–130.

Spender Q, Salt N, Dawkins J, Kendrick T & Hill P (2001). *Child Mental Health in Primary Care.* Abingdon: Radcliffe Medical Press.

United Nations General Assembly (1989). *United Nations Convention on the Rights of the Child.* New York, NY: United Nations.

Utting D, Monteiro H & Ghate D (2006). *Interventions for Children at Risk of Developing Antisocial Personality Disorder: Report to the Department of Health and Prime Minister's Strategy Unit*. London: Policy Research Bureau.

Voigt RG, Llorente AM, Jensen CL, Fraley JK, Berretta MC & Heird WC (2001). A randomized, double-blind, placebo-controlled trial of docosahexaenoic acid supplementation in children with attention-deficit/hyperactivity disorder. *Journal of Pediatrics*, **139**, 189–196.

Wales Audit Office/Health Inspectorate Wales (2009). *Services for Children and Young People with Emotional and Mental Health Needs*. Cardiff: Auditor General for Wales.

Webster-Stratton C (2005). The Incredible Years: a training series for the prevention and treatment of conduct problems in young children. In PS Jensen & ED Hibbs (eds), *Psychosocial Treatments for Child and Adolescent Disorders: Empirically Based Strategies for Clinical Practice*, 2nd edition. Washington, DC: American Psychological Association.

Wolpert M, Fuggle P, Cottrell D, Fonagy P, Phillips J, Pilling S, Stein S & Target M (2006). *Drawing on the Evidence: Advice for Mental Health Professionals Working with Children and Adolescents*, 2nd edition. London: CAMHS Evidence-Based Practice Unit. Available from: www.annafreudcentre.org [accessed 18 January 2010].

WHO (World Health Organisation) (2004). *Promoting Mental Health: Concepts; Emerging Evidence; Practice*. Geneva: WHO.

WHO (World Health Organisation) (2007). *International Classification of Disease, 10th Revision (2007 Version)*. Geneva: WHO. Available from: www.who.int [accessed 12 February 2010].

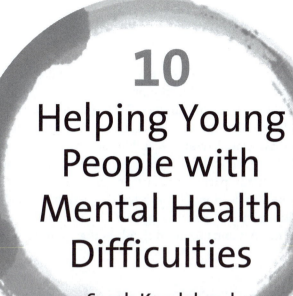

10
Helping Young People with Mental Health Difficulties

Sarah Kendal and Steven Pryjmachuk

What will I learn in this chapter?

This chapter follows on from the last chapter and aims to provide an overview of those mental health difficulties that are more common in older children.

After reading this chapter, you will be able to:

- explain the notion of 'adolescence' and its association with 'transition';
- outline the common mental health difficulties that young people may have;
- recognise the key role that nurses can play in helping young people with mental health problems and identify the skills required to do so;
- identify the interventions that are commonly used with young people with mental health problems and their evidence base.

Introduction

Because young people aged 12–18 are legally children, much of the background and policy discussed in the previous chapter applies as much to this age group as it does to the under-12s. There are, however, some specific issues that affect older children much more than younger children – many of which are associated with the ambiguous state of being neither a child nor an adult – and we will focus on these issues in this chapter. We will look, for example, at the impact of a young person's environment on their mental health and the implications this has for the design and delivery of suitable mental health services for young people, the transition from child to adult services, and those mental health difficulties that seem to affect young people in particular.

The psychological, physiological and social context

Table 10.1 lists some of the factors that might make a young person vulnerable to mental health problems.

TABLE 10.1 Factors in young people's vulnerability to mental health problems (adapted from CAMHS Review, 2008)

Domain	Vulnerability from:
Psychological	Having behavioural, emotional and social difficulties
	Having learning difficulties and disabilities
	Having special educational needs (SEN)
	Having autistic spectrum disorder
	Having communication difficulties
	Being sexually, physically or emotionally abused
	Misusing substances or having parents/carers who misuse substances
	Being bereaved
Physiological	Having Down's syndrome
	Having a life-threatening condition (such as cancer)
	Having a chronic illness (such as diabetes)
	Having a physical disability
	Having a specific genetic condition (such as neurofibromatosis)
	Having a sensory disorder (such as those who are deaf)
Social	Being in care
	Being contact with the youth justice system
	Being lesbian, gay, bisexual or transgender
	Being black or from a minority ethnic group

TABLE 10.1   (Continued)

Domain	Vulnerability from:
	Having housing difficulties
	Seeking asylum
	Not being in education, training or employment
	Being a carer
	Being a 'runaway'

Note that this list does not distinguish between the causes and effects of mental health problems in young people; psychosocial stress, physical illness, depressive illness, substance abuse and poor coping can both affect and be a consequence of a young person's emotional and social wellbeing. Looking at the list should help explain why the mental health of young people matters: as the National Institute for Health and Clinical Excellence (NICE, 2009) points out, good social and emotional wellbeing protects young people against psychological problems, violence and crime, teenage pregnancy and the misuse of drugs and alcohol; it also helps them learn and achieve academically, affecting their long-term social and economic wellbeing (their quality of life) in the process. As such, in order to help young people the most, nurses need to be aware of the complex interplay between the various psychological, physiological and social factors that impact on the mental health of young people.

Adolescence and transition

Part of the reason why we use the term 'young person' in this chapter is that 'adolescence' is a far from simple concept. There are arguments that it is merely a socio-historical creation confined to Western societies. It does not exist in all societies (in some tribal peoples children become adults almost overnight through a rite of passage), and it did not exist in modern-day Britain until the turn of the twentieth century. As Lesko (2001) puts it: 'Adolescence was created ... when child labor laws, industrialization, and union organizing gutted apprenticeships, which had been the conventional way for youth to move from dependency to independence' (p. 7).

From a biological point of view, it is the movement through **puberty** that separates childhood from adulthood. In Western cultures, puberty is often taken as the point at which adolescence starts. But where does it end? You might argue that it ends when the social, legal, economic, political and sexual rights and responsibilities of adults are adopted or obtained – yet these vary across societies and have varied across time. In France and Greece you can legally have sex at 15, but in the UK, not until 16; in most of the USA you can drive at 15, but in the UK not until 17; you can drink when you are 18 in the UK but you have to wait until you are 21 in most of the USA; and it wasn't until 1970 that the age of majority in the UK was reduced from 21 to 18.

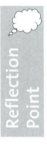

Reflection Point

Adolescence

When you think of terms such as 'adolescent' and 'teenager' what images come into mind? Are they largely positive or negative? What about the media's portrayal of adolescence? How much does that influence society's view of the adolescent? How much do you think it influences your own view of adolescence?

The stereotypical view of adolescence – the moody teenager who takes risks, gets into trouble and is at loggerheads with the adults around them – has also been questioned. Coleman and Hagell (2007) argue that the empirical evidence shows that the majority of young people navigate this stage of life with relatively little trauma. This is not to say that **some** young people do not have major problems (including mental health problems) – they do – but then, so do **some** adults. Why this turbulent and stressful view of adolescence persists could be down to a number of reasons. It could be attributed to those voices in the media that see society degenerating, subsequently blaming young people for such degeneration. Alternatively, it could be due to a bias towards what Ayman-Nolley and Taira (2000) call the 'dark side of adolescence' in the research literature, perhaps because studying topics such as risk taking, emotional turmoil and burgeoning sexuality in young people is more interesting to researchers (especially psychiatrists and psychologists) than topics like emotional stability or good educational attainment. Or it could be because adolescence may be the first time that individuals encounter a significant **transition** in their lives. Indeed, when thinking about healthcare provision for young people, it is perhaps best to focus on this transition period rather than worry about how to define adolescence. Services that focus on the distinctions between childhood and adulthood at the expense of young people's needs often create problems for young people. For example, they may be kept in a children's service longer than is really appropriate, transferred to adult services hastily and abruptly or they may leave healthcare altogether, either voluntarily or by default (RCN, 2004). In addition, many young people with ongoing mental health problems have difficulty adjusting to the environment of mental health facilities designed for adults (Office of the Children's Commissioner, 2007). And those who leave local authority care often need support to find suitable housing, live independently and develop life skills such as managing money, cooking and paying bills. The transition to adult services, therefore, needs to be managed as seamlessly as possible.

The Policy Context

The vast majority of generic childcare policy that we looked at in the previous chapter is as applicable to young people as it is to children. Notwithstanding this, one policy issue affecting young people with mental health problems in particular is the provision of inpatient care.

In the past, young people requiring hospitalisation for a serious mental health problems were often hospitalised in adult mental health wards. The reasons for this were many and varied but it often came down to a lack of appropriate provision for young people. In 2007, the Office of the Children's Commissioner (for England) published a report on the practice – *Pushed into the Shadows* – which found that young people's experiences of adult mental health wards were largely negative. The law subsequently changed in England such that the Mental Health Act 2007 now specifies that children and young people must be treated in **an environment suitable for their age**. For those under 16, this essentially means a Tier 4 CAMHS service (see Chapter 9) but 16–17-year-olds can be treated in adult mental health wards if their needs can be met there. McDougall et al. (2009) summarise the Royal College of Psychiatrists' guidance on this, which is, that to be placed on an adult ward, a 16-or 17-year-old's needs have to be **overriding** (because of risks to their safety or the safety of others, for example) or **atypical** (because, for example, the young person prefers to be treated on an adult ward).

Elsewhere in the UK, guidance (rather than a legal requirement) stating that young people under 18 should not be admitted to adult mental health wards was issued by the Mental Welfare Commission for Scotland in 2006 (MWCS, 2006) but, despite this guidance, the Commission reported a 'deeply concerning' increase in admissions to adult wards in 2009 (MWCS, 2009).

The position is similar in Wales, in that adult mental health (and paediatric) wards were still being inappropriately used for the care of young people with mental health problems in 2009 (Wales Audit Office/Health Inspectorate Wales, 2009). In 2008, the Northern Ireland Assembly announced funding for a new young people's unit in Belfast to tackle similar problems in Northern Ireland (DHSSPS, 2008).

Discussion Point

In a young person's best interests?

Adam, a young man of 16 living in a children's home, was admitted to an adult psychiatric intensive care unit (PICU) after a series of aggressive incidents which the staff at the home couldn't manage. He was presumed to be psychotic. On the PICU he was extremely withdrawn, monosyllabic and appeared angry. He was preoccupied with ideas and rituals about dirt and cleanliness and frequently made derogatory remarks about himself. He was judged to be vulnerable on the PICU because he was a minor and so was accompanied by staff at all times 'for his own protection'.

After staying on the PICU for two months, a bed in a secure young people's unit 200 miles away became available.

Do you think Adam should be transferred to the young people's unit or stay on the PICU? How can you be sure that, whatever action is taken, it is in Adam's best interests?

Typical Mental Health Difficulties in Young People

Young people are affected by many of the same mental health problems that affect adults but there are some problems that are especially significant in young people, notably **anxiety disorders, depression, psychosis, self-harm** and **eating disorders**.

Anxiety disorders and depression were discussed briefly in the previous chapter and in detail in Chapters 4 and 5. It is worth mentioning, however, that depression is often linked to self-harm which is considered in depth in this chapter. We will also look briefly at the controversy over the use of 'SSRI' antidepressants in young people. For psychosis, you will find relevant material in Chapters 6 and 7, but there are one or two issues that relate specifically to young people that we will pick up in this chapter. When relating the material in the chapters focusing on adults (Chapters 4 to 7), it is important to remember that young people are **not** adults and that, as such, some elements of care described in those chapters may be inappropriate for young people.

Psychosis

While schizophrenia and bipolar disorder are relatively rare before the age of 13, it's quite likely that you will meet young people with psychosis during your nursing career, especially since as many as 40% of men and 23% of women with schizophrenia first develop the disorder before the age of 19 (Cullen et al., 2008). Developing schizophrenia during the teenage years is often called **early onset schizophrenia**. There has been some recent debate over the role that illicit drugs – especially certain types of cannabis – might play in the development of schizophrenia in young people (see the next chapter). As such, you may well hear the phrase **drug–induced psychosis** used in practice. Before using the term yourself, you should ask whether it is value-laden or pejorative (a student nurse we once taught asked her fellow students whether they would openly use the phrase 'greed–induced heart attack' in coronary care!).

Given the stigma associated with psychosis, care needs to be taken to ensure that young people are not misdiagnosed with psychosis, especially since the symptoms for first episode schizophrenia and depression are often the same (Häfner & Maurer, 2006). Indeed, common **prodromal** symptoms of psychosis – those symptoms acting as 'early warning signs' of an impending psychotic episode – include 'dysphoric' symptoms such as depressed mood, withdrawal and sleep and appetite problems (Birchwood et al., 2000), symptoms that are remarkably similar to those of depression.

Self-harm

Self-harm affects at least 7% of young people in the UK, females in particular (Hawton et al., 2002). It is a major public health issue, so much so that a national inquiry was established in 2004 by two charities – the Camelot Foundation and the Mental Health Foundation – with the inquiry reporting two years later (see NISHYP, 2006).

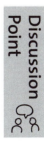

Defining self-harm

Hawton et al. (2002) define **deliberate self-harm** as:

> An act with a non-fatal outcome in which an individual deliberately did one or more of the following: initiated behaviour (for example, self cutting,

(Continued)

(Continued)

jumping from a height) which they intended to cause self-harm; ingested a substance in excess of the prescribed or generally recognised therapeutic dose; ingested a recreational or illicit drug that was an act that the person regarded as self-harm; ingested a non-ingestible substance or object. (p. 1208)

Can you see any limitations in the above definition of self-harm? In particular, think about:

- The use of the word **deliberate** when describing self-harm (is it useful? pejorative? value-laden?)
- Accidental overdoses of drugs taken for 'kicks'
- **Repeated** self-harm against one-off attempts
- Risk taking in young people.

For young people, the most frequent form of self-harm in the UK is **self-cutting**, although burning, scalding and scratching the body and self-poisoning are also relatively common (NISHYP, 2006). Self-poisoning is the most common form of self-harm seen in a hospital setting (Harrington, 2001).

For most young people self-harm is merely a one-off response to some temporary difficulties (Harrington, 2001). However, around 10–20% of young people who self-harm make **repeated** attempts (Kerfoot & McHugh, 1992; Harrington, 2001). Since individuals with a history of repeated self-harm – females especially – are more likely to go on to complete suicide (Zahl & Hawton, 2004; Cooper et al., 2005), these young people are often those for whom mental health professionals have the greatest concerns. In addition, young people who repeatedly self-harm are often more disturbed (e.g. in terms of depression and suicidal ideation) and are more likely to have substance misuse problems than those who make a single, non-fatal attempt (Harrington, 2001; Hawton et al., 2002; Aglan et al., 2008).

Eating disorders

In its communications to the general public, the Royal College of Psychiatrists (2008) describes eating disorders as 'eating styles' that are driven by an intense fear of becoming fat. They affect mainly the 15–25 age group and are far more common in girls than boys. Around eight times more young women than young men will experience eating disorders (NCCMH, 2004a). The two most common eating disorders are **anorexia nervosa** and **bulimia nervosa** (which are often just abbreviated to 'anorexia' and 'bulimia'). Anorexia affects around 8 in 2,000 young women and around 1 in 2,000 young men; bulimia affects around five times as many young people (NCCMH, 2004a). In both conditions there is constant worry about weight but in anorexia, unlike bulimia, weight may drop below a 'safe' weight (that is, below 85% of normal weight or below a body mass index of 17.5 kg/m²; NCCMH, 2004a). In view of this, anorexia should be considered a potentially **life-threatening** disease.

A young person with anorexia will eat less, often having ritualised behaviours attached to food (such as cutting food into small pieces). To most independent observers, the excessive weight loss will be obvious but the young person may try to conceal this with baggy clothes and they will usually deny that they are underweight or have any problems. Physical signs might include: constipation; dizziness; fine, downy hair on the skin (called **lanugo**); dry, rough skin; and a loss of interest in sex. Additionally, in women, **amenorrhoea** (a loss of periods) may be present.

Bulimia is harder to detect because the young person doesn't usually lose weight and so the physiological features associated with extreme weight loss (e.g. lanugo, amenorrhoea and dry, rough skin) are often absent. The principal features in bulimia are an urge to eat vast amounts of food (a **binge**), followed by a **purge** through either vomiting or the use of laxatives. Some subsidiary effects of purging include erosion of tooth enamel (through the stomach acid in vomit) and serious bowel problems from the overuse of laxatives.

No one really knows what causes anorexia and bulimia. Body dysmorphic disorder (BDD) – a disorder in which an individual becomes over-concerned with perceived defects in their body image – may underpin some eating disorders (BDD may also underpin excessive exercise, an obsession with cosmetic surgery and extreme bodybuilding in some young people). **Control** is often an issue in eating disorders in that for some young people eating may be the only thing they have control over since (unintentionally) overbearing parents may have decided on which subjects the young person should study at school, which university they should go to, which friends they should have, which careers they should pursue, and so on.

Case scenario: anorexia and family values

Elisha was 16 when she was admitted to a private psychiatric unit with anorexia. She weighed 5 stone (about 32 kg). She was a model pupil at school, achieving high grades in most of her subjects, and was a promising athlete at her local running club.

The treatment regime on this unit was developed from a behavioural model and Elisha was compliant with all the rules concerning eating, being weighed and having bed rest. She made friends with all the nurses and frequently apologised for being a nuisance.

One aspect of the treatment regime was that Elisha and her key nurse ate together and on one occasion her parents, who were visiting, joined them. The nurse observed that Elisha's mother barely ate her food, pushing it around her plate, and describing herself as 'never a big eater'. Elisha's father agreed and said that his wife and daughter were similar in lots of ways, including wanting to stay slim. Her father also said he hoped Elisha would get better soon as they had 'such high hopes for her'.

When reporting on this interaction later, the nurse reflected that Elisha might have been influenced by her mother in her attitude to food, and might have mixed feelings about gaining weight which would block the success of her treatment. She also reflected on whether control might be an issue in the family.

What do you think of the nurse's reflections? Do you agree or disagree? Are there any other aspects of Elisha's life that you feel the nurse should explore in more detail?

There are also 'sociocultural' models of disordered eating that implicate society in general and the media in particular (Halliwell & Harvey, 2006). The argument goes that unrealistic standards set for beauty by Western society (usually with the collusion of the media) mean that most individuals do not match these standards. Those particularly dissatisfied with the mismatch between this 'image-ideal' and reality may try to achieve these standards through pathological dieting (as is more often the case in women) or pathological exercising and body building (as is more often the case in men). Indeed, pathological exercising and body building in men – so-called **muscle dysmorphia** – has also been called 'bigorexia' and 'reverse anorexia'.

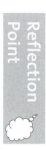

Reflection
Point

Obesity

Obesity seems to be an epidemic sweeping the UK: by 2050, 60% of men and 50% of women could be clinically obese (Foresight, 2007).

The Royal College of Psychiatrists did not include overeating in its definition of eating disorders. Should overeating be considered an eating disorder? Do you think mental health nurses have a role to play in dealing with this so-called epidemic?

Substance misuse

You might recall from Chapter 1 that dependence on alcohol or drugs is not legally a mental disorder. It is important, however, to mention substance misuse when talking about mental health problems in young people for a number of reasons. First, since adolescence is a time of experimentation, substance use – especially alcohol, tobacco and cannabis use – becomes a reality for many young people. Secondly, worrying trends in substance misuse are becoming apparent among young people. Alcohol consumption is a particular worry, with more than 10,000 under-18s being admitted to hospital each year because of their drinking (DCSF, 2009) and a significant number of 11–15-year-olds in both England and Scotland have admitted to drinking on a regular basis (SALSUS, 2006; Fuller, 2009). Thirdly, there appear to be strong connections between substance misuse and mental health problems in some people though the direction of the effect is unclear. While we know that certain substances can exacerbate some mental health problems (see the earlier discussion on cannabis and schizophrenia), many people with mental health problems would argue that they use substances such as alcohol, tobacco and cannabis to alleviate symptoms through 'self-medication'.

While substance misuse is clearly an important issue where young people are concerned, we will not dwell any further on this issue since the issue is better discussed in the next chapter (Chapter 11), which deals with substance misuse.

Engaging and assessing young people with mental health problems

In the previous chapter we saw how we might assess younger children with mental health problems and we touched upon the skills required to carry out

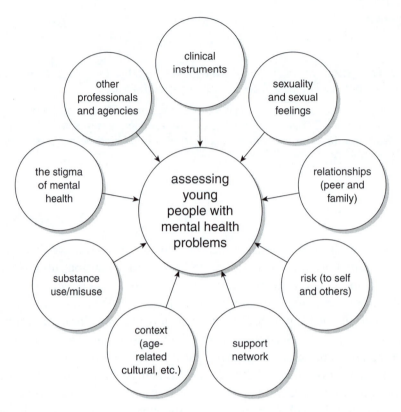

FIGURE 10.1 Things to consider when assessing young people with mental health problems

such an assessment. Figure 10.1 illustrates some of the issues you will need to think about when assessing young people with mental health problems.

Regarding assessment, much of what was described in the previous chapter is as applicable to young people as it is to children but there are, perhaps, a few additional principles that need to be considered. These are summarised in Box 10.1 and discussed in more detail in the ensuing subsections. You might also want to map them onto the skills and capabilities discussed in Chapter 2.

Box 10.1   Some principles for working with young people with mental health problems

- Use your interpersonal skills to build a trusting relationship
- See the young person's point of view and focus on their needs

- Be aware that you might have got it wrong
- Communicate and liaise with colleagues and the family
- Know your roles and responsibilities and recognise your training needs
- Challenge prejudice and stigma

Use your interpersonal skills to build a trusting relationship

The relationship between the nurse and young person is crucial if you are to engage young people and get them to reveal the information you need to help. **Good communication skills** are essential and **respect** is very important. You need to be **courteous**, **listen carefully** and **acknowledge young people's views** about what matters to them. Important **verbal skills** include using language and words appropriate for the individual, taking into account their preferences. It is worth checking how the young person prefers to be addressed; they may, for example, object to an interviewer using a nickname or shortened version of their name, such as Steve instead of Steven. Complicated sentences, nursing jargon and long words can be as patronising as oversimplified, childish sentences. Even worse can be attempts to mimic the language of the young person: using 'street' talk is more likely to sound ridiculous to a young person than put them at ease! Important **non-verbal skills** include using the right body language for the situation – judging how close to sit to the young person, smiling, appearing calm and approachable – and arranging the environment so that it facilitates open conversation. When considering the environment think about whether you can be overheard or seen. Even in a dedicated interview room, the sound might carry to the next room, compromising the privacy of the interview.

You should negotiate with the young person how long an interview will take and what topics are likely to be covered. Importantly, whether a therapeutic encounter lasts five minutes or five months, its **ending** requires forward planning so that it is not unexpected. A young person who is used to rejection or not being taken seriously may interpret the ending of a period of therapy or even the ending of a conversation as a personal rejection. As such, you should explain at the beginning of the encounter how much time you have and indicate during the encounter how much time you have left before you finish.

To be able to help young people, they need to be honest with you, and you with them. This is more likely to be achieved if you are seen as friendly, kind, trustworthy and credible. **Friendliness** implies warmth and respect. Tell the young person a bit about yourself; avoid asking them to tell you things about their problem which they may have already explained to several other professionals; tell them how long you will be able to support them for; tell them when you will be available to them (will you be there when they need you?). **Kindness** can be communicated through being considerate, such as noticing if the young person is distressed or uncomfortable and responding appropriately and tactfully. **Trustworthiness** implies being honest and realistic, especially about maintaining confidentiality (see also the discussion on consent and confidentiality in the previous chapter). Since doubts about confidentiality can prevent young people from talking about their problems (Harbour, 2004) or even accessing healthcare in the first place (Ginsburg et al., 2002), it is important to explain any limits to confidentiality, such as the need to pass on information about risk to others. If you are planning to use an informal style of assessment, it's unfair to proceed without explaining your agenda, so that the young person knows they are being assessed. **Credibility** can be established by demonstrating you have the (nursing) skills and knowledge required for the task. Explain what kind of things you, as a nurse, can offer and do for them. It is helpful to be equipped with knowledge about relevant clinical issues, local services and potential support networks. Poor quality advice and information can be detrimental to the therapeutic relationship and may well discourage a young person from accessing help in the future.

See the young person's point of view and focus on their needs

Unless you understand the young person's perspective, you will not be able to deliver a service that truly reflects their needs. We know, for example, that young people may be less likely to seek healthcare if they think that receptionists and health professionals might embarrass or make judgements about them (Ginsburg et al., 1997).

When assessing a young person's mental state, remember that changes in mental health are often reflected in changed behaviour; difficult and challenging behaviour in a young person may merely be their response to changes in their thoughts or feelings. For example, a young person who is experiencing low mood, anxiety, or troublesome or intrusive thoughts, may become withdrawn or overactive. If withdrawn, they may speak less, interact less, spend time alone, or avoid contact with others. There may be changes in weight (loss or gain), appearance (neglecting their appearance or adopting a new look) and friendship groups. Similarly, low mood or anxiety might lead to over activity and emotional arousal, and agitation may show in overassertive or aggressive behaviour. A young person may attempt to ease uncomfortable mental or emotional states by using drugs or alcohol, risk taking or other distractions to alter their feelings. It is important to remember, however, that mood swings, high adrenalin activities and intense relationships may not be related, either to the use of substances or mental health problems: they could simply be how that person wants to behave at the time. Finally, to understand a young person's mental health, you will need a grasp of the psychological, physiological and social factors affecting them.

Clinical instruments and measures can help you screen for a particular problem and help assess the young person's needs. The use of formal, published and validated instruments is often more helpful than informal, local measures because they tend to be more reliable and accurate and scores can often be compared with wider populations of young people in order to benchmark the young person's problems. Some formal clinical instruments used with young people are listed in Table 10.2

TABLE 10.2   Some clinical instruments used in CAMHS

Name	Abbreviation	Authors
Kiddie Schedule for Affective Disorders	Kiddie-SADS	Kaufman et al. (1997)
Mood and Feelings Questionnaire	MFQ	Costello & Angold (1988)
Child and Adolescent Psychiatric Assessment	CAPA	Angold & Costello (2000)
Strengths and Difficulties Questionnaire	SDQ	Goodman (1997)
Children's Global Assessment Scale	CGAS	Schaffer et al. (1983)

Be aware that you might have got it wrong

Assessing mental health problems in young people is a complicated business. At one end of the spectrum we may be tempted to interpret any challenging behaviour as a sign of disorder, creating a risk of labelling, stigma, shame and inappropriate treatment in the process; at the other end, we may fail to notice when a clinical problem is developing because we assume some challenging behaviour is part of the normal experience of being a young person.

Research into young people's use of healthcare in the UK and elsewhere has demonstrated some of the problems involved in assessment. For example, studies of adolescents and their parents have indicated that each generation may have a different view of what constitutes normality and what constitutes a mental health problem. In addition, some research in primary care has suggested that young people themselves, as well as GPs and parents, may not be able to tell whether a physical problem has a psychological cause, and vice versa (Garralda & Bailey, 1990; Jacobson et al., 2002; Kramer et al., 2004). As such, you should consider each subsequent contact you have with the young person as an opportunity to check that any formulation you have made about the young person remains valid.

Communicate and liaise with colleagues and the family

The quality of care for young people can improve when the skills, knowledge and experience of a multidisciplinary team are brought together to help a young person, provided that, at the same time, the young person and their family/carers are also consulted (though you need to be cognisant of the issue of **consent** in young people, especially in relation to those deemed to be 'Gillick competent' – see the discussion in the previous chapter). Nurses can play a central role here. For example, young people often feel intimidated in a large professional meeting and a skilled nurse can help by supporting the young person to express their views, making sure that their needs are properly understood by all those present and helping to maintain the focus of meetings on agreed priorities, without getting sidetracked by other issues. In complex casework, this can be a considerable challenge.

By talking to other people involved in the care of a young person, you should be able to develop a plan of care that is more appropriate and sensitive to the young person's needs. For example, they might miss appointments because of a problem with housing, money for transport, or physical health, but unless you know something about their general circumstances, you may conclude from their non-attendance that they are reluctant to engage with you. Thus, by communicating effectively with others in the overall care team (which may well include the family, social care and education professionals) you will be in a much stronger position to see how the interplay between their physical, social and psychological lives is impacting on their mental health.

Know your roles and responsibilities and recognise your training needs

The key aspects of a **care pathway** for CAMHS include: recognition of problems; the defining of agency roles and remits; the referral process; assessment diagnosis and treatment; multi-agency work and ongoing care (Appleby et al., 2006). Nurses can be involved in all of these aspects, though assessment, diagnosis and treatment tends to be the remit of the specialist CAMHS nurse. This means that even if you do not see yourself as a CAMHS specialist, you will, as a nurse, still have obligations when it comes to the mental health of young people. Any nurse, for example, should be able to help young people understand the potential impact of any mental health difficulty they have or any treatment they are offered. A young person may worry about how a mental health problem they are experiencing will affect their relationships or school work. Alternatively, a young person who has been prescribed psychotropic medication might be put off taking that medication because they feel ill informed about it or because they are worried about potential side effects. In both of these cases, most nurses will have the skills required to inform and reassure the young person, and help them make positive decisions about the support on offer. If the nurse does not have these skills, then she or he has a professional responsibility to seek guidance on the issue and/or additional training since the NMC Code of Conduct (2008) explicitly states that nurses should keep their skills and knowledge up to date, recognising and working within the limits of their competence.

Challenge prejudice and stigma

Prejudice, stigma and ignorance about mental health issues can make it much harder for individuals to recover from an episode of mental illness. Young people encounter social and personal prejudices in society simply because of their age and appearance. For example, a report on the use of anti-social behaviour orders (ASBOs) revealed that between 1999 and 2001, nearly three-quarters of the ASBOs granted were against people under the age of 21 (Campbell, 2002). The use of dispersal orders to prevent people assembling outside in groups can criminalise what is essentially a normal social activity for young people (Squires, 2006).

Social prejudice can also act as a barrier to help-seeking in mental health. Many people with mental health problems avoid asking for help because prejudiced attitudes from family, friends, colleagues and health professionals have taught them it is better to hide their problems (Mental Health Foundation, 2000). For young people, who may also lack experience, independence and sophisticated social and communication skills, the effect can be even greater.

Evidence-Based Interventions for Young People with Mental Health Problems

Anxiety and depression

As you will recall from the previous chapter, there are no specific NICE guidelines for anxiety in children and young people although, as young people head towards 18, the guidelines for the management of adults with anxiety may be appropriate (NICE, 2007; see also Chapter 5).

TABLE 10.3 Guidelines for depression in young people

Stage	Action	Tier
Detection	Risk profiling/screening	Tier 1
Recognition	Identification in those who present to services	Tiers 2–4
Mild depression	'Watchful waiting'	Tier 1
	Non-directive supportive therapy/group cognitive behavioural therapy/guided self-help	Tiers 1 or 2
Moderate to severe depression	Tiers 1 or 2 brief psychological therapy and/or fluoxetine	Tiers 2 or 3
Depression unresponsive to treatment/recurrent or psychotic depression	Intensive psychological therapy and/or, augmentation with fluoxetine, sertraline, citalopram or an antipsychotic	Tiers 3 or 4

Adapted From the National Institute for Health and Clinical Excellence Clinical Guidance 28 (depression in children and young people; NICE, 2005).

For depression in children and young people, you will recall from the previous chapter that specific NICE guidance exists. Since depression is more common in teenagers than the under-12s, it's useful to revisit that guidance (see Table 10.3).

Medication

As you can see from Table 10.3, the use of an SSRI antidepressant such as fluoxetine, sertraline or citalopram may be helpful in depression that doesn't abate naturally or respond to self-help measures or a brief psychological intervention. Treating children and young people with antidepressants is controversial, however. In a systematic review of both published and unpublished literature, Whittington et al. (2004) found that with the sole exception of fluoxetine there were more risks than benefits when using SSRIs with children and young people. In addition, Goodyer et al. (2007) found no benefit for CBT combined with an SSRI over the use of an SSRI alone. These conflicting results beg the question 'should young people be given antidepressants?' – a question that was, in fact, debated in the *British Medical Journal* in 2007 (see Box 10.2).

Box 10.2   Should young people be given antidepressants?

Yes (Cotgrove, 2007)	No (Timimi, 2007)
Meta-analysis evidence (NCCMH, 2005) shows that SSRIs have a significant benefit over a placebo	Tricyclic antidepressants are not effective with young people and there is no evidence that SSRIs are any better

Yes (Cotgrove, 2007)	No (Timimi, 2007)
A systematic review (Whittington et al., 2004) shows that the benefits of SSRIs (fluoxetine at least) outweigh the risks in young people	The study showing that fluoxetine had benefits (March et al., 2004) was misrepresented and flawed
Alternative treatments such as CBT, interpersonal therapy and family therapy have small effects when compared to SSRIs and, when combined with an SSRI, are no better than an SSRI alone (see Goodyer et al., 2007)	Most childhood distress is self-limiting and does not require extensive intervention
	The abstracts of many antidepressant studies do not state that the primary outcomes were not statistically significant
While there are methodological errors, publication bias and omissions of evidence with SSRI trials, they are, nevertheless, effective and have a role when treating young people	Marketing spin has taken precedence over scientific accuracy
	Antidepressants may have resulted in a small but tragic number of avoidable suicides, and contributed to a trend of inappropriately medicalising common emotional states and experiences

Given the arguments in Box 10.2 and your own personal views, do you think young people should be given antidepressants?

Discussion Point

Cognitive behaviour therapy

Cognitive behaviour therapy (CBT) features heavily in the NICE guidance for both anxiety and depression, as well as some of the other conditions we will look at in a moment. The philosophical underpinnings of CBT were discussed in detail in Chapter 1 but it is important that a few comments are made about CBT with children and young people since one of its pillars – the **cognitive** domain – has a specific age-related characteristic. Thinking shifts from the concrete to the abstract in most children at around 10–12 years; consequently, those over this age are more likely to have sophisticated reasoning powers, social awareness and a more complex sense of morality (Herbert, 2005). CBT with children and young people, as such, needs to be delivered in a flexible way that accommodates the different abilities between older and younger children. Age, gender, social and cultural context, emotional maturity and cognitive level of the young person all need to be taken into account when considering CBT. Moreover, although CBT is often an individual therapy, it can be helpful to involve the family, particularly parents (Verduyn, 2000). And given that many young people are technologically savvy, computerised CBT may be a particularly useful approach for young people. Specific computerised CBT packages with evidence of effectiveness include *Beating the Blues* for mild-to-moderate depression and *FearFighter* for panic and phobia (NICE, 2006). *Stressbusters* (Abeles et al., 2009) is a derivative of *Beating the Blues* that has been designed specifically for young people with depression.

Psychosis

Since psychosis rarely affects those under 15, most of the evidence base for interventions used in psychosis discussed elsewhere in this book (in Chapter 7 especially) is relevant here. There are a few specific comments we need to make relating to psychosis in young people, however. First, inpatient care, as we have seen, requires special considerations. Secondly, family interventions (again, see Chapter 7) may be especially useful to young people with psychosis and to their families. Thirdly, **early intervention** services – services designed to **prevent** the onset of psychosis in those with **prodromal** symptoms and treat those who develop psychosis early on in order to lessen the severity of the psychosis – are commonly offered to this age group, although a systematic review (Marshall & Rathbone, 2006) concluded that there was insufficient evidence to draw any definitive conclusions about the effectiveness of early intervention services.

Self-harm

Remember that in some circumstances (self-poisoning, in particular), self-harm can be an **emergency** situation. Where self-harm is an ongoing problem, a variety of therapies to help young people who self-harm are in common use. The evidence for each of these therapies is summarised in Table 10.4.

As you can see from Table 10.4, there are few therapies that have any robust evidence in relation to self-harm; indeed, the NICE guidance issued in 2004 recommends only DGP for young people under 16 (NICE, 2004b). The NICE guidance also supports 'safe' cutting in those over 16. Safe cutting – or **harm minimisation** – is a strategy advocated primarily by self-harm 'survivors' (see Pembroke, 2006) that allows those who self-harm to cut while at the same time minimising the inherent risks, for example, by providing

TABLE 10.4   The evidence for self-harm interventions (after Pryjmachuk & Trainor, 2010)

Individual therapies

Cognitive-behaviour therapy (CBT)	Has some value in adolescent depression, although Goodyer et al. (2007) found no benefit of combining CBT with an SSRI over the use of an SSRI alone
Dialectical behaviour therapy (DBT; see Linehan & Dimeff, 2001)	A manual-based therapy combining CBT principles with aspects of Eastern meditative practice. There is some emerging evidence (James et al., 2008) that DBT might be useful with young people who self-harm
Nurse-led sociological approaches	Advocated in by Anderson et al. (2004). No formal evidence to support this approach
A 'green card' that allows automatic admission to hospital	Advocated by Cotgrove et al. (1995). Some hints that it may work with those who repeatedly self-harm but the results lacked statistical significance
A formal, written 'no suicide' contract (NSC)	A review by McMyler & Pryjmachuk (2008) found that the only study to demonstrate an explicit link between an NSC and a reduction in self-harm was a relatively weak study undertaken with children and young people

Family therapies

Brief, home-based family intervention (Kerfoot et al., 1995)	A focused and intensive social work approach. A large RCT (Harrington et al., 1998), showed no substantial benefit over routine care
Systemic family therapy	A manual-based form of systematic family therapy is the focus of a major, multi-centre RCT that began in 2009 (the 'SHIFT' trial; see Cottrell et al., 2009)

Psychopharmacological therapies

SSRIs	See the debate in Box 10.2
Depot flupenthixol	Hawton et al (1998) found some promising results for depot flupenthixol in adults; there is no evidence to support its use in young people

Group therapy

Developmental Group Psychotherapy (DGP)	An eclectic approach influenced by CBT, DBT and psychodynamic group psychotherapy. An exploratory trial (Wood et al., 2001) found those who had DGP were less likely to repeat, had better school attendance and a lower rate of behavioural disorder

access to sterile blades and dressings. Safe cutting can be controversial and is rarely used and, indeed, best avoided in young people since it will take an extremely skilled practitioner to be able to explain to anxious parents why their teenage daughter is being allowed to cut herself with the apparent support of those who are supposed to be helping her.

The full NICE guidance report (NCCMH, 2004a) further adds that it is crucial that good relationships between paediatric services (especially paediatric A&E), CAMHS and social care and child protection agencies are established and that those working with young people who self-harm should be appropriately trained and experienced.

Case scenario: self-harm

Kate, a bright A level student, was referred to a specialist self-harm service by her GP after she revealed that she was regularly cutting her arms and legs with a razor blade when she was in the shower. She received six sessions of interpersonal psychotherapy from a nurse therapist, aimed at trying to understand her cutting behaviour and reducing it.

Kate felt guilty about cutting because, as she explained, she had never had a bad enough experience to justify self-harming. She wondered if something had happened to her in the past which she was denying. She told the therapist that she believed she would be able to stop self-harming when she had found the reason for her behaviour. Much of the interaction in the first two sessions between the nurse therapist and Kate circulated around this theme.

The therapist felt stuck, and brought Kate's story to clinical supervision. The supervisor wondered if Kate was using the issue of seeking the underlying cause of her cutting as a diversion from the work of addressing how she was feeling. As such, the therapist started to manage the sessions with Kate so that the focus was on the 'here and now'. Kate consequently began to think about her self-harm in terms of low mood and moderate anxiety. Once she did this, the therapist used a cognitive behavioural approach to help her.

How would you have assessed Kate in the first place? What about relationships, environment (both home and at school), history, current behaviour and Kate's feelings and those of her parents?

Do you think the therapies described in the scenario are appropriate? What's the evidence base for each? What would you have used?

Eating disorders

The NICE guidelines on eating disorders (NICE, 2004b) suggest that most people with anorexia can be managed through **psychological therapies** in primary care so long as the service is **competent at assessing any physical risk**. For those requiring **inpatient care** for anorexia (where the disorder is life-threatening), an environment where skilled **refeeding** and **intensive physical monitoring** can be combined with **psychosocial interventions** is required. With children or young people, **family interventions** that include siblings and that focus on the sharing of information, behaviour management advice and the facilitation of communication, should also be available. In most cases, a specialised Tier 4 service, whether provided by the NHS, or the private or third sector, will be the most appropriate environment.

For people with bulimia, the NICE guidelines recommend using an evidence-based **self-help** intervention or an **antidepressant** as a first step. If these first line interventions don't work, then a **specifically adapted form of CBT** – cognitive behaviour therapy for bulimia nervosa (CBT-BN) – should be used. As with anorexia, family interventions should be available to children and young people with bulimia.

Tier 1 interventions

Young people often find formal CAMHS provision stigmatising and the rigidity of many formal CAMHS services may mean young people having to travel long distances or come out of school to access support. While the professionals operating in Tier 1 are mainly non-mental health specialists, they can have – as is evident from Table 10.5 – an important role to play in enhancing and protecting the emotional and psychological wellbeing of young people, identifying mental health problems in young people and in dealing with some of the 'milder' mental health problems.

TABLE 10.5 Some examples of Tier 1 provision for young people

Where?	Who?	What?
Telephone and Internet	Third sector; NHS	A range of services including the provision of information and advice, helplines and self-help support. Examples: – The Campaign Against Living Miserably (C.A.L.M.) runs a helpline and website as part of a strategy to reduce suicide and depression in young men aged 15–35 – ChildLine, a national service run by the NSPCC, has a number of ways of being contacted: phone, email, online chat and message board posting – NHS Direct helpline and website – Health Freak website

(Continued)

TABLE 10.5 (Continued)

Where?	Who?	What?
Home	Commercial companies, NHS	Computerised CBT for anxiety and depression and self-help booklets for a range of problems and issues. Examples: – Stressbusters – Tracy Alderman's *The Scarred Soul*, a self-help book for self-harm
Schools	School staff, e.g. school nurses and counsellors	Health promotion and education; detection and screening of mental health problems; interventions for mild mental health problems, Examples: – The national Social and Emotional Aspects of Learning (SEAL) initiative – Drop-in clinics – Guided self-help for anxiety and depression (with school professional as facilitator)
Youth centres and youth centred services	Local authorities Third sector Youth workers	Projects and activities that offer a sense of achievement and boost self-confidence, self-esteem, and social and practical skills in young people. Examples: – 42nd street (a mental health charity based in Manchester supporting young people aged 13–25 under stress) – The Dreadnought Centre (Cornwall-based charity supporting children and young people who are facing emotional or behavioural problems) – Youth-Link (Dundee-based, not-for-profit organisation that tackles social isolation in children and young people)

Another advantage of using Tier 1 services and professionals is that these services and professionals are usually part of the normal, everyday experience of young people and are, as such, easily accessible. Since there is evidence that school-based health services are more likely to be used by young people than hospital or clinic-based services (Anglin et al., 1996; Pastore et al., 2001) there is certainly a case for involving schools in the mental health care of young people. Indeed, schools form the backbone of the national strategy for promoting social and emotional wellbeing in young people (NICE, 2009).

Conclusion

Helping young people with mental health problems is more likely to be effective when we think holistically. This means understanding the psychological, physiological and social factors relevant to their mental health and it means looking at promoting mental health in young people as well as looking at evidence-based ways of dealing with any mental health problems that arise.

As we have explained, to work with young people you will need excellent communication and interpersonal skills not only so you can develop therapeutic relationships with the young people in your care, but also so that you can deal with the young person's family and anyone else involved in their care and so that you can deal with the complications, like issues to do with confidentiality and trust, that are often thrown up when we are helping and safeguarding young people.

Above all, we must remember that the central focus of our care is the young person, and not any problem they may have. Their perspective on their own story is always the most important perspective to hear because our therapeutic endeavours are most useful when we work jointly with them to understand what care plans and pathways will be the most helpful.

Further Reading and Resources

See also the further reading and resources listed in Chapter 9.

Key texts

McDougall T, Armstrong M and Trainor G (2010). *Helping Children and Young People Who Self-Harm: An Introduction to Self-Harming and Suicidal Behaviours for Health Professionals*. Abingdon: Routledge.
Written by three Nurse Consultants, this book offers expert guidance and advice on working with children and young people who self-harm.

Spandler H & Warner S (eds) (2007). *Beyond Fear and Control: Working with Children and Young People who Self-Harm*. Ross-on-Wye: PCCS Books.
An interesting and thought-provoking collection of perspectives on self-harm in young people.

Treasure J, Schmidt & van Furth U (eds) (2005). *Handbook of Eating Disorders*. Chichester: Wiley.
A thorough British textbook on eating disorders that covers a variety of interventions, including CBT, family interventions and drug treatments.

RCN (2009). *Mental Health in Children and Young People: An RCN Toolkit for Nurses Who Are Not Mental Health Specialists*. London: RCN. Available from: www.rcn.org.uk.
Is exactly what it says it is! Primarily for non-mental health nurses but useful all the same.

Key policy documents

The Children's Commissioner for England (2007). *Pushed into the Shadows: Young People's Experiences of Adult Mental Health Facilities*. London: Office of the Children's Commissioner.

National Institute for Clinical Excellence (2004). *Eating Disorders: Core Interventions in the Treatment and Management of Anorexia Nervosa, Bulimia Nervosa and Related Eating Disorders*. London: NICE. Available from www.nice.org.uk/CG9

National Institute for Clinical Excellence (2005). *Depression in Children and Young People: Identification and Management in Primary, Community and Secondary Care*. London: NICE. Available from www.nice.org.uk/CG28

National Institute for Health and Clinical Excellence (2009). *Promoting Young People's Social and Emotional Wellbeing in Secondary Education. NICE Public Health Guidance 20*. London: NICE. Available from www.nice.org.uk/PH20

National Inquiry into Self-Harm among Young People (2006). *Truth Hurts: Report of the National Inquiry into Self-Harm among Young People*. London: The Mental Health Foundation.

Web resources

The Site: www.thesite.org
A website run by YouthNet UK, a registered charity, that aims to be the first place all young adults turn to when they need support and guidance through life. Has good sections on self-harm, depression and eating disorders.

Campaign Against Living Miserably (C.A.L.M.): www.thecalmzone.net
A website and national campaign catering specifically for men aged 15–35, those most at risk of suicide.

Participation Works: www.participationworks.org.uk
Six national children and young people's agencies have got together to help organisations such as the NHS and local authorities effectively involve children and young people in the development, delivery and evaluation of services that affect their lives.

NHS Lothian interactive websites: www.depressioninteenagers.co.uk and www.stressandanxietyinteenagers.com
Interactive self-help sites from Scotland, aimed at young people and based on the principles of cognitive behaviour therapy.

References

Abeles P, Verduyn C, Robinson A, Smith P, Yule W & Proudfoot J (2009). Computerized CBT for adolescent depression ('Stressbusters') and its initial evaluation through an extended case series. *Behavioural and Cognitive Psychotherapy*, **37**, 151–165.

Aglan A, Kerfoot M & Pickles A (2008). Pathways from adolescent deliberate self-poisoning to early adult outcomes: a six-year follow-up. *Journal of Child Psychology and Psychiatry*, **49**(5), 508–515.

Anderson M, Woodward L & Armstrong M (2004). Self-harm in young people: a perspective for mental health nursing care. *International Nursing Review*, **51**, 222–228.

Anglin T, Naylor K & Kaplan D (1996). Comprehensive school-based health care: high school students' use of medical mental health and substance abuse services. *American Academy of Pediatrics*, **97**(3), 318–330.

Angold A & Costello EJ (2000). The Child and Adolescent Psychiatric Assessment (CAPA). *Journal of the American Academy of Child and Adolescent Psychiatry*, **39**(1), 39–48.

Appleby L, Shribman S & Eisenstadt N (2006). *Promoting the Mental Health and Psychological Well-being of Children and Young People. Report on the Implementation of Standard 9 of the National Service Framework for Children, Young People and Maternity Services*. London: DES/DH.

Ayman-Nolley S & Taira LL (2000). Obsession with the dark side of adolescence: a decade of psychological studies. *Journal of Youth Studies*, **3**(1), 35–48.

Birchwood M, Spencer E & McGovern D (2000). Schizophrenia: early warning signs. *Advances in Psychiatric Treatment*, **6**, 93–101.

CAMHS Review (2008). *Children and Young People in Mind: The Final Report of the National CAMHS Review*. London: Department for Children, Schools and Families/Department of Health.

Campbell S (2002). *A Review of Anti-social Behaviour Orders: Home Office Research Study No. 236*. London: The Home Office.

Coleman J and Hagell A (2007). The nature and risk of resilience in adolescence. In J Colem and A Hagell (eds). *Adolescence, Risk and Resilience: Against the Odds*. Chichester: Wiley.

Cooper J, Kapur N, Webb R, Lawlor M, Guthrie E, Mackway-Jones K & Appleby L (2005). Suicide after deliberate self-harm: a 4-year cohort study. *American Journal of Psychiatry*, **162**, 297–303.

Costello EJ & Angold A (1988). Scales to assess child and adolescent depression: checklists, screens, and nets. *Journal of the American Academy of Child and Adolescent Psychiatry*, **27**, 726–737.

Cotgrove A (2007). Should young people be given antidepressants? Yes. *British Medical Journal*, **335**, 750.

Cotgrove AJ, Zirinsky L, Black D & Weston D (1995). Secondary prevention of attempted suicide in adolescence. *Journal of Adolescence*, **18**(5), 569–577.

Cottrell D, Boston P, Eisler I, Fortune S, Green J, House A, et al. (2009). *SHIFT Trial. Self-Harm Intervention, Family Therapy: A randomised controlled trial of family therapy vs. treatment as usual for young people seen after second or subsequent episodes of self-harm*. Southampton: NHS National Institute for Health Research Health Technology Assessment Programme. Available from: www.hta.ac.uk/1733 [accessed 11 March 2010].

Cullen KR, Kumra S, Regan J, Westerman M & Schulz SC (2008). Atypical antipsychotics for treatment of schizophrenia spectrum disorders. *Psychiatric Times*, **23**(3). Available from: www.psychiatrictimes.com [accessed 21 January 2010].

DCSF (Department for Children, Schools and Families) (2009). *Consultation on Children, Young People and Alcohol.* London: DCFS.

DHSSPS (Department of Health, Social Security and Public Safety) (2008). Extra funding for health will save lives – McGimpsey [Press Release]. Belfast: DHSSPS. Available from: www.northernireland.gov.uk [accessed 18 January 2010].

Foresight (2007). *Tackling Obesities: Future Choices – Project Report.* London: Department for Innovation, Universities and Skills.

Fuller E (ed.) (2009). *Smoking, Drinking and Drug Use among Young People in England in 2008.* London: NHS Information Centre for Health and Social Care. Available from: www.ic.nhs.uk [accessed 15 May 2010].

Garralda ME & Bailey D (1990). Paediatrician identification of psychological factors associated with general paediatric consultations. *Journal of Psychosomatic Research,* **34**(3), 303–312.

Ginsburg KR, Forke CM, Cnaan A & Slap GB (2002). Important health provider characteristics: the perspective of urban ninth graders. *Journal of Developmental and Behavioral Pediatrics,* **23**(4), 237–223.

Ginsburg KR, Menapace AS & Slap GB (1997). Factors affecting the decision to seek health care: the voice of adolescents. *Pediatrics,* **100**(6), 922–930.

Goodman R (1997). The Strengths and Difficulties Questionnaire: a research note. *Journal of Child Psychology and Psychiatry,* **38**, 581–586.

Goodyer I, Dubicka B, Wilkinson P, Kelvin R, Roberts C, Byford S, Breen S, Ford C, Barrett B, Leech A, Rothwell J, White L & Harrington R (2007). Selective serotonin reuptake inhibitors (SSRIs) and routine specialist care with and without cognitive behaviour therapy in adolescents with major depression: randomised controlled trial. *British Medical Journal,* **335**, 142.

Häfner H & Maurer K (2006). Early detection of schizophrenia: current evidence and future perspectives. *World Psychiatry,* **5**(3), 130–138.

Halliwell E & Harvey M (2006). Examination of a sociocultural model of disordered eating among male and female adolescents. *British Journal of Health Psychology,* **11**(2), 235–248.

Harbour A (2004). Understanding children and young people's rights to confidentiality. *Child and Adolescent Mental Health,* **9**(4), 187–190.

Harrington R (2001). Depression, suicide and deliberate self-harm in adolescence. *British Medical Bulletin,* **57**, 47–60.

Harrington R, Kerfoot N, Dyer E, McNiven F, Gill J, Harrington, V, Woodham A & Byford S (1998). Randomized trial of a home-based family intervention for children who have deliberately poisoned themselves. *Journal of the American Academy of Child and Adolescent Psychiatry,* **37**(5), 512–518.

Hawton K, Arensman E, Townsend E, Bremner S, Feldman E, Goldney R, Gunnell D, Hazell P, van Heeringen K, House A, Owens D, Sakinofsky I & Träskman Bendz L (1998). Deliberate self-harm: systematic review of efficacy of psychosocial and pharmacological treatments in preventing repetition. *British Medical Journal,* **317**, 441–447.

Hawton K, Rodham K, Evans E & Weatherall R (2002). Deliberate self-harm in adolescents: self report survey in schools in England. *British Medical Journal*, **325**, 1207–1211.

Herbert M (2005). *Developmental Problems of Childhood and Adolescence: Prevention, Treatment & Training*. Oxford: BPS Blackwell.

Jacobson L, Churchill R, Donovan C, Garralda E, Fay J & RCGP Adolescent Working Party (2002). Tackling teenage turmoil: primary care recognition and management of mental ill health during adolescence. *Family Practice*, **19**(4), 401–409.

James AC, Taylor A, Winmill L & Alfoadari K (2008). A preliminary community study of dialectical behaviour therapy (DBT) with adolescent females demonstrating persistent, deliberate self-harm (DSH). *Child and Adolescent Mental Health*, **13**(3), 148–152.

Kaufman J, Birmaher B, Brent D, Rao U, Flynn C, Moreci P, Williamson D & Ryan N (1997). Schedule for affective disorders and schizophrenia for school-age children, present and lifetime version (K-SADS-PL): initial reliability and validity data. *Journal of the American Academy of Child and Adolescent Psychiatry*, **36**, 980–988.

Kerfoot M & McHugh B (1992). The outcome of childhood suicidal behaviour. *Acta Paedopsychiatrica*, **55**(3), 141–145.

Kerfoot M, Harrington R & Dyer E (1995). Brief home-based intervention with young suicide attempters and their families. *Journal of Adolescence*, **18**(5), 557–568.

Kramer TL, Phillips SD, Hargis MB, Miller TL, Burns BJ & Robbins JM (2004). Disagreement between parent and adolescent reports of functional impairment. *Journal of Child Psychology and Psychiatry*, **45**(2), 248–259.

Lesko N (2001). *Act Your Age! A Cultural Construction of Adolescence*. London: Routledge.

Linehan MM and Dimeff L (2001). Dialectical behavior therapy in a nutshell. *The California Psychologist*, **34**, 10–13.

March J, Silva S, Petrycki S, Curry J, Wells K, Fairbank J, Burns B, Domino M, McNulty S, Vitiello B & Severe J (2004). Fluoxetine, cognitive-behavioural therapy, and their combination for adolescents with depression. Treatment for adolescents with depression study (TADS) randomized controlled trial. *Journal of the American Medical Association*, **292**, 807–820.

Marshall M & Rathbone J (2006). Early intervention for psychosis. *Cochrane Database of Systematic Reviews*, Issue 4, Article CD004718.

McDougall T, O'Herlily A, Pugh K & Parker C (2009). Young people on adult mental health wards. *Mental Health Practice*, **12**(8), 16–21.

McMyler C & Pryjmachuk S (2008). Do 'no-suicide' contracts work? *Journal of Psychiatric and Mental Health Nursing*, **15**, 512–522.

Mental Health Foundation (2000). *Pull Yourself Together! A Survey of the Stigma and Discrimination Faced by People Who Experience Mental Distress*. London: The Mental Health Foundation.

MWCS (Mental Welfare Commission for Scotland) (2006). *Mental Welfare Commission Guidance on the Admission of Young People to Adult Mental Health Wards*. Edinburgh: MWCS. Available from: www.mwcscot.org.uk [accessed 21 January 2010].

MWCS (Mental Welfare Commission for Scotland) (2009). *Annual Report* 2008–9. Edinburgh: MWCS. Available from: www.mwcscot.org.uk [accessed 21 January 2010].

NCCMH (National Collaborating Centre for Mental Health) (2004a). *Eating Disorders: Core Interventions in the Treatment and Management of Anorexia Nervosa, Bulimia Nervosa and Related Eating Disorders*. London: Gaskell/British Psychological Society.

NCCMH (National Collaborating Centre for Mental Health) (2004b). *Self-Harm: The Short-Term Physical and Psychological Management and Secondary Prevention of Self-Harm in Primary and Secondary Care*. London: British Psychological Society/Royal College of Psychiatrists.

NCCMH (National Collaborating Centre for Mental Health) (2005). *Depression in Children and Young People: Identification and Management in Primary, Community and Secondary Care*. London: British Psychological Society/Royal College of Psychiatrists.

NICE (National Institute for Clinical Excellence) (2004a). *Self-Harm: The Short-Term Physical and Psychological Management and Secondary Prevention of Self-Harm in Primary and Secondary Care*. London: NICE.

NICE (National Institute for Clinical Excellence) (2004b). *Eating Disorders: Core Interventions in the Treatment and Management of Anorexia Nervosa, Bulimia Nervosa and Related Eating Disorders*. London: NICE.

NICE (National Institute for Health and Clinical Excellence) (2005). *Depression in Children and Young People: Identification and Management in Primary, Community and Secondary Care*. London: NICE. Available from www.nice.org.uk/CG28 [accessed 18 January 2010].

NICE (National Institute for Health and Clinical Excellence) (2006). *Computerised Cognitive Behaviour Therapy for Depression and Anxiety [Review of Technology Appraisal 51]*. London: NICE.

NICE (National Institute for Health and Clinical Excellence) (2007*). Anxiety (amended): Management of Anxiety (Panic Disorder, with or without Agoraphobia, and Generalised Anxiety Disorder) in Adults in Primary, Secondary and Community Care*. London: NICE.

NICE (National Institute for Health and Clinical Excellence) (2009). *Promoting Young People's Social and Emotional Wellbeing in Secondary Education. NICE Public Health Guidance 20*. London: NICE.

NISHYP (National Inquiry into Self-Harm among Young People) (2006). *Truth Hurts: Report of the National Inquiry into Self-Harm among Young People*. London: The Mental Health Foundation.

NMC (Nursing and Midwifery Council) (2008). *Code of Professional Conduct*. London: NMC.

Office of the Children's Commissioner for England (2007). *Pushed into the Shadows: Young People's Experience of Adult Mental Health Facilities*. London: OCCE.

Pastore DR Murray PJ & Juszczak L (2001). School-based health center: position paper of the society for adolescent medicine. *Journal of Adolescent Health*, **29**(6), 448–450.

Pembroke, L (2006). Limiting self-harm. *Emergency Nurse*, **14**(5), 8–10.

Pryjmachuk S & Trainor G (2010). Helping young people who self-harm: perspectives from England. *Journal of Child and Adolescent Psychiatric Nursing*, **23**(2), 52–60.

RCN (Royal College of Nursing) (2004). *Adolescent Transition Care: Guidance for Nursing Staff*. London: RCN.

Royal College of Psychiatrists (2008). *Eating Disorders* [Patient Information Leaflet]. London: Royal College of Psychiatrists. Available from: www.rcpsych.ac.uk [accessed 18 November 2009].

SALSUS (Scottish Schools Adolescent Lifestyle and Substance Use Survey) (2006). *National Report: Smoking, Drinking and Drug Use Among 13 and 15 Year Olds in Scotland in 2006.* Edinburgh: ISD Scotland. Available from: www.drugmisuse.isdscotland.org [accessed 15 May 2010].

Schaffer D, Gould MS, Brasic J, Ambrosini P, Fisher P, Bird H & Aluwahlia S (1983). A children's global assessment scale (CGAS). *Archives of General Psychiatry,* **40**(11), 1228–1231.

Squires P (2006). New Labour and the politics of antisocial behaviour. *Critical Social Policy,* **26**(1), 144–168.

Timimi S (2007). Should young people be given antidepressants? No. *British Medical Journal,* **335**, 750.

Verduyn C (2000). Cognitive behaviour therapy in childhood depression. *Child Psychology and Psychiatry Review,* **5**, 176–180.

Wales Audit Office/Health Inspectorate Wales (2009). *Services for Children and Young People with Emotional and Mental Health Needs.* Cardiff: Auditor General for Wales.

Whittington CJ, Kendall T, Fonagy P, Cottrell D, Cotgrove A & Boddington E (2004). Selective serotonin reuptake inhibitors in childhood depression: systematic review of published versus unpublished data. *Lancet,* **363**, 1341–1345.

Wood A, Trainor G, Rothwell J, Moore A & Harrington R (2001). Randomized trial of group therapy for repeated deliberate self-harm in adolescents. *Journal of the American Academy of Child and Adolescent Psychiatry,* **40**(11), 1246–1253.

Zahl D L & Hawton K (2004). Repetition of deliberate self-harm and subsequent suicide risk: long-term follow-up study of 11583 patients. *British Journal of Psychiatry,* **185**, 70–75.

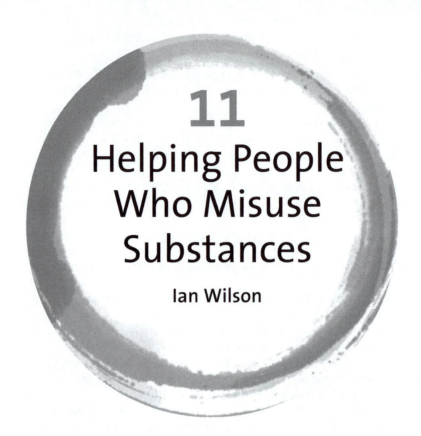

11
Helping People Who Misuse Substances

Ian Wilson

What will I learn in this chapter?

This chapter focuses on the misuse of specific substances, namely alcohol and the so-called 'illicit' drugs. The aim of this chapter is to examine the reasons why people misuse these substances, the prevalence of various types of substance misuse, and the ways in which people who misuse these substances might be helped. In the course of the discussion, the concept of 'dual diagnosis' will also be explored.

After reading this chapter, you will be able to:

- explain the terminology used in substance misuse policy and practice, including the concept of 'dual diagnosis';
- identify the substances that have the potential for misuse and the ways in which they can be categorised;
- describe the most effective ways of assessing those who misuse substances;
- appreciate the evidence-based treatments that are in use in substance misuse practice.

Introduction

Across history, religions and cultures, mind-altering chemical substances have always been used by human beings to change their levels of consciousness. Depending on the time and place, these mind-altering substances have sometimes been legal and sometimes illegal; sometimes socially acceptable and sometimes not. In recent years, however, the undeniable physical, psychological and social harm that can result from the excessive use of some substances (including alcohol and tobacco) means that problematic substance misuse has become a major public health priority in many countries around the world.

As mental health nurses, we need to be knowledgeable and up to date about the substances that our service users choose to take so that we can help them effectively. We also need to know why, despite draconian laws aimed at controlling illicit drugs, changes to the licensing laws for alcohol and a plethora of health promotion initiatives ranging from the frightening to the informative, substance misuse continues to be widespread. Furthermore, we need to be able to have **informed**, **empathic** and **non-judgemental** conversations with our service users about their levels of substance use/misuse. As we have seen in previous chapters, such an approach encourages trust and honesty and may well pave the way for service users to consider the benefits and drawbacks of their current substance use – considerations which may, in turn, lead to healthy conversations about future behaviour change.

Definitions

Definitions of the most commonly used terms in the substance misuse field are summarised in Box 11.1.

Box 11.1   Definitions of terms commonly used in substance misuse

Substance: Any kind of physical matter; a solid, liquid or gas of some sort, normally having a definitive chemical makeup.

(Continued)

(Continued)

Drug: 'Any substance or chemical that alters the structure or functioning of a living being' (WHO, 1981). Drugs can be therapeutic, non-therapeutic or both; have an effect on bodily systems and on behaviour; and include a wide range of prescribed drugs and illegal and socially accepted substances (Rassool, 2009).

Drug (substance) use: The non-problematic use of drugs, usually prescribed medication. Non-problematic does not necessarily equate to harmless since drug use, whether prescribed or not, always carries the potential for adverse effects. Drug use is, however, a socially acceptable concept whereas 'drug misuse' and 'drug abuse' tend to have negative connotations.

Drug (substance) abuse/misuse: Drug abuse and drug misuse are difficult to define and differentiate. The operational use of these concepts is dependent on the culture, practice and ideology of any particular country or society, and is also dependent on the effect of the substance on the individual (Rassool, 1998).

'Drug misuse' can be defined as the use of a drug in a way that harms the individual and/or is socially unacceptable. 'Substance misuse' is the generic term invariably used to denote misuse of alcohol and illicit drugs. 'Drug abuse' is a more value-laden term, usually signifying use associated with dependence and addiction.

(Drug) addiction: 'A compulsion and need to continue taking a drug as a result of taking it in the past' (OED, 1989). Addiction is a more value-laden term than 'dependence'.

(Drug) dependence: A compulsion to take a drug to experience its psychological or physical effects; or to avoid the consequences of not taking the drug (usually known as **withdrawal**). DSM–IV (APA, 2000) sets out seven criteria to judge whether someone is dependent on a substance, three of which need to be present in a 12-month period. These are: (1) tolerance; (2) withdrawal; (3) increased amounts being taken; (4) a desire or unsuccessful attempts to cut down; (5) increased time spent in substance misusing activity; (6) a reduction in social, recreational or occupational activity due to substance use; and (7) the substance use is continued despite knowledge that its continued use is causing harm.

Patterns of drug use in the UK and worldwide

Substance use is a major issue for society throughout the world (Costa e Silva, 2002). About 5% of the world's population (200 million people) between the ages of 15 and 64 use illicit drugs each year (UNODC, 2009), though clearly not all of them are 'problematic' users. The figures for drug use in England and Wales are among the highest in Europe: according to the British Crime Survey 2008/9 (Hoare, 2009), more than a third (36.8%) of 16–59-year-olds have used one or more illicit drugs in their lifetime, around one in ten (10.1%) in the last year. Moreover, as we saw in Chapter 8, alcohol misuse is becoming a particular issue among older people (Dyson, 2006).

Cannabis is the most widely used illicit drug in Europe (EMCDDA, 2009). In the UK, cannabis is also the most commonly used street drug, with approximately 3.5 million users, followed by cocaine, ecstasy and amphetamine. Approximately half of all 15–29-year-olds are said to have tried cannabis at some time. According to the European School Survey Project on Alcohol and Other Drugs (Hibell et al., 2009; data for 2007) the use of illicit drugs amongst 15–16-year-old schoolchildren appears to have stabilised or fallen slightly in the last few years. 'Heavy episodic drinking' of alcohol, however, seems to have increased in this age group, together with a narrowing of the gender gap. Alcohol apart, there appears to be a stabilisation or slight downward trend in the extent of harm from illicit substances. The Drug Harm Index (DHI), which reports on drug-related crime, community perceptions of drug problems, drug nuisance and the health consequences of drug misuse (Home Office, 2009), has shown a year-on-year decline since 2001. The fall in the DHI between 2005 and 2006 is largely due to reductions in drug-related crime and a decrease in drug deaths. The decline in the DHI does not necessarily reflect a decline in substance misuse, however, nor should it make us complacent about the potential impact of substance misuse on the physical, psychological or social wellbeing of the service users we work with.

Why do people take drugs?

People choose to use substances for many different reasons. People may take substances through curiosity and because they are bored. One of the most obvious reasons is that they are enjoyable. Lots of people experience enhanced levels of personal pleasure when under the influence of drugs and alcohol and many social activities revolve around the use of one substance or another. In the UK, for instance, many social occasions and celebrations involve, to a greater or lesser extent, the use of alcohol and the 'dance' or 'club' scene has often been associated with the use of stimulants like ecstasy and cocaine.

Many people use substances because they are a relatively predictable way of changing how they think and feel, particularly if they believe that their use may help them deal with ongoing emotional difficulties. Using substances in this way might be especially attractive to those already experiencing problems in their lives or with their mental health. These people may find that when they take drugs their problems temporarily diminish. For some people, however, the use of drugs may become an established habit and stopping their use can lead to physical or psychological withdrawal.

People also use substances because they are freely available. In most parts of the UK, the price of various illicit drugs, along with alcohol, has been falling steadily, making drugs and alcohol ever-more accessible.

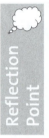

Your own experiences of substance use

Do you drink, smoke or take any illicit or recreational drugs? If not, what are your attitudes towards people who do? If you do, what are the reasons for doing so?

If you take, or have taken, illicit or recreational drugs on a regular basis, do you think that is an asset or a drawback when working with people who may want help in controlling their own substance use?

Classification of substances

There are two main ways of classifying substances: by (a) the **effect** that they have on the physical and psychological condition of the person using them and by (b) their **legal status** (see Table 11.1).

Like most classification systems, these approaches are not without their limitations. Cannabis is problematic for a classification by effect since it has both depressant and hallucinogenic effects. Substances like anabolic steroids (often used illegally by bodybuilders) and solvents (glues) which can produce harmful outcomes in those who misuse them are also difficult to fit into such a classification. Classifying by legal status creates a different set of problems since the 'dangerousness' of a substance – and its subsequent classification – is often determined by societal and political demands rather than by its true potential to cause harm (as you will see explicitly when we come to discuss cannabis in more detail). Sometimes there is a game of cat-and-mouse with the law whereby new substances – 'legal highs' – appear only for these substances

TABLE 11.1   The two principal ways of classifying substances

By effect	By legal status
Stimulants such as cocaine, crack, amphetamine, ecstasy (and to a lesser extent caffeine and nicotine). These substances stimulate the central nervous system and increase brain activity, making users feel more alert and energised	**Class A** includes cocaine, crack, ecstasy, heroin, LSD, magic mushrooms, methylamphetamine. Penalties under the Misuse of Drugs Act 1971 are seven years in prison and/or a fine for possession; life in prison and/or a fine for production or dealing
Depressants such as heroin, alcohol, gamma-hydroxybutyrate (GHB) and (maybe) cannabis. These substances depress the central nervous system and decrease brain activity, reduce pain and often make users feel drowsy and calm	**Class B** includes amphetamine (Class A if prepared for injection), cannabis. Five years in prison and/or a fine for possession; 14 years and/or a fine for production or dealing
Hallucinogens such as ketamine, magic mushrooms, LSD and (maybe) cannabis. These substances affect perception and distort what is seen or heard by the user.	**Class C** includes anabolic steroids, ketamine, GHB, benzodiazepines. Two years in prison and/or a fine for possession; 14 years in and/or fine for production or dealing
	Legal: alcohol, caffeine and tobacco (nicotine)
	'Quasi-legal': solvents.

to be classified illegal once they become popular and/or a tragic case hits the news. Cases in point are the 'dance' drugs GBL (gamma-butyrolactone) and mephedrone. GBL was legal up until the end of 2009 when it became a Class C drug; likewise, mephedrone was legal up until April 2010 when became a Class B drug.

'Legal' drugs

Cigarette smoking (**nicotine**) and the consumption of tea and coffee (**caffeine**) are both forms of substance use, yet these two substances rarely appear in any discussions of substance misuse. Can you think of any reasons why?

Both cigarette smoking and alcohol can have major health implications but only alcohol tends to fall within the remit of the substance misuse field. Again, can you think of any reasons why? Why is alcohol dependence ('alcoholism') generally seen as less socially acceptable than nicotine dependence?

Discussion Point

Policy Context

Overall UK government policy on drugs is contained in a 10-year strategy entitled *Drugs: Protecting Families and Communities* (HM Government, 2008). The strategy, to run from 2008 to 2018, contains four strands of work namely: (1) the **protection of communities** (through tackling drug supply, drug-related crime and anti-social behaviour); (2) the **prevention of harm to children, young people and families affected by drug misuse** (through early intervention and support); (3) the provision of **new approaches to drug treatment and social re-integration** (approaches that involve a whole government approach whereby housing, the benefits system, employment, health and social care work together); and (4) the continued use of **public information campaigns** (building on work such as the national drug information campaign, 'FRANK').

While the strategy contained in *Drugs: Protecting Families and Communities* is a UK-wide strategy, some parts of it are applicable only to England. Scotland, Wales and Northern Ireland are managing their own strategies within this overall framework. The Scottish approach links explicitly to the **recovery model** (see Chapters 1 and 2) and is enshrined in the publication *Road to Recovery* (Scottish Government, 2008). Welsh policy is similarly enshrined in *Working Together to Reduce Harm* (Welsh Assembly Government, 2008). Northern Ireland had established a five-year strategy two years earlier (see DHSSPS, 2006). Though older than the UK national strategy, the focus of Northern Ireland's strategy – notably its five 'pillars' of (1) prevention and early intervention, (2) treatment and support, (3) law and criminal justice, (4) harm reduction and (5) evaluation and research – has clear overlaps with the overarching UK-wide strategy.

For a variety of reasons, government policy on substance misuse is often controversial. Commercial pressures from the manufacturers of legal substances such as the tobacco and alcohol industries and the tax receipts from sales of such substances means that governments are often less than objective about such issues. Imagine making whisky illegal in Scotland, for example! Moreover, governments often pander to media demands to crack down on deviant behaviour among its youth on political grounds rather than on the grounds of the actual risks of harm.

Is cannabis dangerous?

In 2004, the then Home Secretary, David Blunkett, reclassified cannabis from a Class B drug to Class C. However, following concern – especially among the media and some mental health workers – that powerful 'skunk' cannabis was making some young people psychotic, it was reclassified as a Class B drug in early 2009.

The government's Chief Drugs Adviser, Professor David Nutt, publicly opposed this move, stating that the government had ignored the evidence of its own advisory committee (of which he was Chair). Nutt argued that 'to prevent one episode of schizophrenia, we would need to stop about 5,000 men aged 20 to 25 years from ever using the drug', concluding that 'overall, cannabis use does not lead to major health problems' (Nutt, 2009, p. 4). The Home Secretary, Alan Johnson, responded by sacking Professor Nutt from his role as Chair of the Advisory Council on the Misuse of Drugs.

Do you think Alan Johnson was right in the actions he took? When thinking about your answers ask yourself whether you are being objective. For example, are you a cannabis user and, if so, has this affected your views? Do you know someone close to you who has been 'disabled' by cannabis (mis)use? If so, again, has this affected your views? How would you classify cannabis? Would you make it legal?

According to statistics provided by Nutt (2009), alcohol is much more harmful than cannabis. So why is cannabis illegal and alcohol not?

Alcohol Misuse

Alcohol (or, to be more accurate, **ethyl alcohol** or **ethanol**), is a psychoactive substance that depresses the central nervous system through absorption in the mouth, oesophagus and stomach. Alcohol use involves two distinct phases (it is, as such, **biphasic**): initially, small amounts of alcohol leave you feeling relaxed, euphoric and stimulated, with a lowering of inhibitions; at higher and continued levels of consumption, however, there is a marked impairment of cognition, perception and behaviour, with poor physical coordination, slurred speech, poor judgement, insomnia and blackouts.

Alcohol's general social acceptance often masks its potential for harm. According to the World Health Organisation, there are 76.3 million people around the world with diagnosable disorders related to alcohol use

(WHO, 2004). And while alcohol is the UK's most popular substance, UK rates of alcohol misuse appear to be growing at an alarming rate, especially among young people – young women in particular. A recent Parliamentary Committee report on English drinking habits (House of Commons Health Committee, 2010) noted that three times as much alcohol was being consumed per person compared with 1947, that 31% of men and 21% of women were drinking hazardously or harmfully and that the UK rates of liver disease had increased five-fold since the 1970s while, ironically, there had been steep **declines** in the wine drinking countries of Southern Europe.

In the UK, to gauge the risks of harmful drinking and encourage 'responsible' drinking, alcohol is measured in standardised **units**. A unit of alcohol is defined as **8 g** or **10 ml** of **pure alcohol**. Units can also be calculated using the formula in Box 11.2, which also shows the government's recommended safe drinking limits for men and women.

Box 11.2   Calculating a unit of alcohol and safe drinking limits

One unit = Volume (ml) × % Alcohol by Volume (ABV) divided by 1000

330 ml bottle of 5% ABV lager = (330 × 5)/1000 = 1.7 units
Large glass (250 ml) of wine (12% ABV) = (250 × 12)/1000 = 3 units
Double shot (50 ml) of vodka (40% ABV) = (50 × 40)/1000 = 2 units

Safe daily drinking limit for men: 3–4 units
Safe daily drinking limit for women: 2–3 units

Regarding 'safe' drinking, the government also recommended that people should try to have at least two alcohol-free days a week. **Binge drinking** is of particular concern to many societies and governments around the world. In the UK, a 'binge' is defined as the consumption of at least **double the daily recommended units in one day** (ONS, 2007). While most people are aware of the existence of the safe drinking guidelines, the British Medical Association remark that few can accurately recall them or appreciate the relationship between units, glass sizes and drink strengths (BMA, 2008). Moreover, it is clear that a significant proportion of individuals in the UK misuse alcohol by drinking above recommended UK guidelines: the Alcohol

TABLE 11.2 Levels of alcohol misuse (after Babor et al., 2001).

Level	Description
Hazardous	People drinking above safe levels with no current alcohol-related problems but levels of consumption that put them at a specific risk of developing such problems
Harmful	People drinking above safe drinking levels and already experiencing associated problems
Dependent	People drinking above safe drinking levels and experiencing harm and symptoms of alcohol dependence

Needs Assessment Research Project (DH, 2005), for example, found that 7.1 million people in England are drinking harmfully and 1.1 million are dependent on alcohol (see also Table 11.2).

Major problems associated with alcohol misuse

Alcohol is associated with a wide range of problems, including: **severe physical health problems** (see Box 11.3); **social exclusion** and **homelessness**; **high-risk behaviours** (e.g. unprotected sex); **violence** of all kinds (including incontrovertible links to domestic violence, suicidality and self-harm); the **abuse and neglect of children**; and many kinds of **offending behaviour**. Moreover, **death** can sometimes occur from alcohol intoxication. Very high rates of NHS hospital admissions are associated with alcohol use, especially in accident and emergency environments, where 70% of attendances between midnight and 5.00 am at weekends are alcohol-related (DH, 2004).

Box 11.3   Major physical problems associated with alcohol misuse

| Liver disease | Since alcohol is metabolised by the liver, chronic misuse can lead to liver disease. There are three stages of liver disease: (1) **fatty liver** (reversible); (2) **steatohepatitis** (inflamed fatty liver; reversible); and (3) **cirrhosis** (irreversible damage). The health of the liver can be determined via blood-based **liver function tests (LFTs)**, **biopsy** and **ultrasound scan** |

(Continued)

(Continued)

Mental health problems	There are strong links between alcohol misuse and mental health problems (Weaver et al., 2003):
	85.5% of users of alcohol services experience mental health problems the prevalence of alcohol dependence among people with mental disorders is almost twice as high as in the general population people with severe and enduring mental illnesses (e.g. schizophrenia) are at least three times as likely to be alcohol dependent as the general population
Acute emergencies in alcohol misuse	As a central nervous system depressant, alcohol misuse can create a number of emergency situations, including: **acute intoxication** (with a risk of **coma** in severe states); **withdrawal emergencies** (e.g. seizures); **pancreatitis**; **haemetemesis** (vomiting of blood usually due to **oesophageal varices**, which are dilated blood vessels in the lower oesophagus); **cardiovascular problems**; and **hypoglycaemia** (low blood glucose)
Delirium tremens ('the DTs')	Delirium tremens usually occurs 24–96 hours after abrupt alcohol withdrawal and typically lasts 3–5 days. Symptoms include: **hallucinations** (especially visual and tactile hallucinations); **tremor**; and fluctuating **clouding of consciousness** or **confusion**. Delirium tremens has around 5% mortality, which is often due to collapse, hypothermia or hypoglycaemia
Wernicke's encephalopathy and Korsakoff syndrome	Wernicke's encephalopathy is a significantly disabling and potentially lethal condition, characterized by **confusion**, **ophthalmoplegia** (paralysis in the eye muscles) and **ataxia** (lack of coordination); however, it is rare to see all three of these symptoms in any one person
	Korsakoff syndrome is a later neuropsychiatric manifestation of Wernicke's encephalopathy with **memory loss** and associated **confabulation** (the making up of information to cover for memory loss)
	Both conditions are caused by a lack of **thiamine** (vitamin B$_1$), which may be a result of the poor nutritional state seen in many people who misuse alcohol and/or the detrimental effects that alcohol can have on the absorption of thiamine. Wernicke's encephalopathy can be prevented or reversed if the thiamine deficiency is treated early enough.

Assessing for, Detecting and Intervening in Alcohol Misuse

Talking to people about their alcohol use can be tricky. People may perceive that it's not your business to ask questions about alcohol, especially if they are seeing you about something else. They may have a genuine and realistic fear of being judged ('you think I'm an alcoholic') or a fear of records and notes being shared with, for example, their employer or 'social services'. Nurses often have equally strong perceptions of this task. They may fear offending the service user or disturbing any rapport that has been established. They may perceive the service user to have an alcohol intake that is less than or equal to their own which may lead to concerns about their own levels of drinking or to them being blasé about the user's levels of drinking.

One way of overcoming these fears is to use the core capabilities and inter-personal skills outlined in Chapter 2 (and some of the earlier Part II chapters) to **openly** and **honestly** talk about alcohol during routine assessments, regardless of the person's presenting problems.

Interventions for those at risk of harmful drinking

Using these interpersonal skills is the first step in the delivery of **identifica-tion and brief advice** (IBA), an intervention designed for people who are at increasing risk of harm. Alcohol use is **identified** using a screening tool such as the Alcohol Use Detection and Identification Toolkit (Babor et al., 2001) – more commonly known as **AUDIT** – or one of its derivatives. AUDIT is a 10-item questionnaire that takes about two minutes to complete. It is a highly specific and sensitive tool (it correctly identifies levels of drink-ing in around 94% of people) that can be used in a wide variety of clinical settings. If AUDIT identifies harmful or hazardous drinking, then **brief advice** about behaviour change is offered. IBA seems to be an effective inter-vention: for every eight people receiving IBA, one will change their drinking behaviour to a less risky form (by comparison, IBA for smoking cessation has a change ratio of 1:20). Moreover, people receiving IBA are twice as likely to moderate their drinking compared to those who pass through services 'unscreened' and without an appropriate and timely conversation about alcohol (Raistrick et al., 2005).

Interventions for dependent drinkers

If assessment of alcohol use indicates a level of use that suggests dependent drinking, **detoxification** (often abbreviated to **detox**) is normally the main option. In an ideal world, detox should be carefully planned because sudden cessation can cause what is known as a **rebound stimulatory effect**, increasing excitability in the nervous system which, in turn, can lead to potentially fatal seizures.

In the UK, it is common to offer planned detox at home if the person wishes it and if the home environment is judged to be suitable by those involved. Home detox is invariably undertaken by a **community alcohol team**, who will carry out all initial and ongoing assessments and who will subsequently supply medical treatments and carry out all the necessary physical health checks. Regarding medical treatments, the NICE guidelines on alcohol use disorders (NICE, 2010a) currently recommend a quick-acting benzodiazepine such as lorezapam to help protect against seizures, and thiamine supplements to protect against Wernicke's encephalopathy. Since thiamine is often poorly absorbed during the initial, acute phase of detox, thiamine is normally given parenterally (intravenously or intramuscularly) and frequently (3–5 times a day) during this phase. Oral thiamine and B-vitamin complex is given thereafter. Since thiamine is used by the body to metabolize glucose, **intravenous solutions containing glucose should not be given before thiamine therapy has been started** as it can precipitate Wernicke's encephalopathy in those previously unaffected or worsen early forms of the disease. Detox sometimes takes place in specialist residential units, where medical, social and psychological treatments will be given by trained staff. Indeed, the NICE guidelines advocate residential (hospital) treatment for the **vulnerable**, including those who are frail, under 16 or who lack social support. Regardless of where detox takes place, it is vital that a package of follow-up support is negotiated with the service user.

While you should always advise **against sudden cessation** of drinking (for the reasons given above), sudden cessation is sometimes enforced, for instance by committal to a secure facility like prison. Local community alcohol teams can normally offer telephone advice and support in these circumstances. In any case, prophylactic thiamine/B-vitamin complex should always be considered, as should a medical assessment for a benzodiazepine.

The kindling effect and increased risk of seizures

Seizures – such as those seen in epilepsy – normally arise because of over-excitability in the electrical circuitry of the brain. However, in some circumstances electrical or chemical stimuli that are not normally strong enough to induce a seizure can induce a seizure if such stimuli are repeated and intermittent – a phenomenon known as **kindling**. A kindling effect has been seen in those who undergo repeated alcohol withdrawal (Becker, 1998), in that an initial mild withdrawal is often followed by future withdrawals (following a return to drinking) with a greater risk of brain damage or seizure. The explanation behind this is that, initially, abrupt withdrawal from alcohol (which upsets the chemical balance of the brain) causes excitability (the 'rebound stimulatory effect' mentioned above) which is not normally strong enough to induce seizures but the brain becomes sensitized and, in future withdrawals, this excitability increases sufficiently to induce seizure. Becker (1998) argues that because of the kindling effect and because a large number of dependent drinkers return to drinking following withdrawal, each withdrawal episode should not be viewed as an isolated event but **as part of a long-term process**. In any case, it is clear that information about **previous withdrawal attempts needs to be an integral part of the assessment** of dependent drinkers.

 ## Case scenario: alcohol withdrawal

Margaret is a 62-year-old former intensive care nurse who lives alone. She has referred herself to the community alcohol team (CAT) following a relatively minor car accident (no one was seriously injured), but one that left her with a driving ban, a fine and – most shamefully for Margaret – a report in the local newspaper.

As a member of the CAT, you visit her at home to find her tearful and smelling strongly of alcohol. She tells you that her drinking has steadily increased over the past few years, which she puts down to the stress of working in intensive care. She started off having a glass or two of wine at night 'to relax' but admits that this has increased over the years to one or two bottles of wine a day. She has tried to cut down but she says it's still her main way of coping with stress. She tells you that she was 'pensioned off' from her nursing job in a round of early retirements a year ago and at first she liked not having to work and thought that the reasonable pension she had would sustain her. However, she has been spending a considerable amount of money on alcohol and has subsequently run up a substantial debt on her credit cards, a situation which only adds to her stresses.

Margaret says she is determined to stop drinking once and for all and says that – with your support – she is going to stop today.

(Continued)

(Continued)

As part of the assessment process and in order to ensure Margaret remains safe, what are the important things you will need to find out about Margaret and her drinking? (The ABCE assessment strategy for depression and anxiety outlined in Chapters 4 and 5 might have some relevance here. Can you think of any reasons why it might be relevant?)

What plan of action should you and Margaret agree to?

Public health interventions

The interventions for potential and actual alcohol misuse that we have looked at so far have been targeted at the individual. Alcohol misuse is a problem affecting society as a whole – as the media constantly remind us when referring to 'binge Britain' – so it is hardly surprising to find that much of the recent debate has focused on tackling the problem from a wider societal perspective, that is, from a *population* rather than individual perspective. At the time of writing, for example, an Alcohol Bill with major public health aspects is making its way through the Scottish Parliament, and public health guidance for England and Wales is hot off the press from NICE (NICE, 2010b; see Box 11.4 for a summary of the recommendations).

Box 11.4   Public health guidance on alcohol-use disorders

NICE recommend that government and society:

- intervene in relation to the **price** of alcohol
- limit the **availability** of alcohol, whether it be bought for consumption off the premises (shops and supermarkets) or on the premises (pubs, clubs and bars)
- limit the **marketing** of alcohol
- increase resources for **screening** and **brief interventions**
- focus particularly on **children and young people** – for children and young people aged 10–15 years childcare professionals should use their professional judgement to routinely assess for alcohol use/misuse; for young people aged 16 and 17.

> Professionals should routinely screen for alcohol misuse (using a validated tool such as AUDIT), offering extended brief interventions whenever hazardous or harmful drinking is identified
>
> Adapted from the National Institute for Health and Clinical Excellence Public Health Guidance 24 (alcohol use disorders; Nice, 2010b)

The Scottish Alcohol Bill and NICE guidance both recommend setting minimum prices for alcohol and banning 'irresponsible' alcohol marketing, though of course they will have to deal with the inevitable hostility from the powerful drinks industry lobby. The NICE guidance is particularly noteworthy given the brief discussion on substance misuse in the previous chapter on young people since it gives a considerable focus to the detection and prevention of alcohol misuse in children and young people.

Illicit drug use

This section outlines the most frequently used and potentially most harmful substances that people in the UK choose to take and which you can expect to see at some time during clinical practice. 'Illicit' is defined as something 'not sanctioned by law, rule, or custom' (OED, 1989). To this extent, illicit drug use includes not only those substances that are illegal but also – as you will see – those substances that are deemed to be socially unacceptable or used for purposes other than for which they were intended.

Cannabis

Cannabis is the most frequently used illicit substance worldwide. In the UK, over 3.5 million people use it and half of 16–29-year-olds have tried it. Despite its illegality, many people view cannabis as harmless, even beneficial.

Cannabis is derived from the plant *Cannabis sativa*, a member of the nettle family. The plant has been used for a variety of purposes for thousands of years, including the manufacture of hemp for rope, textiles and other products as well as being a medicinal herb and a recreational drug. The drug has many names, some in common usage and some that are specific to a particular place or group of users. The most common are **grass**, **ganja**, **pot**,

dope, **draw**, **smoke**, **weed**, **blow**, **hash**, **puff**. Some names refer to the type of cannabis – **skunkweed** (so called because of its strong smell), **sensi**, **black**, **zero zero**, **red leb**. Some are joke titles or plays on words – **Mary Jane** (marijuana), **wacky baccy**, **Bobby Moore** (draw), **Bob Hope** (dope). Some are esoteric and obscure and quickly fall in and out of fashion.

Cannabis is supplied in herbal form – as dried leaves, flower heads and buds – or as a dark green, brown or black resin (**hashish**). In the UK and throughout Europe it is usually smoked in cigarettes (often known as **joints** or **spliffs**) or in pipes and 'bongs'. It can also be eaten, sometimes in cakes and biscuits (**hash brownies** or **space cakes**). When smoked, it is easier to control the amount absorbed and the effects are more immediate and short-lived. If eaten, cannabis can be unpredictable: it can take a long to time to reach full effect, can be more hallucinogenic and can last for several hours before gradually wearing off. The strength of cannabis can vary widely. Generally, though not always, resin (hashish) is less strong than herbal cannabis, while some forms of herbal cannabis – those usually referred to as skunkweed – are stronger than others.

There are as many as 60 active compounds and 400 different chemicals in cannabis. The main psychoactive compounds in cannabis, however, are the **tetrahydrocannabinols (THCs)** delta-9-THC and delta-8-THC, **cannabidiol (CBD)** and **cannabinol**. The THCs are the main psychoactive compound in cannabis, mimicking the action of **anandamide**, the brain's own natural cannabinoid. Delta-8-THC has a lower psychotropic potency than delta-9-THC. CBD is a significant component of cannabis but is psychoactively different from the THCs and is thought to have analgesic (pain relieving) and possibly even antipsychotic properties. Cannabinol is only mildly psychoactive. THCs are absorbed into the bloodstream via the lungs (if smoked) or the stomach (if eaten) and carried to the brain to produce the familiar 'high'. The mechanism by which cannabis affects the brain is complicated but it is known to affect areas of the brain that are involved in **pleasure**, **balance**, **perception** (of time, sounds and colour in particular), and **appetite** (hence the phenomenon known as 'the munchies').

Cannabis can have some pleasant effects. After using it, people may feel relaxed, calm and happy and may experience colours and music more intensely. However, it can also have some untoward effects. Up to 15% of users report some degree of **confusion**, **hallucinations**, **anxiety**, **panic** or **paranoia**, often called 'the horrors'. It can also have depressant effects and may lead to reduced motivation. Regular users quickly build up a tolerance for cannabis, which means that they have to smoke more to gain the same effects. There is also a growing awareness of a distinct withdrawal syndrome, which is both physical and psychological: physical withdrawal effects may include insomnia or hypersomnia, aches and pains, headaches and increased bodily restlessness; psychological withdrawal signs may include cravings, increased irritability, anxiety and depressed mood.

Cannabis and psychosis

As we saw in the discussion point earlier in this chapter, there is some controversy over the possible links between cannabis usage and the onset and course of schizophrenia. Skunkweed (which may have up to three times the amounts of THC than 'traditional' cannabis), in particular, has been linked to symptoms such as the acute paranoia seen in psychosis. Several studies (e.g. van Os et al., 2002; Arsenault et al., 2002; Zammit et al., 2002) and a recent systematic review (Moore et al., 2007) have suggested a causal link between the use of cannabis – especially if started at an early age – and the subsequent development of psychosis, and it now appears clear that the use of cannabis by people with a vulnerability to psychosis can be a risky behaviour. Some people seem to be 'super-sensitive' to even quite small amounts of the drug (Rassool, 2006). Families and carers of young people who have developed psychotic symptoms often report that the young person experienced problems with thoughts, feelings and behaviours at the same time that it was first noticed that cannabis was being used. Nevertheless, these observations have to be balanced against the Advisory Council on the Misuse of Drugs' view that 'cannabis use does not lead to major health problems' (Nutt, 2009).

Amphetamines

Amphetamines are a group of synthetic drugs that act as central nervous system stimulants. Both legitimate (prescribable) and illicitly manufactured forms of the drug exist. In the UK, only two legitimate amphetamines are available: **dexamphetamine** (marketed as Dexedrine) and **methylphenidate hydrochloride** (marketed as Ritalin). Both are used with children diagnosed with ADHD (see Chapter 9) and for the sleep disorder **narcolepsy**. In the past, dexamphetamine was often used as a slimming aid but it is no longer licensed for this use. **Methylamphetamine** (**crystal meth**) is a common illicit form of the drug and currently one of its strongest forms.

The most common street name for the amphetamines is **speed**, an apt description since the drug 'speeds you up'. It is available in powder or pills and is also known as **buzz**, **Billy** or **Whizz** (after the cartoon character Billy

Whizz), **white** or **yellow** (depending on its appearances in powder form), **amphet**, **sulph** (after amphetamine sulphate), **dexie**, **base** or **paste** (the last two street names describe a less processed and stronger variety of the drug). Methylamphetamine comes with its own set of street names, usually imported from the United States where its use is more common than in Europe. Its crystal form, usually smoked, is known as **ice**, **meth**, **crystal**, **glass**, **crank**, **ice cream** and '**Nazi**' (possibly because of the sometimes terrifyingly violent actions that users occasionally commit). In its powder form it is often known as **methedrine**.

Amphetamines are similar in chemical structure to a chemical called **nor-epinephrine** (or **noradrenaline**) which occurs naturally in the brain. The drug artificially stimulates the body's central nervous system in a similar way that adrenaline affects the body when we are under great stress or facing an emergency. When faced with a crisis, adrenaline floods into the system: breathing and heart rate increase, pupils in the eye dilate (get bigger) and appetite is suppressed. The amphetamine user gets the same 'rush', feeling more energetic and alert. Feelings of increased confidence and enhanced mood usually occur. For a short period, nothing seems boring, tiredness vanishes and everything seems very exciting. With higher doses, an intense feeling of exhilaration has often been reported. Ideas (especially creative ones) flow freely and people report that they feel able to undertake huge physical and mental tasks. It is hardly surprising that some people (particularly if their 'normal' lives are boring, limited and predictable) find these experiences pleasurable and rewarding.

Amphetamine use, however, has some severe adverse effects. **Anxiety**, **irritability** and **restlessness** are common. Amphetamines are a powerful appetite suppressant (hence their use as slimming aids in the past) and some users neglect to eat properly. If the person taking the drug is vulnerable to certain types of mental illness (such as schizophrenia or bipolar disorder), amphetamine use can be extremely harmful and unpleasant, with symptoms including **acute paranoia** and **hallucinations**. When the user 'comes down' they are left feeling tired, sad, irritable and distant from friends and family. This sudden onset of tiredness and loss of strength should be dealt with by allowing the body to rest and recover in its own time. Unfortunately, many people feel so worn out and weary that they take more amphetamine in order to feel better more quickly. This only delays the inevitable time when they have to stop the drug (because they may have run out of money or supplies) and then the comedown is likely to be even worse. Severe physical problems caused by amphetamine use are reasonably rare. However, because amphetamines raise blood pressure, body temperature and heart rate, if the user is unlucky enough to have an underlying defect or weakness within their circulatory system, heart attacks and strokes have been known to occur. There have been documented cases of such a physical catastrophe occurring during a user's first experience of experimenting with amphetamines. In addition, many users feel very thirsty during an amphetamine high and there is the risk of physical collapse through dehydration.

Ecstasy

Ecstasy or MDMA (or 3,4-methylenedioxymethamphetamine, to give it its chemical name) is an amphetamine derivative known also as **E**, **XTC**, **doves**, **New Yorkers**, **disco burgers** and a myriad of ever-changing names largely deriving from the symbols on the pills containing it. It produces a euphoric and energising effect about 30 minutes after use which lasts between four and six hours. Some users report that ecstasy makes them feel more empathic towards those around them and this leads to feelings of warmth and openness that has proved to be very popular, especially at the height of the 'rave' culture in the late 1980s and early 1990s. Ecstasy can also produce some mild hallucinogenic effects. It is now a reasonably cheap drug (partly because it is out of fashion) though the purity of the tablets currently available is often very low – seized tablets, when analysed, often turn out to include hardly any of the substance, containing instead amphetamine, caffeine or other stimulants.

The adverse effects of ecstasy use are similar to those of other stimulant drugs. **Tiredness**, **anxiety**, **low mood** and **insomnia** are common following use and these symptoms become worse if the use is heavy or prolonged. It may also cause **paranoia** and **confusion**. There is growing concern that long-term use may result in neuronal damage within the brain, especially affecting the transmission and uptake of the neurotransmitter **serotonin**. Tolerance may develop, leading to some users taking more and more to gain the desired effect. Some people may become psychologically dependent on it and lose their confidence in being able to enjoy themselves in social situations without its use.

Cocaine and crack cocaine

Cocaine, a Class A substance, also known as **coke**, **Charlie**, **snow**, **C**, **blow**, **Colombian marching powder** and many other names, is usually sold as a white powder and is available for use by snorting (sniffing up the nose through a tube, often a rolled bank note) or by injecting. Its more potent form, known as **crack**, is a synthesised crystalline version of the drug (often known as **rock** because of its appearance) and this is usually smoked in improvised pipes over a bed of cigarette ash or injected, sometimes with heroin in a technique known as **speedballing**.

Cocaine is a stimulant that gives users a feeling of wellbeing, with an increase in confidence and alertness. It acts on the brain's reward and pleasure centres and prevents the reabsorption of the 'pleasure' neurotransmitter **dopamine**, resulting in a dopamine build-up that, in turn, leads to feelings of euphoria. This effect lasts for less than 30 minutes and the user then gets cravings for more of the drug in order to restore dopamine levels. The comedown from cocaine leaves the user feeling tired and depressed. Cocaine also disrupts the reuptake of the stress hormone norepinephrine, which results in an increased stimulation of the sympathetic nervous system which, in turn, leads to tachycardia, hypertension, dilation of the pupils, sweating and sometimes a tremor and general shakiness. It is also strongly linked to **serious psychological problems** if used in frequent and/or high doses. **Disturbed sleep patterns**, **depression**, **hallucinations** (including **parasitosis**, the hallucination of small bugs crawling either on or just below the skin), **paranoia** and other delusional beliefs are all features of cocaine use.

Cocaine is psychologically habit-forming (with crack cocaine being particularly difficult to resist among regular users). It can also cause heart problems and chest pains, especially if the user has high blood pressure. It can cause convulsions, confusion and restlessness. Snorting may damage the inside of the nose, while smoking crack is potentially very harmful to the lungs because of the pollutants added during its manufacture or added by unscrupulous dealers to increase profitability.

It appears that cocaine is becoming ever-more freely available and popular among drug users, as well as being cheaper in price, making it no longer the 'rich person's drug' of recent popular mythology. However, there is also recent evidence that the actual percentage of cocaine being detected in police drug seizures has reduced, with some finds now having as little as 2% of actual cocaine when tested. Similarly, the purity of crack cocaine also appears to have been reduced. This may be a reflection of a 'two-tier' drug market in the UK with cheaper, low-quality illicit drugs of all kinds – but cocaine in particular – being available alongside more expensive, higher-quality drugs that are marketed and sold to a different client group (DrugScope, 2007).

Khat

Khat (alternatively spelt qat, qhat or kat) is an evergreen shrub that grows almost exclusively in Ethiopia, Somalia and the Yemen. Its leaves are chewed, usually in social situations where it acts as a 'social lubricant' much as alcohol does in European cultures. It is a stimulant drug with similar effects to those of the amphetamines, though usually to a lesser degree. Users chew the fresh leaves, often for hours at a time, swallowing the juices that are extracted. As chewing leads to dry mouths, large quantities of drink are also imbibed at the same time, usually tea or soft drinks. The effects of chewing begin to be felt after about 15 minutes of use and can continue to be felt up to two hours after stopping. There seems to be some anecdotal evidence linking heavy use of khat to psychosis, particularly in first onset episodes. However, its use is widespread among the Somali and Yemeni populations and most users do not seem to have any major problems arising from its use. The use of all other psychoactive substances within these communities, including alcohol, is very low. Khat is legal in the UK but not in the United States.

Opiates (heroin, associated substances and heroin substitutes)

Heroin (diacetylmorphine or diamorphine), a Class A substance, is the most harmful illicit substance misused in the UK (Nutt et al., 2007) and is the substance that takes up most of the effort of our drugs services. Heroin is from the family of drugs known as **opiates** and, in contrast to stimulants, is a central nervous system **depressant**. The opiates – including **morphine**, **codeine** and **pethidine** – are obtained from the scored seed head of the opium poppy (hence 'opiates'). Heroin, which is refined from morphine by adding acetic anhydride, makes up, by far, the bulk of the UK's opiate market. It is estimated that in any one year, less than 0.1% of the 16–59-year-olds in England and Wales have used heroin and the lifetime use of heroin seems to be around 0.7% of the population (Hoare, 2009). The picture is similar in Northern Ireland, where lifetime use is around 0.5% (NACD/PHIRB, 2008). Scotland may have a particular problem with heroin, as the lifetime heroin use figures appear, at around 1.2%, to be double that of England, Wales and Northern Ireland (ISD Scotland, 2007).

Most of the illicit heroin originates in Afghanistan, Pakistan and Iran. It usually comes in powder form and may be white, yellowish or reddish brown. It has many street names, including **brown** (due to its distinctive appearance),

junk, **H**, **smack**, **gear**, **skag** and **dragon** (after a method of smoking it called 'chasing the dragon'). Heroin can be smoked, injected, or snorted.

Using heroin gives people a sense of warmth and well-being. It can lead to drowsiness and people report feeling very relaxed. Although there is evidence of controlled heroin use that is not associated with significant problems and which may go unrecorded and well hidden for many years (Rassoul, 2009), many heroin users experience a range of severe physical, psychological and social problems associated with its use. This includes the major problem of **addiction** and, as tolerance develops, the user needs to take more and more to get the same effect and/or to feel normal. The drug, as such, often ends up dominating users' lives. As a depressant drug, it leaves the user feeling sick, sleepy, constipated and detached from the world around them.

Injecting can lead to numerous problems, including **blood-borne viruses** (especially hepatitis B and C and HIV), **collapsed veins** due to over-injection, **pulmonary embolisms**, local **infections**, **abscesses**, **circulatory problems**, **thrombosis**, infections in heart valves and whole system infections. There is also a high risk of overdose, which can lead to death if not treated immediately since heroin's effect on the respiratory centre in the brain can lead to respiratory and cardiac arrest. Most of these adverse effects are a direct result of, or partially attributable to, the adulterated nature of the street heroin available to most users, or to unsterile and unsafe injecting techniques.

Regardless of how it is administered, heroin enters the bloodstream very quickly. The sense of extreme wellbeing and relaxation is caused by the binding of the morphine molecule to opioid receptors in the brain, which in turn then detect the body's own opiate-like substances, called **endorphins**. The body responds to heroin by reducing and sometimes stopping production of endogenous endorphins, thus causing dependence on it. **Withdrawing** from heroin can be very uncomfortable, with severe aches and pains, influenza-like symptoms, diarrhoea, tremor, sweating, muscular spasms, yawning and very low mood. Withdrawal from heroin typically occurs around six hours after the substance is last taken.

Methadone

Methadone is a synthetic opiate – known as **doll**, **juice** or **script** – used therapeutically as a painkiller but much more widely as a heroin substitute. Methadone maintenance is commonly used as a drug treatment for opiate addiction in the UK because it has similar effects to heroin. Methadone is also a Class A drug. It is considered the best method of substitute prescribing because it is long-acting, with a half-life of over 24 hours, meaning it can be administered once a day. It usually comes as an oral syrup (coloured green) but it is also available as ampoules to be injected or as tablets. Most users take between 60 and 120 mg daily. Like heroin, methadone has its own withdrawal symptoms, which include nausea and vomiting, high temperature, tremor, chills, sneezing and tachycardia. Methadone may also lead to overdose if taken in quantities above prescribed levels and if mixed with alcohol, heroin or other depressants such as benzodiazepines.

Hallucinogens

Hallucinogens (or hallucinogenic drugs, as they are often called) are a group of drugs, both natural and synthetic, that induce an alteration of perception, thought, emotion and levels of consciousness. The most common known hallucinogens in the UK are **lysergic acid diethylamide** or **LSD** (a synthetic drug based on the naturally produced substance ergot) and 'magic mushrooms' (**psilocybin**) also called 'liberty caps' because of their similarity in shape to the bonnets worn by French revolutionaries. Other substances less freely available and well known in the UK include **mescaline** (from a cactus found in Mexico and the Southwestern states of the USA) and **PCP** (phencyclidine). More common drugs, such as ecstasy and cannabis, which we have already discussed, may be considered to have hallucinogenic effects, especially if taken in large quantities.

Hallucinogenic drugs are not a homogenous group. They include a wide variety of substances that act in a bewilderingly different way on the brain. However, they can be grouped together because of their similarity of effect, especially on the levels of human consciousness. The history of hallucinogenic drug use is a fascinating and complicated one. They have been used for millennia by cultures across the world, often in religious or spiritual contexts. However, their popularity reached a peak in the 1960s and again in the late 1980s. They are less popular today but are still to be found, including in newer and more worrying forms such as **ketamine**, a tranquiliser used in veterinary medicine that appears to be becoming increasingly popular on the dance and club scene.

LSD, a Class A drug, is derived from ergot, a fungus that grows on rye. It is colourless, odourless and tasteless and usually comes in tablet, capsule or liquid form. It is also commonly found soaked into blotting paper, which often has intricate and esoteric designs printed onto it. It is known as **acid**, **microdots**, **dots**, **tabs**, **windowpane** (all of these names are to do with the manner of its production) or by colourful names – often associated with rock music – such as **purple haze** and **strawberry fields**. Each dose is usually known as a 'trip'. It is taken in extremely small doses, between 50 and 250 micrograms, and is possibly the most psychoactive substance yet discovered. LSD takes between 30 and 45 minutes to take effect following ingestion and each trip can last up to 12 hours.

Although there was early interest in the therapeutic potential of LSD to treat mental disorders and even by the military (who experimented with it as a truth drug and also as a means to disorientate the enemy, with little success) most people have taken LSD experimentally – to change their consciousness or as a means of enhancing pleasure in social situations. The effects of the drug are mainly dependent on the set and setting[1]; what the mood or expectations of the person taking it are, and where and when it is taken. The sought-after effects are alterations in mood and perceptions, with colours seeming more vivid and perceptions being distorted. The user may experience **synaesthesia**, where colours can be heard as sound or where smells may be experienced as tastes or physical sensations. Adverse effects are always possible: impulsive, risky behaviours might result from its use, though recorded incidents of serious harm arising from such incidents are, thankfully, very rare. A 'bad trip' may result in unpleasant feelings of paranoia, anxiety, fear and even panic attacks. Physiological effects may include tiredness and exhaustion, increased heart rate, raised body temperatures, sweating, loss of appetite, insomnia and tremors. Increased tolerance to LSD is rarely seen because most users do not choose to use it regularly. Physical withdrawal symptoms do not appear to exist.

Solvents

Some carbon-based compounds produce effects that can be compared with alcohol or anaesthetics when the vapours these products give off are inhaled. The most common name given for this form of substance taking is **glue sniffing,** though healthcare workers and allied professionals are more likely to refer to **volatile substance abuse** (VSA) or **solvent abuse**. The range of common and easily available products that can be abused is vast; indeed, solvents can be found in almost every home. The main types of solvent open to misuse are summarised in Table 11.3.

---

[1]A term coined by the 1960s 'counterculture' icon Timothy Leary meaning the mindset and physical setting for drug experiences.

TABLE 11.3 Main categories of solvent abuse

Type of solvent	Method of administration
Solvent based glues: Impact adhesives of the type used to stick down laminate surfaces or vinyl floor tiles	Either sniffed directly from their containers or poured into plastic bags or other receptacles before being sniffed
Liquid solvents: Includes volatile substances such as document correction fluid, paints and paint removers, nail polish and nail polish remover, some fire extinguishers, car anti-freeze and petrol	Substances are poured into a plastic bag and then inhaled by opening the bag as widely as possible to let in air. A kind of balloon is then made by holding the top of the bag tightly and the vapour-laden air is then squeezed from the balloon into the user's mouth
Liquid petroleum gases (LPGs): Includes butane and propane found in many aerosols, camping gas cylinders and gas refills for lighters	The gas is often sprayed directly into the mouth

Adapted, with kind permission of Jessica Kingsley Publishers, from Emmett and Nice (2006) *Understanding Street Drugs*. 2nd edition. Jessica Kingsley Publishers, London and Philadelphia.

All solvents are potentially dangerous, especially since the effects of different solvents can be unpredictable. For example, there is a danger of **sudden death** due to over-stimulation of the muscles of the heart. Another real and common danger is that **asphyxiation** may be caused either by the user's throat swelling or by choking on vomit. Users also make themselves vulnerable to dangerous situations (like being knocked down by a car or by taking unusual risks) while they are either hallucinating or intoxicated to the point where they are not able to make sensible decisions. **Short-term memory loss**, longer-term **cognitive impairments** and even, in some instances, **changes in personality**, have been known to result from solvent abuse. There have also been reports of long-term damage being caused to nerves in the body leading to **uncontrollable twitching** and **shakiness**.

As many as 10% of secondary school children will have tried solvents at least once (DrugScope, 2001). The numbers appear to be higher in Scotland. In the United States, the National Drug Survey puts the figure as high as 25% (Dennison, 2003). Solvent abuse isn't in itself illegal; however, the situation regarding the sale of volatile substances is complex. The Intoxicating Substances Supply Act 1985, which applies to England and Wales, makes it an offence for anyone to supply, or offer to supply, to someone under 18 a substance 'if he/she knows or has reasonable cause to believe that the substance or its fumes are likely to be inhaled for the purpose of causing intoxication'.

Northern Ireland has similar legislation, while Scotland has a slightly different common law offence of 'recklessly' selling solvents to children knowing that they are going to be inhaled. Additional legislation to regulate the sale of solvents is to be found in an amendment to the Consumer Protection Act, the Cigarette Lighter Refill (Safety) Regulations 1999. This amendment, which covers the whole of the UK, made it an offence to supply 'any cigarette lighter refill canister containing butane or a substance with butane as a constituent part to any person under the age of eighteen years'.

Gammahydroxybutyrate

Gammahydroxybutyrate (GHB) is a central nervous system depressant that has recently become increasingly popular as a drug of misuse, particularly on the UK club scene. It is known by many street names, including **GBH** and **liquid ecstasy**. It is a Class C drug and currently retails at about £15 for a 30 ml plastic container. It is a colourless and odourless liquid with a slightly salty taste. Because the potency of the substance seems to vary considerably from batch to batch, it is very difficult for a user to accurately predict how much has been taken at any time. The sought-after effects of GHB are similar to those of alcohol: disinhibition, relaxation, exhilaration and sedation. However, there are a range of adverse effects associated with its use. GHB use can cause unconsciousness, coma and, occasionally, death. Even regular, experienced users are at risk from death by intoxication. Taking these drugs with alcohol or other sedative drugs adds to the risk of harm.

The misuse of prescribed and other medicines

Some prescribed drugs that have useful therapeutic properties are regularly misused by people for whom they have not been prescribed. This list is too numerous to include in full but the most popularly misused prescription medicines are the **benzodiazepines,** such as diazepam, lorazepam and chlordiazepoxide. These drugs are marketed and prescribed as a short-term treatment for anxiety (and, as we have seen, in alcohol detoxification) and are highly addictive. There is a large black market for these drugs, both as a substance of misuse in their own right and as an adjunct to stimulant use where they are used to help cope with the comedown. The heroin substitute **methadone** is known to be misused by people for whom it has not been prescribed and, as a powerful central nervous system depressant, methadone can be a dangerous drug for anyone who is not used to its effects.

An equally bewildering range of over-the-counter medicines is used for non-medical effect. Stimulants that are commonly bought over-the-counter for their energising effects include Mercocaine lozenges, Sudafed and Sinutads; depressants include Gee's Linctus, kaolin and morphine, Collis Brown Mixture and codeine linctus (Rassool, 2009). Many pharmacists will be aware that these drugs are open to misuse and will refuse to serve customers if they are suspicious about the intentions of the user. However, people will go to considerable lengths, sometimes travelling to other parts of cities or from town to town, to obtain their desired substance.

The **alkyl nitrites**, amyl nitrite and butyl nitrite, are stimulants similar to nitrous oxide (laughing gas). These drugs, known as **poppers**, are not illegal are often on sale in sex shops, pubs and bars and are mainly, though not exclusively, used by the gay community. Medically, amyl nitrite is used as a treatment for angina. The effects are short lived, less than 5 minutes, and produce a rush that is especially utilised to enhance sexual pleasure.

Anabolic steroids are often used without prescription by athletes and bodybuilders to enhance muscle growth during training. They are taken orally, via skin patches or injected. They are a Class C drug with well-reported adverse effects. Because of their close chemical link to male hormones, women may have an increase in body hair, deepening voice and a decrease in breast size. Men may experience a reduction in sperm production and testes size. Liver damage, including jaundice and cancers, oedema, increase in blood lipids (high cholesterol) and high blood pressure have all been reported. The misuse of steroids has also been linked to paranoia, aggressive and violent behaviour, and sudden and unpredictable mood swings. Because some users inject anabolic steroids, there is the associated risk of injecting blood-borne viruses, especially since many steroid misusers eschew the services of needle exchanges as they do not see themselves as conventional drug misusers. Drug services have become aware of this and have successfully attempted to reach out to steroid users and make them aware of needle exchanges and options for the safe disposal of injecting paraphernalia.

Assessing for, detecting and intervening in illicit drug misuse

Health and social care workers in primary and secondary care settings are often the first point of contact for clients with developing or existing illicit drug misuse problems. As with alcohol misuse, we need to be aware of these problems and how to detect them and carry out adequate assessments.

Furthermore, we need to be able to offer identification and brief advice (IBA) or, at the very least, have a working knowledge of when and how to refer to specialist services. Again, as with alcohol misuse, the key to effective practice here are the core capabilities and interpersonal skills outlined in Chapter 2.

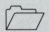

Case scenario: drug-induced psychosis

Jack, a 19-year-old university student, is brought to A&E by his girlfriend, Zoë. She was advised to take him to A&E after she telephoned a drugs helpline because she was worried about his behaviour. Zoë explains to the junior doctor assessing Jack that he is convinced the police have planted electronic bugs in his skin to 'monitor him' and that she is especially worried now because he has tried to remove one of the 'bugs' with a pair of kitchen scissors. He hasn't done any serious damage (there is just a bit of bruising and a small superficial cut to the top of his left arm) because she was able to reassure and placate him. Zoë says his behaviour became increasingly bizarre after a weekend-long party a few weeks ago that involved substantial amounts of speed (amphetamine). She adds that this is not the first time that she and Jack have taken speed but, as she says, it is perhaps the first time they have 'overdone' it. Throughout all of Zoë's conversation with the doctor, Jack remains passive and smiling, commenting every now and then that 'she [Zoë] doesn't believe anything I say'.

The junior doctor involved says it's a simple case of 'drug-induced psychosis' and arranges for Jack to be admitted to an acute mental health ward for further assessment.

How helpful is the 'diagnosis' of 'drug-induced psychosis'? Are there any problems with using this term? Do you think admission to an acute mental health ward is appropriate?

As the nurse on the acute ward responsible for admitting Jack, what could you do to reassure Jack and his girlfriend and ensure Jack's safety? How would you go about assessing Jack? (You might find that the assessment strategies outlined in Chapters 6 and 7 have some relevance here.)

Evidence-based guidelines for the clinical management of drug misuse and dependence were published in 2007 by the English Department of Health

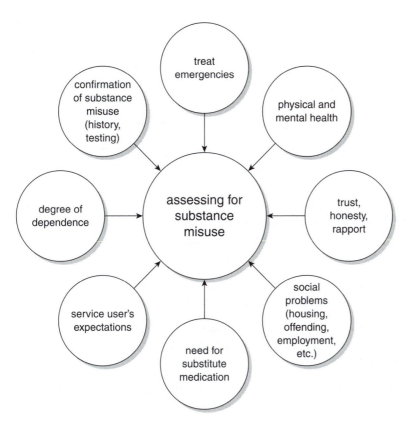

FIGURE 11.1 Things to consider when assessing for drug misuse (after DH (England) and the devolved administrations, 2007)

and the devolved administrations in Scotland, Wales and Northern Ireland (DH (England) and the devolved administrations, 2007). There is only room in this chapter for a brief summary of this very comprehensive document, but it is worth noting that it offers some robust and general guidance for both the assessment of drug misusers and the ways in which health and social care professionals might intervene. As with alcohol misuse, your interpersonal skills are of paramount importance in establishing rapport, trust and honesty. Figure 11.1 outlines some other factors you will need to consider when assessing substance misusers and Box 11.5 outlines best practice guidelines for intervening in illicit drug use. Rassool (2009) also provides comprehensive clinical and practical advice on substance misuse interventions, management and education.

Box 11.5   Best practice guidelines for intervening in drug misuse (after DH (England) and the devolved administrations, 2007)

Treatment packages should be **comprehensive** and **multifaceted** and should involve:

- A **psychosocial** component, especially for cocaine and other stimulants, cannabis and hallucinogens (where there is no effective substitution agent)
- The provision of drug-related **advice**
- **Harm-reduction strategies** (such as the provision of needle exchanges and strategies for reducing the risk of overdose)
- Interventions to increase **motivation** and **prevent relapse**
- A good **therapeutic alliance** with substance misuse professionals

Methadone, buprenophine and lofexidine are all effective in opioid detoxification and methadone and buprenophine in maintenance therapy.

There is a strong evidence base for **contingency management** (where vouchers or tokens are used to reward) and **family and couples interventions,** but neither is commonly used in the UK.

Self-help and **mutual aid** approaches, especially 12-step approaches, have been found to be highly effective for some individuals, and patients seeking **abstinence** should be signposted to such services.

Co-existing Substance Misuse and Mental Health Problems

There is growing awareness about the issues affecting people with co-existing substance misuse and mental health problems (often referred to as a **dual diagnosis**). Traditional services offered by mental health and drug and alcohol agencies have sometimes been restrictive and non-inclusive, leading to lost opportunities for accurate detection and assessment of problems, pessimistic and unhelpful attitudes of individual members of staff and poor engagement with services by some service users given a dual diagnosis. As such, some of the most chaotic and vulnerable clients have received inadequate services.

There is no uniform and agreed definition of what 'dual diagnosis' actually means and there is no formal medical diagnostic category of dual diagnosis. A simple working definition of dual diagnosis is: 'a mental health problem and a substance misuse problem, both of which require some form of intervention and may or may not have been medically diagnosed' (Alcohol Concern, 1999).

Alternatively, it has been defined as 'the combination of severe mental illness (usually psychotic) and problematic substance use' (Holland & Midson, 2003). Indeed, some prefer the term **co-existing problems** because, as Cooper (2008) notes, the term dual diagnosis 'encourages a focus on two distinct problems that may lead to inaccurate case formulations and inappropriate interventions, or, no intervention at all' (p. 1).

There is a growing evidence base of effective interventions for clients with co-existing problems, based on comprehensive, integrated approaches that deal with all aspects of their complex lives. Early studies in this field examined the application of conventional 12-step style substance misuse interventions that had abstinence as the intended outcome. A Cochrane Review (Ley et al., 1999) found that these studies produced disappointing results for clients with co-existing problems. Later research used comprehensive packages of interventions to address interrelated issues. These programmes used the principles of comprehensiveness, **assertive outreach**, **health behaviour change** using a **motivational interviewing** approach (Miller & Rollnick, 2002) and took a **long-term perspective** with clients who may not acknowledge that they have a substance misuse or a mental health problem or that there are connections between the two.

Much of the research into effective treatments for clients with co-existing problems has been carried out in the United States, and has included staged interventions using assertive outreach, psychoeducation delivered in a collaborative and empowering style, and integrated care based on case management principles. A randomised controlled trial has been carried out in the UK with promising results (Barrowclough et al., 2001; Haddock et al., 2003) and a much larger study – MIDAS – has been funded as a consequence. MIDAS is a large, multi-site, randomised controlled trial into the efficacy of motivational interviewing and cognitive behavioural therapy using a collaborative approach to address the connections between mental ill health and substance use. Although outcomes from this study on integrated treatment have yet to be published, data on recruitment and retention indicate that drop-out rates are low for this treatment and that most of those receiving the treatment attended a substantial number of treatment sessions (Barrowclough et al., 2009).

Conclusion

In this chapter you will have seen how the misuse of substances has affected societies for many years and how health and social care professionals can help with current problematic substance misuse.

Those who misuse substances are not 'someone else's problem': they form a major part of the daily working lives of many health and social care professionals. Knowledge of substance misuse is, as such, an essential part of pre-and post-registration nurse education and training. As a mental health nurse, you need to be able to detect underlying substance misuse issues in the service users you work with and this means having a working knowledge of the extent and types of substance misuse in our communities, keeping up-to-date with local and national trends in substance misuse and developing an awareness of available treatments and services.

You should try to be optimistic, empathic and non-judgemental in your dealings with substance misusers, not just because this is what your professional code of conduct may say but because this is the most effective way of engaging and working with these clients. You may sometimes find yourself out of your depth when attempting to address complex substance use issues, but as you will have gathered from this chapter, information, advice and support are now freely available and easily accessible, both for you and the service users you work with. Using the principles of harm reduction, empowering health advice and timely and appropriate interventions, nurses can play a major part in the management of substance misuse in all areas of clinical practice.

Finally, if what you have learnt from this chapter makes you worried about your own levels of substance use or of those close to you, remember that confidential support services for students are provided by most universities. Information and advice is also available from the organisations listed under Web resources below.

Further Reading and Resources

Key texts

Rassool GH (2009). *Alcohol and Drug Misuse: A Handbook for Students and Health Professionals.* Abingdon: Routledge.
A comprehensive textbook that offers a global perspective on substance use, misuse and treatments. It also provides guidance in the skills that students and practitioners need to deal effectively with substance misuse.

Rassool GH (2006). *Dual Diagnosis Nursing.* Oxford: Blackwell.
A comprehensive textbook that addresses a wide range of contemporary approaches to working with dual diagnosis service users.

Miller WR & Rollnick S (2002). *Motivational Interviewing: Preparing People for Change,* 2nd edition. New York: Guilford Press.

This is a key text from the leaders in the field for anyone wanting to learn about motivational interviewing (MI). The spirit that underpins MI is given as much emphasis as the techniques, which are supported by detailed case examples.

DrugScope (2007). *The Essential Guide to Drugs and Alcohol.* London: DrugScope. *Formerly known as Drug Abuse Briefing. 'Gives you the basic information on all the most widely used licit and illicit drugs … covering the whole of the UK'.*

Key policy documents

Department of Health (England) and the devolved administrations (2007). *Drug Misuse and Dependence: UK Guidelines on Clinical Management.* London: Department of Health (England), the Scottish Government, Welsh Assembly Government and Northern Ireland Executive.

HM Government (2008). *Drugs: Protecting Families and Communities. The 2008 Drugs Strategy.* London: Central Office of Information.

National Institute for Health and Clinical Excellence (2010). *Alcohol Use Disorders: Diagnosis and Clinical Management of Alcohol-Related Physical Complications.* London: NICE. Available from www.nice.org.uk/CG100

National Institute for Health and Clinical Excellence (2010). *Alcohol-Use Disorders: Preventing the Development of Hazardous and Harmful Drinking [NICE Public Health Guidance 24].* London: NICE. Available from www.nice.org.uk/PH24

Web resources

DrugScope: www.drugscope.org.uk
The UK's leading independent centre of information and expertise on drugs. DrugScope provides quality information about licit and illicit drugs, promotes effective responses to drug use, undertakes research, advises on policy-making and good practice and encourages informed debate.

FRANK: www.talktofrank.com
The UK's government-backed national drugs information campaign.

UK Harm Reduction Alliance: www.ukhra.org
'A campaigning coalition of drug users, health and social care workers, criminal justice workers and educationalists that aims to put public health and human rights at the centre of drug treatment and service provision for drug users.'

UK Drug Policy Commission: www.ukdpc.org.uk
An independent body providing objective analysis of UK drug policy.

Alcohol Identification and Brief Advice e-Learning Course: www.alcohollearningcentre. org.uk/eLearning/IBA/
A free online course supported by the Royal College of Nursing, Royal College of Physicians and Royal College of General Practitioners.

References

Alcohol Concern (1999). *Fact Sheet on Alcohol and Mental Health*. London: Alcohol Concern.

APA (American Psychiatric Association) (2000). *Diagnostic and Statistical Manual of Mental Disorders, 4th Edition* (Text Revision) (DSM-IVR) Arlington, VA: APA.

Arseneault L, Cannon M, Poulton R, Murray R, Caspi A & Moffitt TE (2002). Cannabis use in adolescence and risk for adult psychosis: longitudinal prospective study. *British Medical Journal*, **325**, 1212–1213.

Babor T, Higgins-Biddle JC, Saunders JB & Monteiro MG (2001). *AUDIT, the Alcohol Use Disorders Identification Test: Guidelines for Use in Primary Care*, 2nd edition. Geneva: World Health Organisation.

Barrowclough C, Haddock G, Beardmore R, Conrod P, Craig T, Davies L, Dunn G, Lewis S, Moring J, Tarrier N & Wykes T (2009). Evaluating integrated MI and CBT for people with psychosis and substance misuse: recruitment, retention and sample characteristics of the MIDAS trial. *Addictive Behaviors*, **34**, 859–866.

Barrowclough C, Haddock G, Tarrier N, Lewis S, Moring J, O'Brien R, Schofield N & McGovern J (2001). Randomised controlled trial of MI, CBT and FI for patients with co-morbid schizophrenia and SUD. *American Journal of Psychiatry*, **158**, 1706–1713.

BMA (British Medical Association) (2008). *Alcohol Misuse: Tackling the UK Epidemic*. London: BMA.

Becker HC (1998). Kindling in alcohol withdrawal. *Alcohol Health & Research World*, **22**(1), 25–33.

Cooper PD (2008). Editorial. *Mental Health and Substance Use: Dual Diagnosis*, **1**(1), 1.

Costa e Silva JA (2002). Evidence based analysis of the worldwide abuse of licit and illicit drugs. *Human Psychopharmacology*, **17**, 131–140.

Dennison SJ (2003). *Handbook of the Dually Diagnosed Patient*. Philadelphia, PA: Lippincott, Williams and Wilkins.

DH (Department of Health) (England) and the Devolved Administrations (2007). *Drug Misuse and Dependence: UK Guidelines on Clinical Management*. London: Department of Health (England), the Scottish Government, Welsh Assembly Government and Northern Ireland Executive.

DH (Department of Health) (2004). *Choosing Health: Summary of Intelligence on Alcohol*. London: DH.

DH (Department of Health) (2005). *Alcohol Needs Assessment Research Project (ANARP): The 2004 National Alcohol Needs Assessment for England*. London: DH.

DHSSPS (Department for Health, Social Security and Public Safety) (2006). *New Strategic Direction for Alcohol and Drugs (2006–2011)*. Belfast: DHSSPS.

DrugScope (2001). *Drug Abuse Briefing: A Guide to the Non-Medical Use of Drugs in Britain*, 8th edition. London: DrugScope.

DrugScope (2007). DrugScope Street Drug Trends Survey 2007: Two tier cocaine market puts drug in reach of more users [press release]. Available from www.drugscope.org.uk [accessed 5 January 2010].

Dyson J (2006). Alcohol misuse and older people. *Nursing Older People*, **18**(7), 32–35.

EMCDDA (European Monitoring Centre for Drug & Drug Addiction (2009). *2009 Annual Report on the State of the Drugs Problem in the European Union*. Brussels: EMCDDA.

Emmett D & Nice G (2006). *Understanding Street Drugs*, 2nd edition. London: Jessica Kingsley.

Haddock G, Barrowclough C, Tarrier N, Moring J, O'Brien R, Schofield N, Quinn J, Palmer S, Davis L, Lowens I, McGovern J & Lewis S (2003). Cognitive behavioural therapy and motivational intervention for schizophrenia and substance misuse – 18 month outcomes of a randomised controlled trial. *British Journal of Psychiatry*, **183**, 418–426.

Hibell B, Guttormsson U, Ahlström S, Balakireva O, Bjarnason T, Kokkevi A & Kraus L (2009). *The 2007 ESPAD Report: Substance Use among Students in 35 European Countries*. Stockholm: The Swedish Council for Information on Alcohol and Other Drugs.

HM Government (2008). *Drugs: Protecting Families and Communities. The 2008 Drugs Strategy*. London: Central Office of Information.

Hoare J (2009). *Drug Misuse Declared: Findings from the 2008/09 British Crime Survey, England and Wales* [Home Office Statistical Bulletin]. London: The Home Office.

Holland M & Midson V (2003). Substance misuse and mental illness. In T Ryan & J Pritchard (eds), *Good Practice in Mental Health*. London: Jessica Kingsley.

Home Office (2009). *Measuring the Harm from Illegal Drugs: A Summary of the Drug Harm Index 2006*. London: The Home Office.

House of Commons Health Committee (2010). *First Report of Session 2009–10: Alcohol*. London: TSO.

ISD Scotland (2007). *Drug Misuse Statistics Scotland 2007*. Edinburgh: ISD Publications. Available from www.drugmisuse.isdscotland.org [accessed 5 January 2010].

Ley A, Jeffery DP, McClaren S & Seigfried N (1999). Treatment programmes for people with both severe mental illness and substance misuse [Cochrane Review]. Cochrane Library, Issue 2. Oxford: Update Software.

Miller WR & Rollnick S (2002). *Motivational Interviewing: Preparing People for Change*, 2nd edition. New York: Guilford Press.

Moore TH, Zammit S, Lingford-Hughes A, Barnes TR, Jones PB, Burke M & Lewis G (2007). Cannabis use and risk of psychotic or affective mental health outcomes: a systematic review. *Lancet*, **370**, 319–328.

NACD/PHIRB, National Advisory Committee on Drugs/Public Health Information and Research Branch (2008). *Drug Use in Ireland & Northern Ireland 2006/2007 Drug Prevalence Survey: Regional Drug Task Force (Ireland) & Health and Social Services Board (Northern Ireland) Results*. Dublin: NACD.

NICE (National Institute for Health and Clinical Excellence) (2010a). *Alcohol Use Disorders: Diagnosis and Clinical Management of Alcohol-Related Physical Complications*. London: NICE. Available from www.nice.org.uk/CG100 [accessed 30 July 2010].

NICE (National Institute for Health and Clinical Excellence) (2010b). *Alcohol-Use Disorders: Preventing the Development of Hazardous and Harmful Drinking [NICE Public Health Guidance 24]*. London: NICE. Available from www.nice.org.uk/PH24 [accessed 5 January 2010].

Nutt D, King LA, Saulsbury W, & Blakemore C (2007). Development of a rational scale to assess the harm of drugs of potential misuse. *Lancet*, **369**, 1047–1053.

Nutt D (2009). Estimating drug harms: a risky business? [Eve Saville Lecture 2009] *Centre for Crime and Justice Studies Briefing Paper 10*. Available from: www.crimeandjustice.org.uk [accessed 5 January 2010].

OED (Oxford English Dictionary) (1989). Available from: www.oed.com [accessed 6 January 2010].

ONS (Office for Nationals Statistics) (2007). *Health Related Behaviour. Alcohol: More Men Than Women Exceed Recommended Daily Limit*. Available from www.statistics.gov.uk [accessed 5 January 2010].

Raistrick D, Heather N & Godfrey C (2005). *Review of the Effectiveness of Treatment for Alcohol Problems*. London: National Treatment Agency.

Rassool GH (1998). Contemporary issues in addiction nursing. In GH Rassool (ed.), *Substance Use and Misuse: Nature, Context and Clinical Interventions*. Oxford, Blackwell Science.

Rassool GH (2006). *Dual Diagnosis Nursing*. Oxford, Blackwell.

Rassool GH (2009). *Alcohol and Drug Misuse: A Handbook for Students and Health Professionals*. Abingdon: Routledge.

Scottish Government (2008). *The Road to Recovery: A New Approach to Tackling Scotland's Drug Problem*. Edinburgh: The Scottish Government.

UNODC (United Nations Office on Drugs and Crime) (2009). *World Drug Report 2009*. Vienna: UNODC. Available from: www.unodc.org [accessed 4 January 2010].

van Os J, Bak M, Hanssen M, Bijl RV, de Graaf R & Verdou H (2002). Cannabis use and psychosis: a longitudinal population study. *American Journal of Epidemiology*, **156**, 319–327.

Weaver T, Charles V, Zenobia Carnwath Z, Madden P, Renton A, Stimson G, Tyrer P, Barnes T, Bench C & Paterson S (2003). Co-morbidity of substance misuse and mental illness in community mental health and substance misuse services. *British Journal of Psychiatry*, **183**, 304–313.

Welsh Assembly Government (2008). *Working Together to Reduce Harm: The Substance Misuse Strategy for Wales*, 2008–2018. Cardiff: The Welsh Assembly Government.

WHO (World Health Organisation) (1981). Nomenclature and classification of drug and alcohol related problems: a WHO memorandum. *Bulletin of the World Health Organisation*, **59**(2), 225–242.

WHO (World Health Organisation) (2004). *Global Status Report on Alcohol, 2004*. Geneva: WHO.

Zammit S, Allebeck P, Andreasson S, Lundberg I & Lewis G (2002). Self reported cannabis use as a risk factor for schizophrenia in Swedish conscripts of 1969: historical cohort study. *British Medical Journal*, **325**, 1199–1203.

12

Helping People with Mental Health Problems Who Come into Contact with the Criminal Justice System

John Baker, Michael Coffey and Mike Doyle

What will I learn in this chapter?

The aim of this chapter is to introduce you to the specialty of forensic mental health and to explore the ways in which nurses can help people with mental health problems who come into contact with the criminal justice system.

After reading this chapter, you will be able to:

- explain some of the key concepts in forensic mental health such as risk, dangerousness and personality disorder;
- appreciate the policy context of forensic mental health care across the UK;
- understand the reasons why individuals may require forensic mental health care, their needs and the range of options available to meet those needs;
- identify the main interventions used in forensic mental health care and the evidence base for those interventions.

Introduction

Forensic mental health is the area of mental health practice that perhaps generates the greatest anxieties among the general public, if not also among those working in mental health. This may, in part, be due to misunderstandings of the meaning of the word **forensic**, which means 'related to courts of law'. Forensic is, as such, a term that can be associated with **any** crime and not just those deemed serious or those perpetrated by 'dangerous' offenders. However, given that forensic mental health services tend to deal with the more serious crimes or offenders, it is entirely understandable that the general public might associate the word forensic with dangerousness.

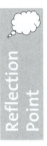

Some loaded terms?

The words 'forensic', 'dangerousness' and 'criminal' occur throughout this chapter. What images do these words conjure up? Do they generally have negative or positive connotations? Is there any value in using related terms like 'criminal justice', 'public protection' and 'offender' as alternatives?

It is important to bear in mind, however, that while the business of forensic mental health is essentially the care and management of offenders with a mental disorder,[1] or **mentally disordered offenders** (MDOs) as they are known, not all mentally disordered offenders are a danger to society. Indeed, forensic mental health could be said to have two inter-related branches: (1) the care of those in prison (regardless of the severity of the crime) who have, or who subsequently develop, mental health problems; and (2) the care and management of those with mental health problems who commit serious crimes. The former is on the agenda because there has, in recent years, been considerable concern expressed about the levels of mental ill health in the general prison population (Edgar & Rickford, 2009; SCMH, 2009). Indeed, one survey suggested that the prevalence of mental ill health among the prison population could be as high as 90% with 70% suffering two or more conditions (Singleton et al., 1998). The latter has been on the agenda for centuries

---

[1] We use 'mental disorder' here rather than 'mental health problem' because it has – as you will recall from Chapter 1 – a specific legal meaning.

and is related to the arguments over whether such people are 'mad' (and so **care** is appropriate) or whether they are 'bad' (and so management – or even **punishment** – is appropriate).

The 'mad vs. bad' debate

From historic and cultural perspectives 'madness' and 'badness' have been seen as both separate and the same thing. At times some symptoms of madness have been accepted as a form of divine intervention, the person being seen to have the special gift of healing or spiritual insight (Screech, 1985). At other times (especially during the sixteenth and seventeenth centuries when there was a widespread fear of witchcraft), mental illness was often construed as a form of demonic possession, with a need for the demons to be recanted or purged, often by extreme forms of what could now only be called torture (Jones, 1983). Moreover, religious ideology has often associated 'sin' and 'sickness' in a way which suggests a direct causal link – a person is sick because they've sinned. In many societies, including our own, mental illness is often coupled with societal and cultural responses to the 'otherness' (or strangeness) of the mentally ill, responses that fashion an almost innate fear of being 'mad' and not 'normal'. Furthermore, when mental illness is coupled with the commission of serious criminal offences, society has deep-rooted concerns about whether the behaviours are the result of ill-health, criminal intent or badness (Aubert & Messinger, 1958).

There is, of course, a continuum of seriousness among offences ranging from petty public nuisances to crimes such as serious assault and murder. We may be able to understand some of these crimes in the context of a mental illness but, instinctively, the label of 'madness' may be an insufficient explanation for the more serious crimes. Psychiatry is often called upon to determine the presence of mental disorder in someone who has committed a crime, the question being: 'are they deliberately and wilfully breaking the law or is their behaviour a symptom of some underlying madness?' Many workers in the mental health, social care or criminal justice systems are required to make such judgements about others all of the time and, in struggling to understand deviant behaviour, it may be easier to resort to a 'badness' category – possibly because when serious offences are committed, we often find ourselves feeling emotions such as frustration, anger and disgust. As such, when we are horrified by acts that are almost impossible for us to comprehend, we may see those acts as wicked and the perpetrator as evil. Our judgements are not helped much by the media, who frequently sensationalise stories and, in the process, negatively influence public perceptions of mental illness (Berlin & Malin, 1991). Moreover, in particularly newsworthy or controversial cases, the media often see the 'mental illness defence' as a soft option or as an attempt to undeservedly limit culpability. This makes working in forensic mental health additionally complex and requires workers to monitor their own values and beliefs about mental illness, serious offences and where any blame should lie.

'Schizophrenic killer'

In September 2009, London's *Evening Standard* ran a story entitled 'Black cab drivers' fury over wife killer'. The story explained how around 100 black cab (taxi) drivers in Islington had protested against plans to allow a 'schizophrenic killer' to train for 'the Knowledge', a prerequisite for a London taxi licence. Here are some of the quotes from the protesters:

> "How can a schizophrenic who has killed before be allowed this level of trust?" "We are the best taxi drivers in the world, but having a killer with a licence will affect us all." "I was talking to a passenger ... and she was absolutely terrified that someone like that should be driving a black cab." (*Evening Standard*, 11 September 2009, p. 18)

Do you agree with the taxi drivers? If so, why? If not, why not? Do you think it would have made any difference if a 'schizophrenic' hadn't been the killer?

Psychiatry itself is also unsure of what to do with such people; there are, as such, differing views on whether treatment, punishment or both are warranted for different conditions. The current consensus seems to support the 'diversion' of MDOs from the criminal justice system into the mental health system (DH/Home Office, 1992; DH, 2009). Despite this, people with mental illness are still disproportionately represented in the criminal justice system (DH, 2009). This fact would not surprise those sociologists (see, for example, Lowman et al., 1987; Conrad, 1992) who claim that the criminal justice and mental health systems are both societal mechanisms for controlling those deemed to be 'deviant'. Moreover, the process of 'transcarceration' (the routing of MDOs between the two systems) serves only to trap MDOs as it does not give them the flexibility to vary their roles or renegotiate their identities to be anything other than 'mad' or 'bad' (Arrigo, 2001).

Policy Context

A major milestone in the development of forensic mental health policy was the **Reed Report** (DH/Home Office, 1992), a report that reaffirmed the policy that MDOs should, as far as possible, be cared for by health and social services rather than the criminal justice system. The Reed Report identified a number of principles that should underpin forensic health and social care (see Box 12.1 for a summary). These principles have been a significant driving force in service development over the past decade or so, influencing, for example, reviews of high security provision, the development of local secure services and the development of community-based aftercare.

Box 12.1   Principles of care for MDOs from the Reed Report (DH (Department of Health)/Home Office, 1992)

MDOs should be cared for:

- with regard to the quality of care and individual need
- in the community, as far as possible, rather than in institutional settings
- under conditions of no greater security than is justified by the degree of danger they present to self or others
- in such a way as to maximise rehabilitation and their chances of sustaining an independent life
- as near as possible to their own homes or families if they have them

---

Fifteen years after the Reed Report, the government remained concerned about the number of people in custody who had mental health problems, especially since incarceration greatly enhances the risk of self-harm and suicide in those with severe mental health problems. The government therefore asked Lord Bradley, a former Home Office Minister, to look at the situation again in late 2007. The subsequent **Bradley Report** (DH, 2009) contended that, while the issues identified in the Reed Report were as relevant in 2009 as they were in 1992, the political and social context had changed significantly over the years. In particular, during the intervening years, **prison healthcare had been transferred from the Prison Service to the**

NHS, the **social exclusion** agenda had emerged, a **new Mental Health Act** had been approved, and there was a new focus on **safeguarding the public** following some high-profile cases of such as those of Christopher Clunis (see Ritchie et al., 1994), John Barratt (see NHS London, 2006) and 'Mr C' (Health Inspectorate Wales, 2008). The Bradley Report takes a broad-brush approach to the whole criminal justice process, covering early intervention, arrest, prosecution, the courts, prison, community sentences and resettlement; some of the most relevant recommendations (which are to a large extent complementary to those from the Reed Report) are summarised in Box 12.2. One particular theme emerging from the Bradley Report is the **convergence** of the criminal justice and mental health systems, in terms of legislation and policy as well as practice (Rutherford, 2010).

Box 12.2 Some of the recommendations of the Bradley Report (DH (Department of Health), 2009)

- Mental health awareness training should be offered to relevant staff including school staff, primary care staff, the police, prison and probation staff and the judiciary.
- Youth offending teams should include qualified mental health workers.
- There should be joint (health and police) protocols on the use of Sections 135 and 136 of the Mental Health Act 2007.
- Mental health facilities rather than police stations should be used as places of safety.
- Healthcare in police custody suites should be the business of the NHS.
- Primary care health services should promote wellbeing in prison via a range of health and non-health activities.
- Inreach teams should focus on prisoners with severe mental illness.
- Services for prisoners with dual diagnosis should be improved urgently.
- An inter-departmental (health and criminal justice) strategy for personality disorder should be created and the evidence base for the interventions used to help people with personality disorder should be established.
- The Care Programme Approach (CPA) is as applicable to prisoners as it is to non-prisoners and needs enhancing.
- A comprehensive mentoring programme for people leaving custody with mental health problems should be established.

- There should be a national model for criminal justice mental health teams (CJMHTs) with agreed standards for liaison with community services, screening and assessment, information management, joint training and active service user involvement.
- CJMHTs should give special consideration to people with learning disabilities, women, children and young people, and black and ethnic minorities who come into contact with the criminal justice system.

Legislation relating to MDOs

Mental health legislation for the four countries of the UK was discussed in some detail in Chapter 7. MDOs, however, are considered separately in all three sets of legislation: in Part III (Sections 35–55) of the **Mental Health Act 1983** (as amended by the **Mental Health Act 2007**); in Part III (Articles 42–61) of the **Mental Health (Northern Ireland) Order 1986**; and in Part 8 (Sections 130–136) of the **Mental Health (Care and Treatment) (Scotland) Act 2003**. Part 8 of the Scottish Act essentially alters Part 6 of the Criminal Procedure (Scotland) Act 1995 which is the core Scottish legislation dealing with MDOs.

Across all three pieces of legislation, detention orders (compulsory treatment or assessment orders) for MDOs often come with additional safeguards. These include **restriction orders** or demands that a patient[2] be recalled to hospital even after being discharged or, as is the case in Scotland, demands that offenders be returned to prison once treatment has ended.

As we mentioned in Chapter 7, it's important that you are familiar with the key elements of the relevant parts and sections of the legislation applicable to the country you are practising in (see Tables 12.1 and 12.2). A general textbook like this can, however, give only a superficial overview of the legislation. Consequently, you should look elsewhere for more definitive information and guidance: for example, from expert practitioners, specialised texts on mental health law and government guidance such as the Codes of Practice (see Scottish Executive, 2005; DH, 2008).

---

[2]Although we have tried to limit the use the term 'patient' throughout this book, its use in this chapter is unavoidable since it is the term used in the legislation.

TABLE 12.1 Sections of the legislation dealing with MDOs for England, Wales and Northern Ireland (after Puri et al., 2005; DH, 2008)

Name	Title	Notes (England and Wales)
Section 35 *NI: Article 42*	Remand to hospital for medical report	Magistrates or Crown Court can apply Section lasts 28 days although it can be renewed (for a maximum of 12 weeks) Not able to have Section 17 leave
Section 36 *NI: Article 43*	Remand to hospital for treatment	Crown Court only can apply Similar to a Section 2 in that it lasts 28 days in the first instance although it can be renewed (for a maximum of 12 weeks)
Section 37 *NI: Article 44*	Hospital order	Magistrates or Crown Court can apply Applies following conviction for an imprisonable offence where a mental disorder is identified Similar to a Section 3 in that it lasts 6 months in the first instance but can be renewed indefinitely
Section 37/41 *NI: Articles 47 and 48 deal with restriction orders*	Hospital order with restrictions	Crown Court only can apply Section 41 order obtained if there is **significant** risk to others The restrictions affect leave of absence, transfer between hospitals, and discharge, all of which require Ministry of Justice permission. Patients are also subject to recall once discharged from hospital
Section 38 *NI: Article 45*	Interim hospital order	Magistrates or Crown Court can apply. 12 weeks in the first instance Used where there is doubt whether a Section 37 order is necessary
Section 47 *NI: Article 53*	Transfer to hospital from prison	Ministry of Justice approval required Occurs post conviction and/or sentencing This section lasts 6 months in first instance and can be renewed indefinitely
Section 48 *NI: Articles 54 and 58*	Transfer to hospital from prison whilst on remand	Ministry of Justice approval required Prisoner must be in **urgent** need of treatment Essentially the same as Section 47 though occurs before conviction and/or sentencing
Sections 47/49 and 48/49 *NI: Articles 56 and 57*	Transfer to hospital with restrictions	Ministry of Justice approval required The restrictions are the same as for Section 41 Also allows transfer back to prison once treated

'Sections' refer to the Mental Health Act 1983 (as amended by the Mental Health Act 2007) and cover England and Wales; 'Articles' refer to the Mental Health (Northern Ireland) Order 1986.

In England and Wales, the Ministry of Justice (previously part of the Home Office), through the Mental Health Unit of its National Offender Management Service, have responsibility for overseeing the care of, and restrictions imposed on, patients by Sections 41 and 49 of the Mental Health Act. The Ministry of Justice employs case workers to review multidisciplinary team

TABLE 12.2 Sections of the legislation dealing with MDOs in Scotland (after Scottish Executive, 2005)

Section	Title	Notes
Pre-trial court appearance		
CPA S.52D	Assessment order	Court refers to hospital for assessment. **Restricted status** (the patient is subject to certain restrictions which only the Scottish Ministers can vary)
CPA S.52B	Assessment order for those on remand	Only the Scottish Ministers can apply for a hospital assessment order. Restricted status
CPA S.52M	Treatment order	Court refers to hospital for treatment. Person can subsequently stand trial. Restricted status
CPA S.52L	Treatment order for those on remand	Scottish Ministers apply for a hospital treatment order Restricted status
Pre-trial court appearance or after trial has commenced		
CPA S.54(1)	Person found 'insane in bar of trial'	An examination of the facts (Section 55) determines whether beyond reasonable doubt the person committed the offence (subsequently leading to a **disposal** in the case of insanity) or acquits on grounds other than insanity
Trial (including post-conviction, pre-disposal orders)		
CPA S.54(6)	Acquittal on the grounds of insanity	May be subject to a disposal listed below
CPA S.52D or S.53 or MHA S.200	Conviction requiring assessment pending disposal	Restricted status
CPA S.52M	Conviction requiring treatment pending disposal	Restricted status
CPA S.53	Interim compulsion order	Restricted status
CPA S.200	Remand for enquiry into physical or mental health	Seldom used. No authority to treat
Post-conviction disposals		
CPA S.57A	Compulsion order	Can be for community or hospital-based treatment. Restrictions under Sections 57A and 50 may be added
CPA S.59A with MHA S.210/215	Hospital direction followed by revocation	Person is ordered to hospital for treatment in addition to being sentenced. Revocation of this order by the Scottish Ministers (MHA Section 210) or the Scottish Mental Health Tribunal (Section 215) means the person goes to prison to serve his or her sentence
MHA S.230	Probation with condition of treatment	Can be community or hospital treatment
CPA S.58(1A)	Guardianship order	Person returns to the community under guardianship (long term legal authority for someone to act on the person's behalf)
CPA S.60B	Intervention order	Person returns to the community under intervention (short term or one-off legal authority for someone to act on the person's behalf)

CPA = Criminal Procedure (Scotland) Act 1995; MHA = Mental Health (Care and Treatment) (Scotland) Act 2005 documentation, checking on risk status prior to granting approval for periods of leave (whether supervised or unsupervised) and for eventual discharge. At the time of writing, justice matters in Northern Ireland were in the process of being devolved to the Northern Ireland Assembly. Once these powers are devolved, it is expected that the Northern Ireland Minister for Justice will take over responsibility for the oversight of restriction orders (Articles 47 and 48) under the Mental Health (Northern Ireland) Order 1986 from the Secretary of State for Northern Ireland. Since decision making in Scotland is undertaken collectively by members of the Scottish government, it is the 'Scottish Ministers' rather than any single individual or department who are the ultimate authority in Scotland in relation to MDOs.

Forensic Mental Health Service Provision

Earlier, we mentioned that there were essentially two branches to forensic mental health: the mental health care of those in prison; and the care of those MDOs for whom prison is deemed inappropriate.

Prison provision

There are over 90,000 prisoners in UK prisons (Walmsley, 2009; 2008 figures) and, as we mentioned earlier, the majority of these may suffer some form of mental health problem. Typically, the experience of prisoners (and ex-prisoners) is one characterised by **exclusion** (Murray, 2007). When incarcerated, prisoners are excluded from the wider community and from access to healthcare of their own choosing. The life experience for many prisoners will have been one of lifelong social exclusion: poor numeracy, literacy and coping skills, long periods of unemployment, and being placed in care are all more likely in the prison than the non-prison population (Social Exclusion Unit, 2002; Shepherd, 2010). Since having mental health problems can exacerbate and compound these problems, mental health problems often serve to further cement social exclusion in place.

There have been attempts to address this. Following the UK-wide decision to transfer prison healthcare from the various prison services to the NHS (see, for example, DH, 2003; PHAB, 2007), a central principle of prison healthcare provision is that prisoners should receive the same standard of care as the non-prison population. For mental health, one way of achieving this principle is though **inreach** services, services designed specifically to assess, detect and treat serious mental ill-health in prisons. In many ways, inreach teams are similar to community mental health teams (Emslie et al., 2005), in that their explicit purpose is the identification of those with a diagnosable mental illness and the provision of ongoing care until they are transferred or released from prison (Armitage, 2003). The duties of inreach workers can be many and varied but they often include the facilitation of regular multidisciplinary **reviews of medication**, liaison with care coordinators regarding the **ongoing management** of the prisoner, the **facilitation of early NHS transfers**, liaison with NHS staff regarding **continuity of care for those prisoners discharged back into prison**, liaison with key external agencies in relation to **pre-release planning** and the **provision of support to families**. Inreach workers may also be involved in **direct therapeutic interventions** so that prisoners avoid admission to a prison inpatient unit and so remain in the main part of the prison. For instance, psychological and social support might be combined through relapse awareness training and ensuring that meaningful activities are available.

While the growth in inreach teams is to be welcomed, service provision has tended to be somewhat inconsistent with wide regional variations, largely because the services have been underfunded (SCMH, 2009). As such, inreach teams often find that they have to prioritise those with severe, complex and enduring mental health problems, that is, those with **psychoses**, **severe depression**, **personality disorder**, a **dual diagnosis** of co-morbid mental health problems and substance misuse, and those requiring interventions under the various UK mental health laws. Whether the remit of inreach teams should be as narrow as this is open to debate but the Bradley Report (Box 12.2) does suggest the principal focus of inreach teams should be those with severe mental health problems.

Secure provision

The alternative for those MDOs for whom prison is deemed inappropriate is some sort of secure accommodation. Since the advent of community care in the 1970s and 1980s, there has been a considerable reduction in the number of inpatient beds in the UK (Bell & Lindley, 2005). There has, however, been a resurgence in bed provision in recent times and most of that resurgence has been in secure beds: there are now almost 5,000 medium or high secure beds in the UK (Rutherford & Duggan, 2007).

The rise in secure beds

Why do you think the provision of secure beds has risen so much in the last decade? Is it down to a failure of community care? Has society become more violent? Was there always a hidden need which has only surfaced because of media attention on a few high-profile cases? Is it the private sector spotting 'a gap in the market'?

Security

One of the most common things that students notice and comment on when first working in secure environments are the security measures that are in place. This is a key feature of these environments and reflects the variety of systems and processes needed to keep both users of forensic services and staff safe. Taylor and Dunn (2009) argue that there are essentially five aspects to security (Figure 12.1).

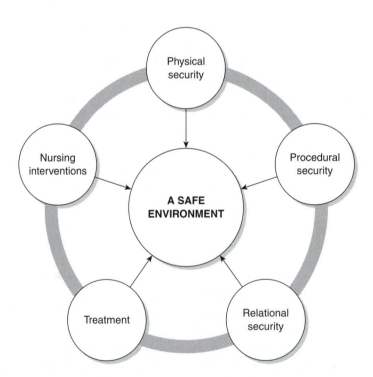

FIGURE 12.1   Aspects of security in forensic mental health

Regarding **physical security**, secure units are designed with a clear purpose in mind and are subject to very clear criteria regarding the way that buildings are designed and organised. Features of physical security may include fences, airlocks (double sets of doors where one set will open only when the other set is closed), individual rooms, seclusion facilities and CCTV cameras. Probably the most noticeable feature of these environments is locked doors. As the keys for these doors need to be securely attached to a belt, nurses and other members of the multidisciplinary team are sometimes seen as jailers. The very act of possessing these keys is an explicit statement of power and those holding keys should take care not to openly reinforce this power imbalance by, for example, swinging or jingling the keys.

Procedural security relates to the checks, searching and screening that occurs in secure environments. These aspects are designed to improve the general security within a service. Examples include random searches of individuals and locations (wards, bedrooms, etc.), counting of sharp objects such as knives and forks at mealtimes, and the banning on wards of items that have the potential to cause harm, such as sharp items, alcohol and lighters, cameras (which could be used to take photographs of security and layouts which in turn, could aid absconding), and glue and Blu-Tak (which can be used to copy keys or jam locks). Policies that emphasise procedural security might include escorted access policies, visiting policies and the role specifications of the nurse with a specific responsibility for security.

The ability of the multidisciplinary team to engage with the service user and assess and understand any warning signs of relapse or of escalating risk is the principal feature of **relational security**. Relational security often requires nursing staff to closely observe and monitor patients and necessitates higher staff–patient ratios than those found in 'standard' mental health settings.

The **treatments** and **interventions** provided by forensic services are another dimension to the maintenance of security in that anything that improves the mental health of service users will tend to reduce the risks. We will look at treatments and interventions later on but it is worth noting the **nursing** and nurses can play a significant role in the maintenance of security because of the unique contact and relationships they have with service users and because they are frequently the agents – and sometimes the architects – of therapeutic intervention.

Levels of secure care

High secure facilities are provided for people who demonstrate particularly dangerous behaviours and who require a level of security that is otherwise unavailable within mental health services. The highest level of care has traditionally been provided by the 'special' hospitals. Three English hospitals currently provide high-security inpatient care for England and Wales, with approximately 800 beds: **Ashworth** in Merseyside, **Rampton** in Nottinghamshire and **Broadmoor** in Berkshire. There is also a high-security hospital at **Carstairs**, near Edinburgh (officially called 'The State Hospital'), that serves both Scotland and Northern Ireland. The special hospitals are large, regionally distant institutions, which are reminiscent of Victorian mental institutions combined with prison-like levels of security. The considerable criticisms levelled at these institutions have led to the development of medium and low secure services which are geared more towards rehabilitation and eventual return to the community (McMurran et al., 2009).

Medium secure units were envisaged as a 'step-down' provision for service users moving from higher to lower levels of secure care with the aim of providing rehabilitation and preparation for eventual community return within a few years of admission. Following the Reed Report recommendations, a significant number of regional medium secure units have been built. Medium secure units account for roughly three-quarters of secure provision (Rutherford & Duggan, 2007). Provision can be both short- and long-stay and care is provided according to the supervision and security needs of the person rather than the offending behaviour. The growth in demand for medium secure beds is thought to have resulted from pressures in acute and community mental health services, the need to move service users away from high security services, and high levels of mental ill-health among the prison population (MHA Commission, 2008). Interestingly, the private sector provides a considerable portion of medium secure services in the UK; in 2005, it was estimated to account for approximately 40% of medium secure bed provision (MHA Commission, 2008).

There are also a number of **low secure services** beginning to emerge at local level which can be used as a further step towards eventual discharge. These include **Psychiatric Intensive Care Units** (PICUs) and **Low Secure Units** (LSUs). PICUs are often managed as part of general inpatient provision, and can provide a safe and intensive period of care for those who are too disturbed for acute mental health wards yet do not require medium secure provision. LSUs tend to be part of a forensic service and provide short- to medium-term treatment and rehabilitation in a setting that has security features additional to those of a PICU. To some extent, the use of low secure units reflects a stepped care approach (cf. stepped care in primary care in Chapter 4) to the eventual return of MDOs to the community, except that the 'risk escalator' is downwards rather than the upwards one you might see in the treatment of, say, anxiety and depression (Heyman et al., 2004).

Community provision

Not all people with mental health problems who come into contact with the criminal justice system are dealt with in an institutional setting. Community care and support is an option not only for those discharged from prison or the secure services but also for those who are given some sort of community disposal following conviction, such as a community compulsion order in Scotland or a community sentence with a mental health treatment requirement (MHTR) in England and Wales (interestingly, less than 0.5% of community sentences in 2006 included a MHTR; DH, 2009).

In England, many people leaving forensic settings for return to community living return on a **conditional discharge order** (under Section 37/41). Based on actuarial[3] assessments of the risk to the general public from those discharged, conditional discharge appears to be an effective approach to safely reintegrating those discharged from secure services. Gibbens and Robertson (1983), for example, conducted a 15-year follow-up study of male offenders receiving hospital orders in 1963 and 1964 in order to determine the rates of re-offending, convictions, hospital admissions and death. Fifteen years later, there were 249 men alive and of these 42% had had no court appearances, 28% had one or two court appearances and 30% had had three or more. Of those who re-offended two had committed homicide, one had committed arson, six wounding with intent or grievous bodily harm (GBH) and 24 aggravated bodily harm (ABH). Half of all convictions were within 12 months of leaving hospital. Gibbens & Robertson concluded that the 'results do not suggest that hospital orders failed to protect the public from dangerous offenders' (p. 368). More recent reports by Kershaw et al. (1997), Street (1998) and Johnson and Taylor (2002) have presented data on the numbers of recalls to hospital, the number of admissions under Part 3 of the Mental Health Act and the number of conditional discharges. The general consensus of these reports is that conditional discharge works; it protects the public and it ensures that problem behaviours are detected and addressed promptly. From this viewpoint, the return to community living appears to be one that is uncomplicated and effectively managed.

However, a focus on recidivism and counting the number of incidents tends to obscure some real concerns about the challenges people leaving

---

[3]Actuaries are specialists in the statistics of *risk*; they work mainly, though not exclusively, in business and finance, especially in the insurance industry.

forensic facilities face in re-establishing themselves as viable community citizens. Indeed, there are few studies of how people achieve successful community reintegration and what helps or hinders this process. One obvious challenge is that potentially dangerous behaviours may have to be managed in the relatively uncontrolled environment of wider society. A less obvious challenge is how to engage service users as partners in care when they are subject to legislation that may well exert a degree of control and compulsion on them and when governments may well be more concerned with populist demands over public safety than with the individual rights of service users (Beresford, 2001). As Moon (2000) notes, (specific and dramatic) failures in the supervision of the mentally ill living in the community have now given rise to a renewed 'discourse of confinement' targeted at those seen to be the most unpredictable and dangerous. Community mental healthcare might aspire to a utopian and libertarian ideal of collaborative and independent living; the reality for many people with mental illness, however, may be one of swapping one type of institution – the mental hospital – for more subtle forms of supervision and scrutiny within the wider community (Cohen, 1985; Steadman & Morrissey, 1987; Armstrong, 1995).

The Profile of Those Seen in Forensic Mental Health Services

Around 5% of people forcibly detained under mental health legislation require a forensic service, a figure that has been pretty stable over the past few years (NHS Information Centre, 2008). In 2007–8, this translated into around 1,400 court and prison decisions each year under Part III of the Mental Health Act, including approximately 300 people detained under Section 37 with a restriction order (i.e. Section 37/41).

Type of offence

Rutherford & Duggan (2007) report that the most common offence committed by people referred to forensic mental health services is **violence against the person** (which includes murder), accounting for approximately 36% of admissions, followed by **criminal damage** (14%; mostly arson) and **robbery** (10%). Violence against the person is more common in the over-40s; robbery is more common in those under 40. The number of people admitted to forensic mental health services with murder convictions rose 65% (from 62 to 102) between 2000 and 2004.

Demographic characteristics

The majority of those in forensic mental health services are **males** aged between 26 and 40; women comprise about 1 in 8 of the population and there are proportionately more women in forensic mental health services than in prison (Rutherford and Duggan, 2007). Rutherford and Duggan also report that proportionally more women in forensic services have a 'psychopathic disorder' (see the next subsection) than men. The levels of security required for women in forensic services and the particular needs of such women are different from those of men; as such, it is not surprising to find that specific services for women have been developed in recent years – the National High Secure Healthcare Service for Women at Rampton and a number of 'Women's Enhanced Medium Secure Units', for example (McMurran et al., 2009).

Black and ethnic minorities are overrepresented in both the prison and forensic mental health services (Rutherford & Duggan, 2007).

Type of disorder

Since the Mental Health Act 2007 changed the definition of mental disorder to a single condition (see Chapter 1), official statistics no longer contain data on the types of disorder that come into forensic services. Prior to the 2007 Act, the majority of those detained in hospital were categorised as having 'mental illness' while around 13% were identified as having **psychopathic disorder** (Ministry of Justice, 2007). 'Psychopathic disorder' – defined in Section 1(2) of the Mental Health Act 1983 as 'a persistent disorder or disability of mind ... which results in abnormally aggressive or seriously irresponsible conduct on the part of the person concerned' – is a **legal** rather than medical term that encompasses many of the so-called **personality disorders**. In contrast to England and Wales, Scotland has retained a categorised definition of mental disorder (Section 328 of the Scottish Act), one of the categories being personality disorder.

Personality disorder

Personality disorder is a controversial concept. It is beyond the scope of this chapter to give you any more than a brief overview of some of the arguments behind the controversy but, if interested, extended critiques are readily available (see, for example, Manning, 2000). Ostensibly, personality disorders are conditions that describe some deviation from a 'normal' personality state; yet psychology has no clear-cut view of what 'personality' is – let alone 'normal

TABLE 12.3   DSM-IVR classifications of personality disorder (APA, 2000)

Cluster	Type	Description
Cluster A: Suspicious	Paranoid	Suspicious of other people; sensitive to rejection and holds grudges
	Schizoid	Prefers own company to that of others; has a rich fantasy world
	Schizotypal	Has odd ideas and difficulty with thinking; 'eccentric'
Cluster B: Emotional and impulsive	Antisocial	The commonly held view of the 'psychopath': doesn't care about the feelings of others or feel guilty; impulsive; finds it hard to have close relationships; often involved in crime
	Borderline (or emotionally unstable)	Finds it hard to control emotions; feels bad about his or her self; often self-harms; can form relationships quickly but easily loses them
	Histrionic	Overdramatic and self-centred; worries about appearance; craves excitement
	Narcissistic	Feels important and dreams of success, power and status; craves attention; tends to exploit others
Cluster C: Anxious	Obsessive–compulsive (or anankastic)	Perfectionist; cautious; finds it hard to make decisions; sensitive to criticism
	Avoidant (or anxious/avoidant)	Anxious and tense; worries a lot; feels insecure and inferior; wants to be liked; sensitive to criticism
	Dependent	Relies on others to make decisions; feels incompetent finds it hard to cope with daily tasks; easily feels abandoned by others

personality' – having many theoretical perspectives on the subject, ranging from behavioural to psychodynamic to statistical (where what the majority do is 'normal'). Many of the traits that describe a personality disorder (see Table 12.3) are normal human traits that are exaggerated or used in environments or circumstances that are not especially adaptive. In addition, psychiatry – forensic psychiatry in particular – has spent many years attempting to intervene in personality disorder (and with only limited success) despite its being implicit in the 1983 Mental Health Act that personality disorder is untreatable.[4]

---

[4]Section 3(2)(b) of the Act implied that, in the case of psychopathic disorder, treatment was merely about alleviating or preventing a deterioration of the condition rather than 'curing' (or treating) it.

Personality disorder

After looking through the descriptors for the various personality disorders in Table 12.3 you may well be thinking 'Do I have a personality disorder?' This in itself is a criticism of the concept of personality disorder: that normal human behaviour ends up being labelled deviant when it doesn't suit a particular context or environment or when it gets exaggerated or extreme.

Do you think it's better to think of personality *extremes* rather than personality disorder? What about the usefulness of giving someone the label of personality disorder? Is it helpful or unhelpful?

Do you think there are any circumstances when some of the descriptors in Table 12.3 would be adaptive rather than maladaptive? In war? In business? In the arts and creative industries?

People with a diagnosis of personality disorder have traditionally had a mixed response from mental health services. Often they are rejected by services, or they themselves choose to reject services (NCCMH, 2010). They may be seen by staff as a difficult or unpopular patient (Stockwell, 1972) or they might be characterized as in a constant struggle for control with staff (Breeze & Repper, 1998).

While there may be a conceptual debate over personality disorder, the concept remains important in forensic mental health since those working in forensic services will undoubtedly have contact with people labelled or diagnosed with one form of personality disorder or another (though, more often than not, it will be anti-social personality disorder). In particular, forensic services will deal with those whose personality disorder is deemed to be dangerous and/or severe. And this is perhaps the real issue in forensic mental health: not whether people have a specific personality disorder but whether they have a history of, or the potential to be, **dangerous**. This isn't an easy subject to tackle, especially when debates over dangerousness are often coupled with legal and ethical debates over whether society has the right to deny people their liberty for fear of what they might do in the future rather than on the basis of what they have done in the past (Roberts, 2006). Clearly relevant to these debates is the notion of **risk** and whether it is possible to **predict** such risk – issues we will discuss in more detail later.

Assessment in Forensic Mental Health Services

Robust assessment in forensic services is based around a number of princi-ples, especially those that relate to **holistic**, **person-centred** and **recovery-focused** care. Holistic care means that the large multidisciplinary teams involved in forensic care – teams involving forensic psychiatrists, clinical psychologists, forensic psychologists, nurses and nursing assistants, occupa-tional therapists, pharmacists and social workers – need to work together when assessing and treating individual service users. Person-centred care means that the service user's strengths and assets are identified as well as their needs and any identified risks, that interventions are planned **collabora-tively** with service users, and that family and carer involvement is encour-aged and maintained. A recovery-focused approach means that there should always be **hope** and that the emphasis should be on **social inclusion** rather than exclusion.

Nursing is a crucial component of the mental health recovery process in forensic mental health care. In community forensic settings, nurses often act as the care coordinator for service users, a role that involves regular and comprehensive assessments of needs and risks. In institutional forensic set-tings, nurses are often involved in 24-hour observation and are, as such, a major source of clinical information regarding a service user's needs and risks. Moreover, the 24-hour contact nurses have often gives them a greater opportunity than other professionals to develop relationships with service users and their families. Since nurses working in secure services will have to constantly judge the level of need and risk to and/or from service users, manage crises as they arise, control freedom of movement within and out-side the institution and maintain safe levels of supervision and observation, nurses who work in forensic services require exceptional interpersonal and clinical decision making skills.

Holistic nursing assessments

Nursing assessments in forensic mental health need to be comprehensive and holistic, considering a range of physical, psychological, social and political strengths and needs, together with a full consideration of the risks to self and to others.

Figure 12.2 provides an overview of some of the things nurses need to consider when undertaking an assessment in forensic mental health services. Doyle & Dolan (2007) also provide a useful five-step framework for clinical

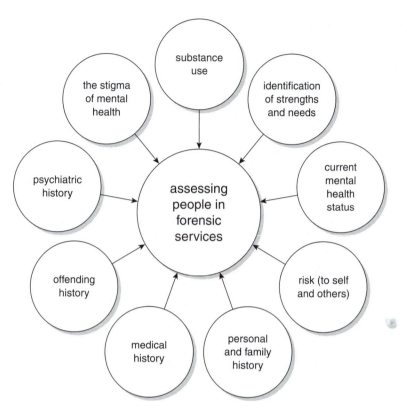

FIGURE 12.2 Things to consider when assessing in forensic mental health services

risk assessment, formulation and management that is comprehensive, holistic and recovery orientated (Box 12.3).

Box 12.3   A framework for assessment, formulation and management in forensic mental health (Doyle & Dolan, 2007)

1 Gathering case information
2 Identifying strengths and needs
3 Assessing risk to self and others
4 Formulating strengths, needs and risks
5 Devising a collaborative management plan

TABLE 12.4   Areas to consider when assessing in forensic mental health

Area	Details
Personal history	Early developments, childhood experiences, schooling, jobs, marital/ relationship history, sexual history, children, social situation, religious/ spiritual/cultural influences
Family history	Parental contact, siblings, socio-economic status, family history of mental/physical illness, next of kin, significant others, visitors
Medical history	Illness or operations, accidents, smoking behaviour (see also substance use), medical treatments received
Forensic history	Index offence, previous arrests, imprisonment, details of offending
Personality	Friendships, socialising, hobbies, sensitive, reserved, shy, suspicious, jealous, resentful, explosive, irritable, impulsive, angry, self-centred, rigid, relationship with others, attitudes, beliefs
Substance use	Substance use history, alcohol consumption, prescribed drug use, illicit drug use, treatments received, detox, average use per week, criminal activities linked to substance use
Psychiatric history	Background to current contact with service, insight, satisfaction, first contact with mental health/learning disability services, chronological record of contact, legal status, nature and course of illness, suicide, self-harm, vulnerability, violence
Current mental state, recent behaviour and functioning	Appearance and behaviour, speech, mood, thought, perceptions, insight, risk to self/others, recent progress, violent ideation and/or threats, antisocial acts, non-compliance

Gathering case information

It is important to gather a thorough picture of the service user's history, current mental state, behaviour and functioning. A detailed list of areas to consider when gathering case information can be found in Table 12.4. Methods of gathering this information include **interviews with the service user**, **interviews with the family/carer** or a person who knows them well, a **review of records**, **behavioural observations**, **physical observations** and findings from **structured tests or assessments**. This information must be documented clearly and concisely and the adequacy of the reports and their sources will need to be evaluated. In some cases, access to historical information may be limited. In these circumstances, mental health nurses still need to assess individuals on the best available information, and limitations in the information available must be communicated and documented.

Identifying strengths and needs

Once the background information has been gathered, the physical, psychological, social and political **strengths and needs** of the service user can be identified. For the **physical** domain this includes, but is not restricted to, physical health, substance misuse, pharmacology, sleep and personal hygiene; the **psychological** domain includes mental and emotional state, impulse control, attitudes, conduct, insight and coping; the **social** domain includes social skills, relationships, occupation, recreation and social support; while the **political** domain includes, finance, benefits, access to services, education and the legal aspects of care including service users' rights and their relationships with the criminal justice system. The START (Short-Term Assessment of Risk and Treatability; Webster et al., 2009) is a nurse-led structured, clinical guideline that can assist nurses in identifying and assessing strengths and needs as well as risks.

Assessing risk to self and others

Based on the historical information obtained and a strengths and needs assessment, identified risks to and from the service user will need to be assessed. Whether assessing risk to self or others, it is important to consider the past history of risk behaviour, any current clinical risk factors and the contextual factors that may increase risk before considering factors that may be protective and minimize risk to self and others (see Table 12.5).

TABLE 12.5   Factors influencing risk to self and others

	Past history of	
	Violence	**Self-harm**
Clinical risk factors *Consider: recency, severity, frequency, patterns in risk behaviour*	Emotional instability (anger) Impulsiveness Hostility Paranoia Substance misuse Lack of insight	Suicide plan, intent thoughts Low mood with agitation Hopelessness and helplessness Impulsiveness Substance misuse Recent loss/anniversary of loss Victim of bullying and/or exploitation
Contextual risk factors *Consider: recency, severity, frequency, patterns in risk behaviour*	Lack of professional and social support Non-compliance Stressful life events Peer group	Changes in support network Lack of professional and social support Non-compliance Imprisonment or recent incarceration Stressful life events
Protective factors	Good social networks and valued home environment Compliant and responding to treatment Good insight Good rapport and therapeutic alliance with staff Regular contact with services No interest in, or knowledge of, weapons	

Although the focus here is on risk to self and others, often other risks need to be assessed in areas such as escape, fire-setting, sex offending and child protection. There are a number of formal, structured tools around that can assist with assessing specific risks, for example **violence risk** (the HCR-20; Webster et al., 1997), **suicide risk** (the ESR-20; Polvi, 1997) or **physical, relational and procedural security risks** (the SNAP; Collins & Davies, 2005).

Formulating strengths, needs and risks

At this stage, the strengths, needs and risk assessment are summarised and formulated in an attempt to gain a better understanding of the service user's current presentation. A concise formulation of the origin, development and maintenance of a person's needs and risk, and any changes in those needs and risk should inform the care plan (Doyle & Dolan, 2002; DH, 2007).

Devising a collaborative management plan

The evidence-based formulation of strengths, needs and risks should be used to inform any management interventions that might be employed. Any such interventions should be aimed at responding to and managing need and risks while enhancing any strengths and protective factors (Doyle & Dolan, 2006). Interventions are considered in more detail in the next section.

 Case scenario: admission to a medium secure unit

Kim is a 31-year-old woman with a 15-year psychiatric history that has variously described her as having depression, bipolar disorder, borderline personality disorder and anti-social personality disorder. She has been admitted under Section 37 of the Mental Health Act to the Laurels, a privately run, medium secure unit for women, after being convicted of grievous bodily harm on her next door neighbour. Kim claims her neighbour taunted her about her mental health problems so she retaliated by punching her neighbour and breaking her nose. She has never been convicted of such a serious offence before, but she has a history of low-level and nuisance offences including shoplifting, being drunk and disorderly, and breach of the peace. She has been admitted to the acute inpatient unit of her local psychiatric hospital several times in the past but never to a secure unit.

Kim is pretty upset at being admitted to the Laurels: she arrived on the unit quite aggressive, kicking out, shouting and very tearful. As the admitting nurse, you manage to calm her down a little and she tells you that she's upset because she had done everything everyone had told her. She had cooperated with her probation officer in relation to a pre-sentence report and she had pleaded guilty yet she had still ended up being sent to the Laurels under a section of the Mental Health Act when she thought she might just get a fine.

What will be the important elements of any nursing assessment you carry out with Kim? What will be the main priorities for her care? How might you deal with her view that compulsory admission to the Laurels is somehow unfair?

Intervening in Forensic Mental Health Care

The main purpose of forensic services is to assess those individuals perceived as dangerous or a risk to others as a result of their disorder and/or behaviour and provide the care, treatment and management they require (Doyle, 2000). As you will have most likely gathered by now, the principal risks are those relating to **aggression** and **violence**, either to the self or to others.

In intervening to prevent or manage aggression and violence, it's worth using as a framework the three stages of the **forensic clinical pathway** (after Novaco, 1975; Doyle, 2000; NICE, 2005; Byrt & Doyle, 2007; Fluttert et al., 2008; MHA Commission, 2008). These are: (1) **early recognition and prevention**; (2) **secondary interventions**; and (3) **ongoing care and management**. In considering each of these stages, we will also look at the evidence base for the interventions that are typically used. It is worth noting, however, that in relation to **psychosocial interventions**, there are still relatively few studies or reviews conclusively showing what works in reducing violence (Harper & Chitty, 2005; Rubin et al., 2008) and that the evidence base for **nursing interventions** is relatively weak and in need of further good quality studies (Woods & Richards, 2003). Despite the lack of robust evidence, however, there is relevant NICE guidance. The guidance on the **short-term management of disturbed and violent behaviour**, published jointly with the Royal College of Nursing (NICE, 2005) and the guidance on the **care of people with antisocial personality disorder** (NICE, 2009) are especially relevant to forensic settings.

Early recognition and prevention

Here, members of the multidisciplinary team use their interpersonal skills to build rapport, develop therapeutic relationships and ensure regular one-to-one time with service users in order to facilitate the early identification of risk and the reduction of any such risk.

Systematic risk assessment (using formal tools such as the HCR-20) and proactive, negotiated risk management plans are helpful. **Advance directives** may also be useful (NICE, 2005). These actions, taken together, can help with the **de-escalation** of aggression and violence. Indeed, NICE recommend that the use of such **de-escalation** techniques should always be the primary intervention in managing aggression and violence (NICE, 2005). Other approaches that can help in early recognition and prevention include **motivational interviewing** (a technique designed to help people work through their ambivalence to change; see Coffey, 2000 and also Chapter 11) and a **collaborative** approach to care planning that actively involves service users, their families and other relevant agencies.

Secondary interventions

If initial preventative measures are unsuccessful and the situation becomes volatile then attempts at de-escalation should continue while maintaining effective communication between staff and the service user. Agreed crisis plans and advance directives can be implemented and, if necessary, **physical restraint** may be used so long as staff are trained. Short periods of isolation from others may help de-stimulate the individual and, if absolutely necessary, **seclusion** in a fit-for-purpose facility can be implemented. **Rapid tranquillization** in accordance with an agreed protocol may also be useful. While the NICE guidance (2005) states that there is a lack of evidence in relation to physical restraint, seclusion and rapid tranquillization, it does acknowledge that these interventions may have a place. At the same time, however, the guidance advises caution in their use: they should only be used if de-escalation fails to calm the service user and only with a number of safeguards in place, for example, adequate training in basic life support and adequate equipment.

Ongoing care and management

Once the acute stage of an incident has subsided and the immediate risk has reduced then there are a number of strategies for ongoing care and management that can be considered. Since most of these strategies have been developed in non-forensic mental health settings, their applicability to a forensic setting may be questionable. However, as we have seen, the evidence base for forensic interventions is somewhat limited so it is worth considering those strategies that have shown promise elsewhere. For example, **coping strategy enhancement**, **family interventions** and **relapse prevention plans** (interventions that were discussed in Chapter 6) are all worthy of consideration. Indeed, all of these elements can be rolled into a collaboratively agreed relapse prevention or 'Staying Safe' plan (see Box 12.4).

Box 12.4   Elements of a Staying Safe plan

Identify:

- a relapse signature (the thoughts, feelings and behaviours that act as warning signs)
- stress triggers
- at risk situations
- personal coping strategies that help prevent violence

Collaboratively involving:

- the service user
- families, carers and significant others
- forensic mental health staff
- other relevant agencies

The NICE guidance on antisocial personality disorder (NICE, 2009) suggest that group-based **cognitive and behavioural interventions** such as 'Reasoning and Rehabilitation' (Ross et al., 1988) be tried with those with a history of offending behaviour. Such group-based programmes can provide the individual with consistent relationships, help the person to learn to cope with crises and so help manage risks to the person and others (Byrt et al., 2005). Anger management programmes may also be used, but as the NCCMH (2010) point out, the evidence for its use with offenders is limited since most of the anger management studies have been conducted on college students.

Aside from its use in rapid tranquilization, **medication** may also have a role to play in the longer-term management of forensic service users. For example, some **atypical antipsychotics** (see Chapter 7) may have an effect on the level of aggression (Krakowski et al., 2008). However, the full NICE guidance report on antisocial personality disorder (NCCMH, 2010) does **not** recommend the routine use of medication for treating aggression and anger although it certainly recommends that psychotropic medication be used to treat any co-morbid mental health problems. Of course, wherever medication is involved, nurses have a crucial role to play in terms of motivating and encouraging service users to adhere to any regimes, monitoring side-effects and supporting service users in any self-medication regimens.

Integrated programmes

For the more serious offenders, there are a number of specific multi-agency programmes. These programmes are structured and co-ordinated, encompassing not only service provision but also a research and training agenda. Examples include the **Dangerous and Severe Personality Disorder Programme** (DSPDP; see www.dspdprogramme.gov.uk), a joint initiative between the Ministry of Justice's National Offender Management Service and the Department of Health in England and Wales, and the **Risk Management Authority** (RMA; see www.rmascotland.gov.uk) in Scotland. The DSPDP is underpinned by a portfolio of largely cognitive and behavioural approaches, including schema therapy (Young et al., 2003), dialectical behaviour therapy (Linehan & Dimeff, 2001) and cognitive analytical therapy (Ryle & Kerr, 2002). Many of these therapies are subject to ongoing research and, as such, the evidence base for them is currently unclear. Tyrer et al. (2010), however, claim that the costs of the DSPD 'experiment' (as they call it) are not justified given that it has failed to produce positive outcomes for the majority of those labelled with DSPD and that the label (diagnosis) of DSPD is in itself suspect.

Conclusion

In this chapter we have provided the reader with a broad introduction to some aspects of forensic mental healthcare. This included an overview of the development and current configuration of inpatient and community services across the UK, aspects of relevant policy and the legal frameworks in which forensic mental health services exist. We have highlighted some of the security issues and risks associated with working with this user group and we have looked at the possible assessments and clinical interventions open to those working in forensic services.

Above all, we have highlighted the crucial role of nurses in forensic mental health. Nurses are, to a large extent, the backbone of the service and ensuring that those nurses have exceptional interpersonal and clinical decision making skills will also ensure that those people with mental health problems who come into contact with the criminal justice system can be helped in their goals to become valued and integrated members of society.

Further Reading and Resources

Key texts

Chaloner C & Coffey M (eds) (2000). *Forensic Mental Health Nursing: Current Approaches*. Oxford: Blackwell.
  A useful source text for exploring the many aspects of forensic mental health nursing.

Harper G & Chitty C (2005). *Home Office Research Study 291. The Impact of Corrections on Re-Offending: A Review of 'What Works'*, Third Edition. London: Home Office.
  An official publication summarising the evidence base for interventions designed to prevent offenders from re-offending.

The National Forensic Nurses' Research & Development Group (eds) (2006). *Forensic Mental Health Nursing: Interventions with People with 'Personality Disorder'*. London: Quay Books.

The National Forensic Nurses' Research & Development Group (eds) (2007). *Forensic Mental Health Nursing: Forensic Aspects of Acute Care*. London: Quay Books.

The National Forensic Nurses' Research & Development Group (eds) (2008). *Forensic Mental Health Nursing: Capabilities, Roles and Responsibilities*. London: Quay Books.
  A series of books edited by the National Forensic Nurses' Research and Development Group.

Key policy documents

National Institute for Clinical Excellence (2005). *Violence: The Short-term Management of Disturbed/Violent Behaviour in In-patient Psychiatric Settings and Emergency Departments*. London: NICE. Available from www.nice.org.uk/CG25

Rutherford M & Duggan S (2007). *Forensic Mental Health Services, Facts and Figures on Current Provision*. London: Sainsbury Centre for Mental Health.

Department of Health (2009). *Lord Bradley's Review of People with Mental Health Problems or Learning Disabilities in the Criminal Justice System.* London: Department of Health.

National Collaborating Centre for Mental Health (2010). *Antisocial Personality Disorder: The Nice Guideline on Treatment, Management and Prevention [National Clinical Guideline Number 77].* London: British Psychological Society/Royal College of Psychiatrists. Available from www.nice.org.uk/CG77

Rutherford M (2010). *Blurring the Boundaries: The Convergence of Mental Health and Criminal Justice Policy, Legislation, Systems and Practice.* London: Sainsbury Centre for Mental Health.

Web resources

The Dangerous and Severe Personality Disorder Programme: www.dspdprogramme.gov.uk
Website providing details of this joint Ministry of Justice and Department of Health initiative.

The Risk Management Authority Scotland: www.rmascotland.gov.uk
The Scottish public body that ensures the 'effective assessment, management and minimisation of risk of serious violent and sexual offenders'.

Scottish Forensic Network: www.forensicnetwork.scot.nhs.uk
Website of the Forensic Mental Health Services Managed Care Network. Although Scottish, has resources that are useful across the UK.

International Association of Forensic Nurses: www.iafn.org
'The mission of the IAFN is to provide leadership in forensic nursing practice by developing, promoting, and disseminating information internationally about forensic nursing science.'

References

APA (American Psychiatric Association) (2000). *Diagnostic and Statistical Manual of Mental Disorders, 4th Edition* (Text Revised) (DSM-IVR) Washington: APA.

Armitage C, Fitzgerald C & Cheong P (2003). Prison in-reach mental health nursing. *Nursing Standard,* **17**(26), 40–42.

Armstrong D (1995). The rise of surveillance medicine. *Sociology of Health and Illness,* **17**(3), 393–404.

Arrigo BA (2001). Transcarceration: a constitutive ethnography of mentally ill 'offenders'. *The Prison Journal,* **81**(12), 162–186.

Aubert V & Messinger S (1958). The criminal and the sick. *Inquiry,* **1**, 137–160.

Bell A & Lindley P (eds) (2005). *Beyond the Water Towers: The Unfinished Revolution in Mental Health Services, 1985–2005.* London: Sainsbury Centre for Mental Health.

Beresford P (2001). Service users, social policy and the future of welfare. *Critical Social Policy,* **21**(4), 494–512.

Berlin FS & Malin HM (1991). Media distortion of the public's perception of recidivism and psychiatric rehabilitation. *American Journal of Psychiatry,* **148**, 1572–1576.

Breeze JA & Repper J (1998). Struggling for control: the care experiences of 'difficult' patients in mental health services. *Journal of Advanced Nursing,* **28**(6), 1301–1311.

Byrt R & Doyle M (2007). Preventing and reducing violence and aggression. In The National Forensic Nurses' Research & Development Group (eds), *Forensic Mental Health Nursing: Forensic Aspects of Acute Care*. London: Quay Books.

Byrt R, Wray C & 'Tom' (2005). Towards hope and inclusion: nursing interventions in a medium secure service for men with 'Personality Disorder'. *Mental Health Practice*, **8**(8), 38–43.

Coffey M (2000). Developing community services. In C Chaloner & M Coffey (eds), *Forensic Mental Health Nursing: Current Approaches*. Oxford: Blackwell.

Cohen S (1985). *Visions of Social Control: Crime, Punishment and Classification*. Cambridge: Polity Press.

Collins M & Davies S (2005). The Security Needs Assessment Profile: a multidimensional approach to measuring security needs. *International Journal of Forensic Mental Health*, **4**(1), 39–52.

Conrad P (1992). Medicalization and social control. *Annual Review of Sociology*, **18**(1), 209–232.

DH (Department of Health)/Home Office (1992). *Review of Mental Health and Social Services for Mentally Disordered Offenders and Others Requiring Similar Services. Vol. 1: Final Summary Report* [The Reed Report]. London: HMSO.

DH (Department of Health) (2003). *National Partnership Agreement on the Transfer of Responsibility for Prison Health from the Home Office to the Department of Health*. London: DH.

DH (Department of Health) (2007*). Best Practice in Managing Risk: Principles and Evidence for Best Practice in the Assessment and Management of Risk to Self and Others in Mental Health Services*. London: DH.

DH (Department of Health) (2008). *Code of Practice: Mental Health Act 1983*. London: TSO.

DH (Department of Health) (2009). *Lord Bradley's Review of People with Mental Health Problems or Learning Disabilities in the Criminal Justice System*. London: DH.

Doyle M (2000). Risk assessment and management. In C Chaloner & M Coffey (eds), *Forensic Mental Health Nursing: Current Approaches*. London: Blackwell Science (pp. 140–170).

Doyle M & Dolan M (2002). Violence risk assessment: combining actuarial and clinical information to structure clinical judgements for the formulation and management of risk. *Journal of Psychiatric and Mental Health Nursing*, **9**, 649–657.

Doyle M & Dolan M (2006). Predicting community violence from patients discharged from mental health services. *British Journal of Psychiatry*, **189**, 520–526.

Doyle M & Dolan M (2007). Standardized risk assessment. *Psychiatry*, **6**(10), 409–414.

Edgar K & Rickford D (2009). *Too Little Too Late: An Independent Review of Unmet Mental Health Need in Prison*. London: Prison Reform Trust.

Emslie L, Coffey M, Duggan S, Bradshaw R, Mitchell D & Rogers P (2005). Including the excluded: developing mental health in-reach in south west England. *Mental Health Practice*, **8**(6), 17–19.

Evening Standard (2009). Black cab drivers' fury over wife killer. 11 September 2009, p. 18.

Fluttert FAJ, VanMeijel B, Webster C, Nijman H, Bartels A & Grypdonck M (2008). Risk management by early recognition of warning signs in forensic psychiatric patients. *Archives of Psychiatric Nursing*, **22**(4), 208–216.

Gibbens TCN & Robertson G (1983). A survey of the criminal careers of hospital order patients. *British Journal of Psychiatry*, **143**(4), 362–369.

Harper G & Chitty C (2005). *Home Office Research Study 291. The Impact of Corrections on Re-Offending: A Review of 'What Works'*. Third Edition. London: Home Office.

Health Inspectorate Wales (2008). *Report of a Review in Respect of Mr C and the Provision of Mental Health Services, Following a Homicide Committed in October 2006*. Caerphilly: Health Inspectorate Wales.

Heyman B, Shaw M, Davies JP, Godin P & Reynolds L (2004). Forensic mental health services as a risk escalator: a case study of ideals and practice. *Health, Risk and Society*, **6**(4), 307-325.

Johnson S & Taylor R (2002). *Statistics of Mentally Disordered Offenders 2001: England & Wales. Home Office Statistical Bulletin 13/02*. London: Home Office.

Jones WL (1983). *Ministering to Minds Diseased: A History of Psychiatry*. London: Heinemann.

Kershaw C, Dowdeswell P & Goodman J (1997). *Restricted Patients – Reconvictions & Recalls by the End of 1995: England & Wales. Home Office Statistical Bulletin 1/97*. London: Home Office.

Krakowski M, Czobor P & Nolan K (2008). Atypical antipsychotics, neurocognitive deficits, and aggression in schizophrenic patients. *Journal of Clinical Psychopharmacology*, **28**(5), 485–493.

Linehan MM & Dimeff L (2001). Dialectical behavior therapy in a nutshell. *The California Psychologist*, **34**, 10–13.

Lowman J, Menzies RJ & Palys TS (1987). Introduction: transcarceration and the modern state of penality. In J Lowman, RJ Menzies & TS Palys (eds), *Transcarceration: Essays in the Sociology of Social Control*. Aldershot: Gower (pp. 1–15).

Manning N (2000). Psychiatric diagnosis under conditions of uncertainty: personality disorder, science and professional legitimacy. *Sociology of Health and Illness*, **22**(5), 621–639.

McMurran M, Khalifa N & Gibbon S (2009). *Forensic Mental Health*. Uffculme: Willan Publishing.

MHA (Mental Health Act) Commission (2008). *Risk, Rights, Recovery: Twelfth Biennial Report, 2005–2007*. London: TSO.

Ministry of Justice (2007). *Statistics of Mentally Disordered Offenders 2006 England and Wales*. London: Ministry of Justice.

Moon G (2000). Risk and protection: the discourse of confinement in contemporary mental health policy. *Health and Place*, **6**, 239–250.

Murray J (2007). The cycle of punishment: social exclusion of prisoners and their children. *Criminology and Criminal Justice*, **7**, 55–81.

NCCMH (National Collaborating Centre for Mental Health) (2010). *Antisocial Personality Disorder: The NICE Guideline on Treatment, Management and Prevention [National Clinical Guideline Number 77]*. London: British Psychological Society/Royal College of Psychiatrists.

NHS Information Centre (2008). *In-Patients Formally Detained in Hospitals under the Mental Health Act 1983 and Other Legislation, England: 1997–98 to 2007–08.* London: NHS Information Centre. Available from www.ic.nhs.uk [accessed 25 January 2010].

NHS London (2006). *The Independent Inquiry into the Care and Treatment of John Barrett.* London: South West London Strategic Health Authority.

Novaco RW (1975). *Anger Control: The Development and Evaluation of an Experimental Treatment.* Lexington, MA: Heath.

NICE (National Institute for Clinical Excellence) (2005). *Violence: The Short-term Management of Disturbed/Violent Behaviour in In-patient Psychiatric Settings and Emergency Departments.* London: NICE.

NICE (National Institute for Health and Clinical Excellence) (2009). *Antisocial Personality Disorder: Treatment, Management and Prevention.* London: NICE.

PHAB (Prison Healthcare Advisory Board) (2007). *Transfer of Enhanced Primary Healthcare Services to the NHS: Report to Cabinet Secretaries for Health and Wellbeing, and Justice, Volumes 1 and 2.* Edinburgh: Scottish Government.

Polvi NH (1997). Assessing risk of suicide in correctional settings. In C Webster & M Jackson (eds), *Impulsivity: Theory, Assessment and Treatment.* New York: Guilford Press, pp. 278–301.

Puri BK, Brown, RA, McKee HJ & Treasaden IH (2005). *Mental Health Law: A Practical Guide.* London: Hodder Arnold.

Ritchie JH, Dick D & Lingham R (1994). *The Report of the Inquiry into the Care and Treatment of Christopher Clunis.* London: HMSO.

Ross R, Fabiano E & Ewels C (1988). Reasoning and rehabilitation. *International Journal of Offender Therapy and Comparative Criminology,* **32,** 29–35.

Royal College of Psychiatrists (2008). *Personality Disorders: Key Facts.* London: Royal College of Psychiatrists. Available from: www.rcpsych.ac.uk [accessed 28 January 2010].

Roberts M (2006). Excessive compulsion disorder: the Mental Health Bill and the public safety agenda. *Criminal Justice Matters,* **66**(1), 24–25.

Rubin J, Gallo F & Coutts A (2008). *Violent Crime: Risk Models, Effective Interventions and Risk Management* [RAND Europe technical report prepared for the National Audit Office]. Cambridge: RAND Europe.

Rutherford M & Duggan S (2007). *Forensic Mental Health Services: Facts and Figures on Current Provision.* London: Sainsbury Centre for Mental Health.

Rutherford M (2010). *Blurring the Boundaries: The Convergence of Mental Health and Criminal Justice Policy, Legislation, Systems and Practice.* London: Sainsbury Centre for Mental Health.

Ryle A & Kerr IB (2002). *Introducing Cognitive Analytical Therapy: Principles and Practice.* Chichester: Wiley.

SCMH (Sainsbury Centre for Mental Health) (2009). *Briefing 39: Mental Health Care and the Criminal Justice System.* London: Sainsbury Centre for Mental Health.

Scottish Executive (2005). *Mental Health (Care and Treatment) (Scotland) Act 2003: Code of Practice. Volume 3: Compulsory Powers in Relation to Mentally Disordered Offenders.* Edinburgh: Scottish Executive.

Screech MA (1985). Good madness in Christendom. In WF Bynum, R Porter & M Shepherd (eds), *The Anatomy of Madness: Essays in the History of Psychiatry, Volume 1*. London: Tavistock Publications, pp. 25–39.

Shepherd G (2010). A lifetime of exclusion? *The Psychologist*, **23**(1), 24–25.

Social Exclusion Unit (2002). *Reducing Re-Offending by Ex-Prisoners*. London: Social Exclusion Unit.

Singleton N, Bumpstead R, O'Brien M, Lee A & Meltzer H (1998). *Psychiatric Morbidity among Prisoners in England and Wales*. London: Office of National Statistics.

Steadman H & Morrissey JP (1987). The impact of deinstitutionalization on the criminal justice system: implications for understanding changing modes of social control. In J Lowman, RJ Menzies & T Palys (eds), *Transcarceration: Essays in the Sociology of Social Control*. Aldershot: Gower, pp. 227–248.

Stockwell F (1972). *The Unpopular Patient*. London: Royal College of Nursing.

Street R (1998). *The Restricted Hospital Order: From Court to the Community. Home Office Research Study 186*. London: Home Office.

Taylor P & Dunn E (2009). Management of offenders with mental disorder in specialist mental health services. In M Gelder, N Andreasen J Lopez-Ibor Jr & J Geddes (eds), *New Oxford Textbook of Psychiatry, Volume 2*. Oxford: Oxford University Press, pp. 2015–2021.

Tyrer P, Duggan C, Cooper S, Crawford M, Seivewright H, Rutter D, Maden T, Byford S & Barrett B (2010). The successes and failures of the DSPD experiment: the assessment and management of severe personality disorder. *Medicine, Science and the Law*, **50**, 95–99.

Walmsley R (2009). *World Prison Population List*, (Eighth Edition). London: International Centre for Prison Studies, Kings College London. Available from www.kcl.ac.uk [accessed 28 January 2010].

Webster CD, Douglas KS, Eaves D & Hart SD (1997). *HCR-20: Assessing Risk of Violence (Version 2)*. Vancouver: Mental Health Law & Policy Institute, Simon Fraser University.

Webster C, Martin M, Brink J, Nicholls T & Desmaris S (2009). *Short-Term Assessment of Risk and Treatability (START)*. Hamilton, BC: St Josephs Healthcare/BC Mental Health & Addiction Services.

Woods P & Richards D (2003). Effectiveness of nursing interventions in people with personality disorders. *Journal of Advanced Nursing*, **44**(2), 154–172.

Young JE, Klosko JS & Weishaar ME (2003). *Schema Therapy: A Practitioner's Guide*. New York: Guilford.

Select Glossary of Terms

adaptive behaviour   Behaviour that enhances an individual's chances of growth, development and survival. *See also* **maladaptive behaviour**.

advance directive   A set of (usually written) instructions that an individual makes during a period of good health to outline what should happen if his or her health or mental capacity deteriorates to the point of not being able to make decisions. In physical healthcare, the term **living will** is sometimes used.

anxiolytic   Having properties that are anxiety-reducing.

bibliotherapy   Using written materials (such as self-help manuals) to support people with mental health problems.

biopsychosocial   Refers to the interaction between an individual's biological and psychological processes and their social environment. *See also* **psychosocial**.

care pathway   A way of standardising healthcare by identifying the key stages and components of care for a particular disease or disorder, the actions required and who might take responsibility for these actions. Also known as a **clinical pathway**.

clinical psychologist   *See* **psychology**.

clinical supervision   A method of professional support in which caseload and other professional issues and concerns are discussed openly and confidentially, and in a structured way, with an experienced, often senior, colleague.

cognition   Concerned with mental processes such as thinking, perceiving, making judgements and so on. Ultimately, concerned with knowledge in its literal sense of obtaining and processing information about the world.

co-morbid   Jointly occurring diseases. *See also* **dual diagnosis**.

critical ability   A cognitive skill that enables information to be discriminated and analysed, and which underpins the making of decisions or judgements.

delusion   A persistent belief held despite strong evidence to the contrary.

demographic   Relating to the study of human populations. **Demographic data** means data that reflects the ways human populations can be differentiated, e.g. by age, gender or socioeconomic status.

dual diagnosis   Substance misuse problems co-existing with (severe) mental health problems.

eclecticism   An approach whereby practitioners are not loyal to any specific theoretical model but instead use elements from a variety of different theoretical perspectives in order to enhance practice.

effectiveness   How much benefit people get from a real life intervention; i.e., how well the intervention works in practice. Contrast with **efficacy**.

efficacy   How well an intervention works in a clinical trial or laboratory setting. Contrast with **effectiveness**.

empirical research   **Empiricism** is a philosophical approach whereby knowledge is seen to be acquired through experience and observation of the world. Thus empirical research is research, such as experimentation, that involves observation of the real world.

epidemiology   The study of the causes and spread of disease within a community or environment.

evidence-based practice   The process of making decisions about healthcare interventions on the basis of clinical expertise and best available clinical evidence. Compare with **values-based practice**.

formulation   A summary of a service user's problems following clinical assessment that provides a framework for understanding the problem and taking action.

generic   Opposite of specific; applicable to a variety of contexts.

genogram   A type of drawing that shows the relationships between a person and his or her family members.

hallucination   A false perception; seeing, hearing, tasting, smelling or feeling something that isn't really there.

health visitor   A Registered Nurse – this includes Registered Mental Health Nurses – who has extended her or his professional training into public health work. Health Visitors work largely in health promotion and prevention, and frequently (though not exclusively) work with families of the under-5s.

heterogeneity   The state of being different (compare with **homogeneity**).

holistic   Taking into account all aspects of the person when considering their needs. Considering the totality of their physical, psychological, social and spiritual needs.

homogeneity   The state of being the same (compare with **heterogeneity**).

hypnotic   Having sleep-inducing properties.

hypo-   Below (a threshold); lower; low levels.

hyper-   Above (a threshold); higher; high levels.

incidence   How often something (e.g. a particular disease) occurs over a given time period, e.g. the number of cases of a disease that occur within, say, a 6-month or a 10-year period. Contrast with **prevalence**.

intervention   In healthcare, something you do with the intention of improving outcomes for patients or service users. All pharmaceutical, medical and psychological treatments are interventions as such, but things like changing the skill mix in a clinical area or changing a service user's physical environment can also be an intervention.

maladaptive behaviour   Behaviour that reduces an individual's chances of growth, development and survival. For example, while exercising to cope with stress is largely adaptive, smoking or drinking alcohol is largely maladaptive.

meta-analysis   A complex technique for pooling the results of several studies on the same intervention to produce what is essentially one very big study on that intervention.

National Service Framework (NSF)   In healthcare, policies that define national standards of care in relation to a specific healthcare population (e.g. children or older people) or specific disease area (e.g. cancer or mental health).

nature/nurture debate   The debate over whether human behaviour is a product of **nature** (biology, genes, 'inborn', etc.) or **nurture** (environment, upbringing, etc.). Since most human behaviour seems to have both a biological and an environmental element, the debate is largely over but still popular in the media.

neuroleptic   Literally means 'affecting the brain'; used as an alternative term for antipsychotic medication. See also **psychotropic**.

NICE   Acronym for the National Institute for Health and Clinical Excellence (formerly the National Institute for Clinical Excellence, hence 'NICE'). According to the NICE website (www.nice.org.uk), it is 'an independent organisation responsible for providing national guidance on promoting good health and preventing and treating ill health'.

outcome   A change an **intervention** intends to bring about. For example, the outcome of an intervention for depression might be a change in mood whereas an outcome for an intervention for dementia might be improvements in a carer's quality of life.

pathology   The (observable) processes of a disease. **Pathological** means relating to disease or disorder.

polypharmacy   The use of many medications to treat either a single disease or (more commonly) a variety of co-occurring diseases.

prevalence   How often something (e.g. a particular disease) occurs within a given population, usually expressed as a percentage, e.g. '30% of the population suffer from stress'. Contrast with **incidence**.

primary care   Services that people with health problems initially seek out, i.e. **first contact** services. See also **secondary care** and **tertiary care**.

p.r.n. or PRN   Medication that can be given as needed rather than on a regular basis. From the Latin *pro re nata* meaning 'as circumstances arise'.

prodromal   Relating to **prodrome** which is a sign or symptom that a disease process may be starting. **Prodromal symptoms** are the 'early warning signs' of a disease.

psychiatry   A medical specialty that looks at the diagnosis and treatment of mental illness. Psychiatrists have a medical degree (i.e. they train as a doctor) before specialising in psychiatry.

psychoeducation   Helping people with a psychological or mental health problem by supplying them with detailed information and advice about the problem and the ways in which it can be managed. The information and advice is often embedded within a training package of some sort.

psychology   The study of the mind and behaviour. While **abnormal psychology** overlaps to some extent with psychiatry, it is only one aspect of the whole discipline. A **psychologist is** an expert in psychological theory and/or the application of such theory. **Clinical psychologists** are trained experts who apply psychological theory to clinical (medical) practice.

psychometric   The measuring of psychological properties; relating to a psychological test of some sort.

psychomotor   Relating to bodily activity (especially voluntary muscle activity) that is triggered by mental activity.

psychosocial   Refers to the interaction between an individual's psychological processes and their social environment.

psychotropic   Like **neuroleptic**, means affecting the brain and nervous system; usually applied to medication and/or chemical substances designed to have an effect on the brain or nervous system.

publication bias   Because studies with positive results tend to be more interesting than those with negative results, studies with positive results have a greater likelihood of publication. This is the publication bias.

randomised controlled trial (RCT)   The medical/clinical version of the true experiment whereby an intervention is compared across two or more groups (there are often just two groups: an intervention group and a control group). An RCT requires: (a) a **control** group of some sort – a group that does not get an intervention; (b) **random allocation** into the groups being compared; and (c) the measurement of some relevant **outcome** (e.g. mood levels may be an appropriate outcome measure in an RCT of an anti-depressant).

recidividism   Repeating an unwanted behaviour after having been 'treated' for that behaviour. Most often used in the study of crime to describe offenders who continue to offend following intervention from the criminal justice system.

resilience   An ability to be able to cope with stress that arises from a capacity to adapt and overcome adversity.

schema   (pl. **schemata)**   A mental 'map' or 'template' that underpins a way of thinking that is automatic and requires little cognitive effort. It is a key concept of the cognitive school of psychology. If a computer analogy is used, the human body can be thought of as hardware, while schemata are akin to software.

secondary care   Specialised general health care services (often hospital-based) that normally require referral from a primary care practitioner. See also **primary care** and **tertiary care**.

self-efficacy   A person's belief in their own ability to do something. Although **confidence** – the strength of belief in something – is an element of self-efficacy, self-efficacy is more than confidence in that it also assumes the person has insight into their capacity to achieve.

sign   Independently observable characteristics of a disease or illness. *See also* **symptom**.

social capital   Social capital theory argues that social and community networks can be assets – or **capital** – just like money and property can be.

symptom   How a person with a disease or illness describes its characteristics. *See also* **sign**.

syndrome   A collection of signs and symptoms that seemingly form a unique pattern of disease.

systematic review   A formal and rigorous method of reviewing literature, often to draw conclusions about the **effectiveness** or **efficacy** of an intervention.

tertiary care   Very specialised services that are provided for particular disorders or groups of people such as those with cancer or those with eating disorders. *See also* **primary care** and **secondary care**.

third sector   The voluntary or charitable sector. The other two sectors are the public and private sectors.

values-based practice   The process of making healthcare decisions within the context of the differing values held within society. Compare with **evidence-based practice**.

waiting list control   Using those on a waiting list as the control group in an RCT. This helps overcome the ethical obstacle of denying potentially beneficial treatments to those taking part in an RCT since those in the control group also get the treatment, only at a later date.

watchful waiting   Not intervening to any great degree initially but keeping a close eye on signs and symptoms in case they become more severe and/or pronounced, at which point therapeutic action is taken by the practitioner and/or person.

Index

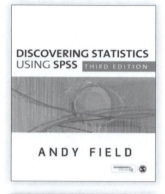
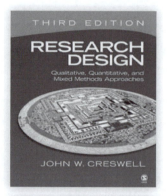
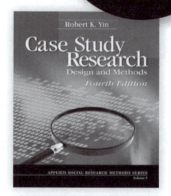
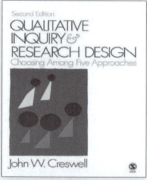
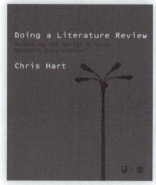
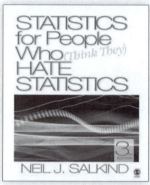
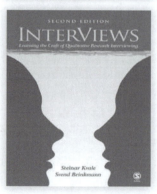
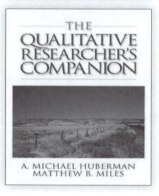
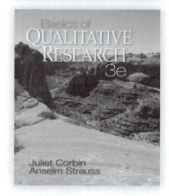
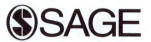

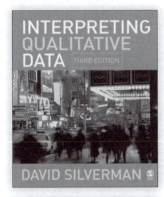
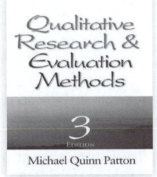
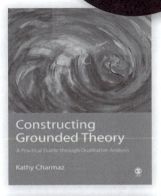
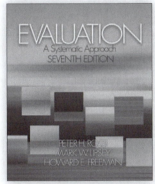
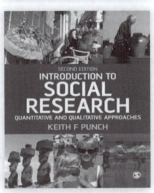
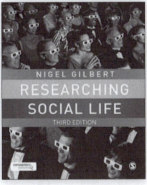
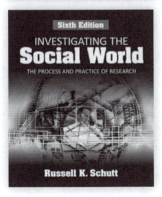
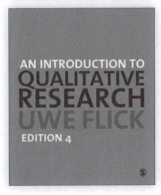
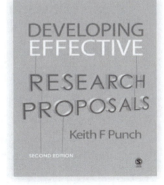
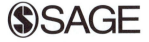

The Qualitative Research Kit

Edited by Uwe Flick

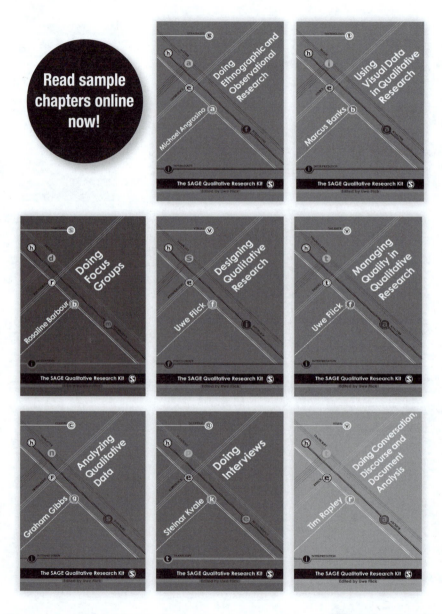

Read sample chapters online now!

Michael Angrosino — Doing Ethnographic and Observational Research — The SAGE Qualitative Research Kit — Edited by Uwe Flick

Marcus Banks — Using Visual Data in Qualitative Research — The SAGE Qualitative Research Kit — Edited by Uwe Flick

Rosaline Barbour — Doing Focus Groups — The SAGE Qualitative Research Kit — Edited by Uwe Flick

Uwe Flick — Designing Qualitative Research — The SAGE Qualitative Research Kit — Edited by Uwe Flick

Uwe Flick — Managing Quality in Qualitative Research — The SAGE Qualitative Research Kit — Edited by Uwe Flick

Graham Gibbs — Analyzing Qualitative Data — The SAGE Qualitative Research Kit — Edited by Uwe Flick

Steinar Kvale — Doing Interviews — The SAGE Qualitative Research Kit — Edited by Uwe Flick

Tim Rapley — Doing Conversation, Discourse and Document Analysis — The SAGE Qualitative Research Kit — Edited by Uwe Flick

www.sagepub.co.uk

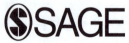

SAGE